APPLIED BIOACTIVE POLYMERIC MATERIALS

POLYMER SCIENCE AND TECHNOLOGY

Recent volumes in the series:

APPLIED BIOACTIVE POLYMERIC MATERIALS

Edited by

Charles G. Gebelein

Youngstown State University
Youngstown, Ohio

Charles E. Carraher, Jr.

Florida Atlantic University
Boca Raton, Florida

and

Van R. Foster

DAP, Inc.
Dayton, Ohio

Springer Science+Business Media, LLC

Library of Congress Cataloging in Publication Data

ACS Symposium on Applied Bioactive Polymeric Materials (1987: New Orleans, La.)
  Applied bioactive polymeric materials / edited by Charles G. Gebelein, Charles E.
Carraher, Jr., and Van R. Foster.
    p.   cm.—(Polymer science and technology; v. 38)
  "Proceedings of an ACS Symposium on Applied Bioactive Polymeric Materials, held
August 30–September 2, 1987, in New Orleans, Louisiana."
  Includes bibliographical references and index.

  1. Biopolymers—Congresses. 2. Drugs—Dosage forms—Congresses. 3. Biopolymers—Physiological effect—Congresses. 4. Biopolymers in medicine—Con-
Gebelein, Charles G. II. Carraher, Charles E. III. Foster, Van R. IV. Title. V. Series.
RS201.B56 27 1987   88-39216
615′.19—dc19   CIP

ISBN 978-1-4684-5612-7   ISBN 978-1-4684-5610-3 (eBook)
DOI 10.1007/978-1-4684-5610-3

Proceedings of an ACS Symposium on Applied Bioactive Polymeric
Materials, held August 30–September 2, 1987,
in New Orleans, Louisiana

© 1988 Springer Science+Business Media New York
Originally published by Plenum Press, New York in 1988
Softcover reprint of the hardcover 1st edition 1988

PREFACE

The biological and biomedical applications of polymeric materials have increased greatly in the past few years. This book will detail some, but not all, of these recent developments. There would not be enough space in this book to cover, even lightly, all of the major advances that have occurred. Some earlier books and summaries are available by two of this book's Editors (Gebelein & Carraher) and these should be consulted for additional information. The books are: "*Bioactive Polymeric Systems*" (Plenum, 1985); "*Polymeric Materials In Medication*" (Plenum, 1985); "*Biological Activities of Polymers*" (American Chemical Society, 1982). Of these three, "*Bioactive Polymeric Systems*" should be the most useful to a person who is new to this field because it only contains review articles written at an introductory level. The present book primarily consists of recent research results and applications, with only a few review or summary articles.

Bioactive polymeric materials have existed from the creation of life itself. Many firmly believe that life could not even exist unless polymeric materials are used to form the basic building blocks. Although this assumption can not be rigorously proven, it is a fact that most, if not all, of the major biochemical pathways involve polymeric species, such as the proteins (including enzymes), polysaccharides and nucleic acids. Among the many reasons for this fact, must be the observation that the natural polymeric materials can be made into an enormous variety of *different*, but inter-related, species. It is now well established that a DNA chain, which only contains four different primary repeating units, can encode an enormous wealth of data permitting not only the replication processes, but protein synthesis and the entire life scheme as well.

It is not surprising, therefore, that many of the applications of bioactive polymeric systems involve interactions with the natural polymeric materials. Likewise, the use of many natural polymers as the base materials for these bioactive systems can hardly be considered a surprise. They are not only readily available, they are also normally more biocompatible and/or biodegradable than the usual synthetic polymer. This book contains several chapters in which natural polymers are the main theme, but there are far more chapters which involve synthetic polymeric materials. There is probably a place for either type of material in the vast realms of biological and/or biomedical applications.

Historically, the earliest "man-made" bioactive polymeric systems utilized a natural polymer (or a modification) in some manner. The advent of the totally synthetic polymers is a more recent innovation. Like many things, however, this pattern appears to be cyclic and we are seeing a renewed interest in the use of natural polymers. This is due, in part, to the perceived need to use renewable resources and, in part, to the desire to eliminate non-biodegradable materials from the environment, whether that environment is medical or biological.

The twenty three chapters of this book largely are concerned with biomedical considerations. This too is a quirk of history; much of the original impetus for the bioactive polymer research was aimed at agricultural applications. Unfortunately, these important applications could not bear the increased cost of the polymeric materials, regardless of whether they were significantly better or not. In the long run, however, many of the pressing environmental concerns may mandate the utilization of bioactive polymeric systems. Fortunately, much of the technology is about the same. A controlled release system could be readily tailored to release a drug or a herbicide. A bioactive polymer could be designed to interact with either the human environment or the biosphere. In short, the knowledge and technology reported herein could be a harbinger of many unexpected future applications.

The design of this book is simple. Chapter 1 (Gebelein, Carraher & Foster) is a summarizing overview of the field and includes several applications not otherwise covered in the book. Chapter 2 (Kurtz & Hassett) considers the use of polymers in pest control, while Chapter 3 (Hirano, et al.) describes the use of chitin and its derivatives as a plant growth activator. Chapters 4 (DiBenedetto, et al.) and 5 (Wang) consider controlled release systems from biodegradable polymers, while Chapter 6 (Pitt, et al.) describes the metal-mediated controlled release of chelating agents. Chapters 7 (Gettings & White) and 8 (Jansen, et al.) cover the release of anti-microbial agents from different types of polymeric systems. Chapter 7 is also mainly concerned with some non-medical applications of this technology. Chapters 9 (Ghosh) and 10 (Kesler) are concerned with bioactive polymeric systems that contain steroidal sex hormones in completely different ways.

The next seven Chapters involve polymers with potential anti-tumor and other medicinal properties. Chapter 11 (Carraher & Strothers) deals with the release of methotrexate and/or chloroplatinate while Chapter 12 (Gebelein, et al.) describes the release of 5-fluorouracil from a biodegradable polymer. Chapter 13 (Matsuzaki, et al.) reviews much research on polysaccharides that have anti-tumor properties, and this theme is enhanced in Chapter 14 (Carraher, et al.) which describes tin-modified polysaccharides. The use of nucleic acid analogs in chromatography is the main theme of Chapter 15 (Inaki, et al.), but these same materials also have potential anti-tumor properties. Poly(ICLC), Chapter 16 (Levy & Bever) is also a nucleic acid analog with some anti-tumor potential. Finally, Chapter 17 (Trombley, et al.) covers polymers with anti-tumor and other medical properties.

Chapter 18 (Singh & Gaber) describes research on polymers that can form bioactive bilayers. Chapters 19-22 report various types of grafted polymers with varied potential medical applications. Thus, Chapter 19 (Daly & Lee) covers grafts of poly(amino acids) onto various proteins while Chapter 20 (Dworjanyn & Garnett) reports on research showing how to prepare grafts using radiation and/or photochemical methods. Chapters 21 and 22 are concerned with preparing anti-thrombogenic polymeric surfaces. In Chapter 21 (Wrobelski, et al.) this is attempted by the modification of poly(methyl methacrylate) with poly(vinylpyrrolidone), which had once been used as a blood plasma extender. In Chapter 22 (Chandy & Sharma) the approach is to graft thrombus lyzing agents or thrombo-resistant proteins onto the polymer surface. The books closes with Chapter 23 (Yannas, et al.) which updates important research on burn wound treatment using collagen modifications which interact with the natural body tissues. This paper by I. V. Yannas was given the Doolittle Award by the Division of

Polymeric Materials: Science & Engineering as the best paper presented in the Division at the American Chemical Society National Meeting, New Orleans, August, 1987.

This is a rapidly changing area of research and new developments will no doubt change some of the conclusions reported in these chapters, but much of this research will ultimately lead to many new applications of polymers in the biological and/or biomedical environments, both of which are of considerable practical human importance. The Editors wish to thank the American Chemical Society Division of Polymeric Materials: Science and Engineering who sponsored the symposium from which this book was derived. Likewise, we wish to thank the individual authors whose excellent research has made this book the challenging volume that it is. Finally, we wish to thank our wives, families and/or friends for their help and patience while we were bring this book into existence. This book was word-processed by CG ENTERPRISES.

Charles G. Gebelein
Charles E. Carraher, Jr.
Van Foster

CONTENTS

OVERVIEW OF SYNTHETIC AND MODIFIED NATURAL BIOACTIVE POLYMERS

Charles G. Gebelein[a], Charles E. Carraher, Jr.[b] &
Van R. Foster[c]

(a) Department of Chemistry
    Youngstown State University
    Youngstown, OH 44555

(b) Department of Chemistry
    Florida Atlantic University
    Boca Raton, FL 33431-0991

(c) DAP, Inc.
    P. O. Box 277
    Dayton, OH 45431

The area of applied bioactive polymeric systems includes
such diverse entities as controlled release systems (erodable
systems, diffusion controlled systems, mechanical systems and
microcapsules), and biologically active polymers, such as
natural polymers, synthetic polypeptides, pseudo-enzymes,
pseudo-nucleic acids and polymeric drugs. The area can also
include immobilized bioactive materials, such as immobilized
enzymes, antibodies and other bioactive agents and the area
of artificial cells. This Chapter reviews the general field
of biologically active synthetic and modified natural macromolecules with an emphasis on their common characteristics,
problems and applications. The areas reviewed include both
medical and non-medical applications for both controlled
release systems and polymers that exhibit direct biological
activity.

INTRODUCTION

Many synthetic and natural macromolecules have some biological
activity, although often inhibitory or toxic in nature. This well known
biological activity of natural proteins (including enzymes), nucleic
acids and polysaccharides actually forms the basis for both plant and
animal life. While some material applications require a lack of biological activity (such as prosthetic hip joints, protective coatings),
other applications require at least some biological activity (e.g., biodegradable materials, which generally require sensitivity to radiation,
moisture, air and/or microorganisms; controlled drug release).[1-3] This
Chapter concentrates on biologically active synthetic and modified
natural macromolecules.

BIOACTIVITY DEFINITION

In this paper, bioactivity will be considered to be the interaction of some chemical agent on a biological system. Examples of bioactivity would include: (1) the action of a drug on a disease center, (2) the action of a herbicide on weeds, (3) the action of an insecticide on insects, and (4) the prevention of conception by a chemical agent. In this sense, an applied bioactive polymeric system is one that utilizes any kind of polymeric material in producing, enhancing or controlling bioactivity.

TYPES OF BIOACTIVE POLYMERS

Many distinctively different types of bioactive polymeric systems exist and some of these are summarized in Table 1. For convenience, these are divided into the three classes of (1) controlled release systems,

Table 1. Classes of bioactive polymeric systems.

CONTROLLED RELEASE SYSTEMS
 	
erodible systems.
diffusion controlled systems:
  a. reservoir
  b. monolithic
mechanical devices.
microcapsules.

BIOLOGICALLY ACTIVE POLYMERS
 	
Natural Polymers:
 	
  proteins
  enzymes
  polysaccharides
  nucleic acids
 	
Synthetic Polymers:
 	
  modified polypeptides
  enzyme-mimetic polymers
  nucleic acid analogs
  polymeric drugs
  polymeric herbicides
  polymeric pesticides

IMMOBILIZED OR ENCAPSULATED BIOACTIVE MATERIALS living cells hemoglobin enzymes hormones antigens antibodies chloroplasts mitochondria plant growth regulators

(2) biologically active polymers, and (3) immobilized or encapsulated bioactive materials. The potential applications of the biologically active polymers are far too numerous to list exhaustively. Some of the applications are summarized in Table 2. It should be noted that any given application could be accomplished by more than one type of bioactive system, and vise versa. For example, cancer might be treated using controlled release systems, bioactive polymers or bound enzymes.

MODIFIED NATURAL BIOACTIVE MACROMOLECULES

Natural polymers have been widely employed as the polymeric matrix for controlled release systems and as a carrier for other bioactive agents. Part of this wide usage is due to three factors. First, the natural macromolecules themselves may exhibit biological activity that could be utilized to make a modified system more specific.[4-7] Second, depending on the specific natural macromolecule, the polymer may exhibit greater biological acceptance or rejection, such as in synthetic skin applications.[8] Third, most biological macromolecules are biodegradable allowing an avenue for controlled release and moderating unwanted concentration buildups.[9] (Controlled release is discussed in the next section.) Synthetic polymers have been used as the carriers in most drug delivery systems, which were designed to be inert and nondegradable, employing diffusion as the primary factor regulating the drug release.[10,11] The study of biodegradable systems is of more recent origin and with added difficulties - namely, specified rates of degradation and biocompatability of the degradation products. Such biodegradable systems have also been referred to as bioerodible and bio-absorbable drug delivery systems.

Poly(lactic acid), PLA, was first described in the literature in 1913 and was reported in 1966 as a material suitable for use in biodegradable surgical implants.[12] The first description of the use of PLA as a biodegradable implant for the delivery of the narcotic antagonists cyclazocine, naltrexone and naloxone was made by Yolles and coworkers in 1971.[13,14] Shortly afterwards, this polymer was tried in a contraceptive system.[15] Following the investigations with PLA, additional hydroxy-containing polypeptides were investigated. Poly(glycolic acid), PGA, has been widely used in surgical sutures, and copolymers of PLA and PGA have been used in delivery systems for drugs, insecticides and fertilizers. Various other copolymers of PLA, PGA, polyamides and polyesters have been synthesized and investigated as delivery systems.[16-19] Bio-lifetimes can be varied from several weeks to over a year.

CONTROLLED RELEASE SYSTEMS

A controlled release system is one which regulates or controls the release of some type of biologically active agent. Most, but not all, of these systems involve some type of polymeric material to restrict the concentration of this agent within a fairly narrow concentration range in order to elicit the desired bioactivity without the potentially dangerous side effects of the agent. Many examples of this behavior can be found in nature. For example, some complex polypeptides release a controlled amount of a subsection of the polypeptide which has some specific biological activity, and this is controlled by the body's chemistry.[20] Recently, hundreds of synthetic polypeptides have been developed, and many have shown biological activity.[5,21,22] Often these polypeptides have been mimics of those that occur naturally.

The basic concepts of controlled release systems will be considered below under the headings: (a) erodable systems, (b) diffusion controlled systems, (c) mechanical systems, and (d) microcapsules. In all cases considered, a polymeric material is used to regulate the bioactive agent.[23,24]

Erodable Systems

An erodable system contains the biologically active agent within some polymeric system which will dissolve or be destroyed by the biological media in which it is placed. Among the oldest medical examples are the

Table 2. Applications of biologically active polymers.

MEDICAL
cancer treatment
disease treatment
transplants
blood replacement
contraception control
narcotic control

AGRICHEMICAL
mildew control
rust & rot control
pest control
weed control
plant growth regulation
seed coating

VETERINARIAN
livestock protection
pets protection
wild animal control

WOOD PRESERVATION
fungus prevention
color protection
pest control

FOOD PROCESSING
enhanced yields
better preservation
flavor enhancement
coloring

HOME USES
pest control
insect control
rodent control
mildew control
furniture preservation
food preservation

enteric coated drugs in which a drug is protected from the stomach fluids and enzymes by a polymer which is then hydrolyzed in the intestines releasing the drug agent. In a similar manner, copper salts have been placed within natural, biodegradable polymers and have controlled barnacles adhering to ships.[25] More recent examples include timed-release capsules for cold and/or headache remedies. The polymers that have been used in this approach include polyacetals, polyesters, poly(orthoesters), polysaccharides, polypeptides and polyketals. The most commonly used synthetic polymers are the poly(lactic acids) and poly(glycolic acids), and their copolymers. Possibly the chief advantage of these systems is that the polymeric material is usually biodegradable and would not have to be removed from a patient. In addition to the enteric coatings and the timed-release capsules, erodable systems have been explored in drug addiction control, contraception, cancer treatment and a wide variety of drug release systems.[10,19,26-28]

Diffusion Controlled Systems

There are two basic types of diffusion controlled systems: (a) the reservior (depot) and (b) the monolithic. Most examples have used a non-degradable polymer, such as poly(dimethyl siloxane), natural or synthetic rubber, a vinyl polymer, or an acrylic polymer, although some examples of devices based on biodegradable polymers have been reported. The release rate of the bioactive agent normally follows first order kinetics in the reservior system, but is proportional to the square root of time in the monolithic systems (Higuchi kinetics). In either case, the specific rates are dependent on the composition of this polymeric material and on the chemical nature of the bioactive agent. In both systems, the release rate shows a steady decrease with time. Both systems usually give a high initial release of the active agent which is termed a "burst effect".[10,11,29,30]

The design of biodegradable implant devices based on PLA and PGA, noted earlier, have been mainly limited to reservoir types where the drug, in suspension or crystalline state, is sealed within a polymeric capsule so that the rate of release is regulated by diffusion characteristics. Another approach involves the use of poly(α-amino acids) in which the drug is encapsulated in polymeric shells, intermixed with the polymer, or covalently bound to the polymer backbone.[31-34]

The difussion based systems have found a variety of non-medical applications such as flea repellant collars, insecticide releasing strips and several agricultural applications. Some medical uses include the release of pilocarpine from a ethylene-vinyl acetate copolymer (Ocusert[R], Alza Corp.) for the control of glaucoma, and the release of progesterone from the same polymer to control fertility (Progestasert[R], Alza Corp.). Diffusion systems have also been utilized to release narcotic antagonists and anti-cancer agents.[35-38] Although most of the early examples of this technology were non-medical, nearly all of the recent emphasis has been in the medical areas. One of major areas of medically related activity is in fertility control and several potential systems are currently in advanced clinical trials, often funded by the World Health Organization. The controlled release of birth control agents has been reviewed recently.[39]

Mechanical Devices

A mechanical device would be one that utilizes any form of control, other than direct diffusion or erosion, to regulate the release of the biologicaly active agent. This catagory includes pumps and extracorporeal devices as well as osmotic pressure powered devices and transdermal membrane systems. Ordinary intravenous devices would also be included under this heading, but will not be considered further.

A number of external or internal pumps have been developed as insulin infusion pumps, or an artificial pancreas, which gives a more precise control over the body's insulin level. These devices normally inject the insulin solution directly into the patient's blood. Many of these "artificial pancreas" devices are able to vary the rate of insulin administration, and much progress has been made to couple these pumps with a microprocessor controlled glucose sensor which would closely approximate normal pancreatic activity. Most of these infusion pumps utilize poly-(dimethylsiloxane).[40,41]

Many devices currently on the medical market are simply a solution of a drug agent enclosed within a semi-permeable membrane. These systems have been reviewed recently.[42,43] Several of these devices operate by allowing water to diffuse into the drug-containing chamber and the diluted solution is forced out through a small orifice by the osmotic pressure that develops. The Oros[R] System (Alza Corp.) is an example.[35,36,44] Some other recent developments include the use of magnetic fields to moderate drug release.[45]

Transdermal patches, which utilize a semi-permeable membrane to regulate the release of a drug directly through the skin into a specified region of the body, have been developed for the administration of nitroglycerine (for treating angina pectoris) and scopolamine (for treating motion sickness).[35,36,42,46,47]

Microcapsules

A microcapsule is a minature membrane system in which the combination of high permeability and large surface area can confer some unusual properties and have made microcapsules of interest for drug release systems and for some artificial organs. Hundreds of different materials have been enclosed within microcapsules for both biomedical and non-medical use. The classic non-medical example would be the carbonless "carbon" papers which are in wide use today. Medically, microcapsules have been used to enclose various enzymes, such as catalase or L-asparaginase (which can be used to treat some forms of cancer), and have been shown to maintain the enzymatic activity for prolonged time periods.[48-50] Microcapsules have been utilized as artificial cells to enclose the beta-cells from the Islets of Langerhans, and such a system can function as a source of insulin (artificial pancreas).[51-55] Other research has centered on the use of such devices for artificial red blood cells.[56]

Market for Controlled Release

At this time, the market for controlled release systems is about $2.16 x 10^9$/year and is growing with an expected market in excess of $3.80 billion by 1991. At the present time, 51% of the controlled release market consists of pharmaceutical and related applications and this is projected to increase to about 63% by 1991. The second largest sector is in industrial applications which is currently about 40%, but is expected to decline to only 29% by 1991. The agricultural and food applications of controlled release is currently only about 9% of the total market and is expected to decline to about 7% by 1991.[57]

This decline in the agrichemical applications is especially interesting to note because much of the early impetus in the field of controlled release technology was in potential agricultural applications. One only has to examine the tables of contents of the papers published at the Annual Meeting of the Controlled Release Society to note a distinct shift in this emphasis. The major reasons for this shift is economics, not the unavailabilty of the technology. The use of any controlled release system will add an expense which can not be tolerated readily in agriculture but can be absorbed in medicine.

In the present markets for controlled release systems, microencapsulation is the dominant technology accounting for about $1.31 billion annually (61%), followed by coatings at $0.55 billion (25%) and polymer/membranes at $0.30 billion (14%). By 1991 these figures are expected to increase to $2.06, $0.69 and $1.05 billion for the microencapsulation, coatings and polymer/membranes, respectively. (The percentages are expected to be 54, 18 and 27, respectively.)[57]

PROTEINS AND ANALOGS

Proteins, enzymes, polysaccharides, and nucleic acids are natural biologically active polymers, but no attempt will be made to review these diverse systems here; several recent books and review articles are available.[20-22,58-60] Synthetic analogs have been prepared of essentially every type of natural macromolecule and many of these have exhibited biological activity. These analogs will be considered briefly in the next several sections.

Samanen and Whiteley have recently reviewed the area of biomedical polypeptides with respect to synthesis, problems and possibilities for developing new drugs.[5,60,61] Sequences can be assigned different roles, such as message sequences, prohormone sequences, and stability sequences. Research in this area illustrates attempts to employ naturally occurring (although typically synthetic) sequences to produce synthetic "nature-like" macromolecules. More than 200 clinical trials have been conducted using such natural peptides and their analogs. Whiteley and Petersen have reviewed the use of proteins and peptides as carriers.[4,6] The research on the endophins and enkephalins is now a classical example of such an effort and artificial derivatives have been synthesized with more than 28,000 times the analgesic activity of the natural materials.[62] Natural polymers, usually polypeptides, have been used as the polymeric matrix or as carrier controlled release systems.[5,6,60]

ENZYMES AND ENZYME-MIMETIC POLYMERS

Hundreds of examples of modified, natural polypeptides have appeared in the literature, many of which have high biological activity.[5,21,22,61] Enzyme-mimetic polymers (also referred to as enzyme-analogs, synzymes, or pseudo-enzymes) have been studied by many workers and these artificial analogs often show some activity, although much less than a typical enzyme.[63-66] This field was pioneered by Overberger,[63] and has been reviewed extensively by Imanishi.[65,66] In some recent research, enzyme activity has been created in otherwise inert protein molecules by chemical modification.[67,68] The potential medical applications of enzyme-mimetic polymers could include the treatment of enzyme deficiency diseases such as as phenylketon uria, tyrosinosis or histidinemia. If the missing enzyme is used to treat the patient, the body rapidly destroys this enzyme as a foreign protein. An enzyme-mimetic polymer might be able to by-pass the body's defense system and treat the enzyme deficient diseases. Enzyme-mimetic polymers might be usable in some manufacturing processes, if the cost can be reduced. The modified proteins are often relatively inexpensive and could have industrial utility. A modified enzyme has been patented recently and could have potential utility in food processing, leather treatment, cleaning applications and metal recovery.[69]

NUCLEIC ACIDS AND ANALOGS

The bioactivity of nucleic acids is also well established and need not be elaborated upon here. Analogous to the enzyme case, selected sequences of bases in DNA and RNA elicit specific responses. A large number of synthetic nucleic acid polymers have been prepared, which usually contain only a single base, and these materials are often biologically active. This topic has been reviewed recently.[70] Recently there have been attempts to mimic selected responses employing nucleic bases attached to vinyl or polypeptide chains. These materials can be called nucleic acid analogs or pseudonucleic acids. Much research has been done on nucleic acid analogs and this research has been reviewed by Takemoto and others.[71-75] Some of these materials have shown anti-viral and/or anti-tumor activities.[74] Some of the synthetic polymeric drugs which contain the anti-cancer agents 5-fluorouracil or 6-methylthiopurine can also be classed as nucleic acid analogs.[76-79]

POLYSACCHARIDES AND ANALOGS

Polysaccharides are widely used in biomedical applications including: demulcents, dental impression materials, dusting powders, hemistatics, plasma replacements, anticoagulants (in solution and as surface treatments on artificial organs), ointments; burn therapy, promoting post-surgery healing, distinguishing normal from malignant cells, in vaccines and adjuvants, body fluids, blood additives, etc. They have been converted into bioactive textiles and/or formed into membranes and hollow fibers for hemofiltration and hemodialysis. With this range of applications, it is hardly surprising that they have been used in drug formulations, drug delivery systems and for targeting drugs to specific sites.[80-82] Analogous to the pseudoenzymes and pseudonucleic acids, there exist pseudopolysaccharides. For example, Usmani and Salyer reacted poly(vinyl alcohol) with sucrose and obtained a product that "tasted" sweet but did not readily hydrolyze.[83]

POLYMERIC DRUGS

Polymeric drugs are macromolecules that contain a drug unit attached to or within the backbone chain or that exhibit drug action in the absence of such a unit. Hundreds of such polymers have been prepared and have been reviewed frequently.[59,84-91] The mode of action of the active polymeric drugs has been summarized. Briefly, these give their activity by one of several methods. Some hydrolyze to release the active drug unit, others enter the cell via endocytosis or indirectly via piggy-back endocytosis using a natural polypeptide, or other agent, as a carrier. A few polymers, such as the divinyl ether:maleic anhydride cyclocopolymer (DIVEMA or "Pyran" copolymer) actually possess drug-like activity without a specific drug unit on the polymer.[94] The DIVEMA polymer appears to interact with the immune system, promoting macrophages formation, which then results in the observed drug action.[95] Some other polymers, often polyanions, appear to increase the interferon concentration in the body.[92,96,97] The potential use of polymeric drugs in cancer therapy has been reviewed.[77,79,98]

One of the major challenges in polymeric drugs, and controlled release technology in general, is the possibility of targeting the delivery of a therapeutic agent to a specific disease site or organ in the body. Much research has been aimed at devising targeted polymeric drugs using liposomes, monoclonal anti-bodies, or other agents. This research has been reviewed.[7,76,84,88,89,93,99-102] Two recent patents (Liposome Technology) may bring the liposome technology nearer to medical usage. These materials are claimed, by the patentee, to meet three critical requirements for successful commercial development. These are: (1) efficient encapsulation of water soluble drugs, (2) an effective extrusion to achieve optimal liposome size and size distribution, and (3) ability to be sterilized at the completion of the manufacturing process.[69]

AGRIPOLYMERS

Parallel to the introduction of drugs within polymeric materials is the introduction of metal containing moieties aimed at the preservation of wood and wood products (e.g., 103). Much effort has been made employing, mainly, tin-containing polymers.[104-112] Many controlled release formulations based on tri-n-butyltin and di-n-butyltin moieties have been developed that permit the wood to resist mildew, rot and salt water deterioration for years. These products exhibit a tolerable toxicity toward mammals and thus may be environmentally acceptable.[113,114] Controlled release systems have found many other applications in the field of agriculture including pest control,[25,115] animal repellants,[116] plant growth regulators,[117] and herbicide control.[118]

Unlike the drug containing systems, few in depth studies have been undertaken and efforts at site specific delivery of bioactive moieties, such as pesticides, have been largely lacking. Part of the reason for this is economics; the greater cost of targeting can be tolerated more readily in medicines than in the lower cost agrichemical products. Evenso, preliminary results are encouraging and demand further investigation. Some unqualified successes (such as the treatment of wood with tin-containing polymers) have already been achieved and others may be forthcoming.

IMMOBILIZED ENZYMES & RELATED MATERIALS

Immobilized bioactive materials, such as enzymes, are beyond the scope of this paper, but the topic has been reviewed often.[67,119-128] Immobilized enzymes have been developed to overcome the limitations of enzymes in many industrial and medical applications. These limitations include cost, difficulty of recovery from a chemical reaction, temperature sensitivity, pH limitations, and the possibility of inactivation by a variety of agents, specially in a biomedical environment. The same techniques used for enzymes have also been used to antibodies, antigens, various cells and/or tissues.[124,125,129]

CONCLUSIONS

Bioactive polymeric systems are a growing field of research that involves several disciplines including chemistry, medicine, biology and engineering. This field of research has mushroomed in the past decade and has already achieved a two+ billion dollar market. Many new techniques and products will probably be placed on the market in the next several years, but most of these will probably be in the biomedical markets because the cost can be more readily absorbed there than in the agrichemical products.

REFERENCES

1. C. E. Carraher, Jr. & C. G. Gebelein, Eds., "*Biological Activities of Polymers*", American Chemical Society, Washington, DC, 1982.
2. C. G. Gebelein & C. E. Carraher, Jr., Eds., "*Bioactive Polymeric Systems*", Plenum Publ. Corp., New York, 1985.
3. C. G. Gebelein & C. E. Carraher, Jr., Eds., "*Polymeric Materials in Medication*", Plenum Publ. Corp., New York, 1985.
4. R. V. Petersen in: "*Bioactive Polymeric Systems*", C. G. Gebelein & C. E. Carraher, Jr., Eds., Plenum Publ., New York, 1985, pp. 151-177.
5. J. Samanen in: "*Bioactive Polymeric Systems*", C. G. Gebelein & C. E. Carraher, Jr., Eds., Plenum Publ., New York, 1985, pp. 279-344.
6. J. M. Whiteley in: "*Bioactive Polymeric Systems*", C. G. Gebelein & C. E. Carraher, Jr., Eds., Plenum Publ., New York, 1985, pp. 345-363.
7. R. L. Juliano, Ed., "*Biological Approaches to the Controlled Delivery of Drugs*", Vol. 507, New York Academy of Science, New York, 1987
8. I. V. Yannas, D. P. Orgill, E. M. Skrabut & J. F. Burke in: "*Polymeric Materials and Artificial Organs*", C. G. Gebelein, Ed., ACS Symposium Series No. 256, American Chemical Society, Washington, DC, 1984, pp. 191-197.
9. C. E. Carraher, Jr. & L. H. Sperling, Polymer News, 13, 101-106 (1988).
10. S. D. Bruck, Ed., "*Controlled Drug Delivery*", Vol. I, II, CRC Press, Boca Raton, FL (1983).
11. A. F. Kydonieus, "*Controlled Release Technologies, Methods, Theory and Applications*", Vol. I, II, CRC Press, Boca Raton, FL (1980).
12. R. Kulkarni, K. Pani, C. Neuman & F. Leonard, "*Poly(Lactic Acid) for Surgical Implants*", Tech. Report 6608, Walter Reed Medical Center, Washington, DC (1966).
13. D. A. Blake, S. Yolles, M. Helrich, H. F. Cascorbi & M. J. Eagan, Acad. Pharm. Sci., San Francisco, March 30, 1971.
14. J. Woodland, S. Yolles, D. Blake, M. Helrich & F. J. Meyer, J. Med. Chem., 16, 97 (1973).
15. T. Jackanicz, H. Nash, D. Wise & J. B. Gregory, Contraception, 8, 227 (1973).
16. A. Schindler, R. Jeffcoat, G. Kimmel, C. G. Pitt, M. E. Wall & R. Zweidinger in: "*Contemporary Topics in Polymer Science*", E. M. Pearce & J. Schaefaer, Eds., Vol. 2, Plenum Publ. Corp., New York, 1977, p. 251.
17. M. C. Bissen & F. Puisieux, "*Proc. Ninth Internat. Symp. Controlled Release of Bioactive Materials*", Controlled Release Society, Ft. Lauderdale, FL, 1982, p. 30.
18. S. Mitra, M. Van Dress, J. Anderson, R. V. Petersen, D. Gregonis & J. Feijen, Polymer Preprints, 20 (2), 32 (1979).
19. N. S. Mason, C. S. Miles & R. E. Sparks, in: "*Biomedical and Dental Applications of Polymers*", C. G. Gebelein & F. F. Koblitz, Eds., pp. 279-291, Plenum Publ., New York (1981).
20. J. J. L'Italien, Ed., "*Proteins: Structure and Function*", Plenum Publ., New York, 1988.
21. C. H. Li, Ed., "*Hormonal Proteins and Peptides*", Vol. 8, Academic

Press, New York (1980).

22. J. Ramachandran, in: "*Biological Activities of Polymers*", C. E. Carraher, Jr. & C. G. Gebelein, Eds., pp. 119-132, American Chemical Society, Washington, DC (1982).

23. Y. W. Chien, "*Novel Drug Delivery Systems*", Dekker, New York, 1982.

24. J. R. Robinson & V. H. L. Lee, "*Controlled Drug Delivery*", Dekker, New York, 1987.

25. N. F. Cardarelli & B. M Cardarelli in: "*Bioactive Polymeric Systems*", C. G. Gebelein & C. E. Carraher, Jr., Eds., Plenum Publ., New York, 1985, pp. 31-92.

26. C. G. Pitt, T. A. Marks & A. Schindler, in: "*Controlled Release of Bioactive Materials*", R. Baker, Ed., pp. 19-43, Academic Press, New York (1980).

27. J. Heller & R. Baker, in: "*Controlled Release of Bioactive Materials*", R. Baker, Ed., pp. 1-17, Academic Press, New York (1980).

28. S. Yolles, R. M. Roat, M. F. Sartori & C. L. Washburne, in: "*Biological Activities of Polymers*", C. E. Carraher, Jr. & C. G. Gebelein, Eds., pp. 233-241, American Chemical Society, Washington, DC (1982).

29. W. R. Good & K. F. Mueller, in: "*Controlled Release of Bioactive Materials*", R. Baker, Ed., pp. 155-175, Academic Press, New York (1980).

30. W. D. Rhine, V. Sukhatme, D. S. T. Hsieh & R. S. Langer, in: "*Controlled Release of Bioactive Materials*", R. Baker, Ed., pp. 177-187, Academic Press, New York (1980).

31. J. Feijen, D. Gregonis, C. Anderson, R. V. Petersen & J. Anderson, J. Pharm. Sci., **69**, 871 (1980).

32. D. Gregonis, J. Feijen, J. Anderson & R. V. Petersen, Polymer Preprints, **20** (1), 612 (1979).

33. W. A. R. Van Heeswijk, G. Brinks & J. Feijen, "*Preprints Internat. Symposium on Polymers in Medicine*", Porto Cervo, Sardinia, Italy, 1982, p. 6.

34. R. V. Petersen, S. W. Kim, J. Anderson, S. Fang, D. G. Gregonis, J. Nelson, D. Coleman, S. Woodward & C. Anderson, "*Development and Testing of New Biodegradable Drug Delivery Systems*", Contract No. 1-HD-2824, Final Report NICHD, (Dec. 14, 1980), p. 1.

35. A. Zaffaroni, in: "*Biomedical and Dental Applications of Polymers*", C. G. Gebelein & F. F. Koblitz, Eds., pp. 293-313, Plenum Publ., New York (1981).

36. A. Zaffaroni, Chemtech, 6, 756-761 (1976).

37. G. W. Duncan, D. R. Kalkwarf & J. T. Veal, in: "*Polymers in Medicine and Surgery*", R. L. Kronenthal, Z. Oser & E. Martin, Eds., pp. 205-212, Plenum Publ., New York (1975).

38. S. Yolles, in: "*Polymers in Medicine and Surgery*", R. L. Kronenthal, Z. Oser & E. Martin, Eds., pp. 245-261, Plenum Publ., New York (1975).

39. D. L. Gardner & B. A. Metz in: "*Bioactive Polymeric Systems*", C. G. Gebelein & C. E. Carraher, Jr., Eds., Plenum Publ., New York, 1985, pp. 93-119.

40. J. V. Santiago, A. H. Clemens, W. L. Clarke & D. M. Kipnis, Diabetes, 28 (1), 71-84 (1979).

41. H. J. Sanders, Chem. Eng. News, Mar. 2, 1981, pp. 30-45.

42. Y. W. Chien in: "*Polymeric Materials in Medication*", C. G. Gebelein & C. E. Carraher, Jr., Eds., Plenum Publ., New York, 1985, pp. 27-46.

43. W. R. Vieth, "*Membrane Systems: Analysis and Design*", Oxford University Press, New York, 1988.

44. F. Theeuwes & B. Eckenhoff, in: "*Controlled Release of Bioactive Materials*", R. Baker, Ed., pp. 61-82, Academic Press, New York (1980).

45. E. R. Edelman, L. Brown, J. Taylor & R. Langer, J. Biomed. Mater. Res., **21**, 339 (1987).
46. S. K. Chandrasekaran & J. E. Shaw, in: "*Controlled Release of Bioactive Materials*", R. Baker, Ed., pp. 99-106, Academic Press, New York (1980).
47. D. A. Jones, Ed., "*Transdermal & Related Drug Delivery Systems*", Noyes Data Corp., Park Ridge, NJ, 1984.
48. B. Sedláček & J. Kahovec, Eds., "*Synthetic Polymeric Membranes*", de Gruyter, New York, 1987.
49. P. Guiot & P. Couvreur, Eds., "*Polymeric Nanoparticles and Microspheres*", CRC Press, Boca Raton, 1986.
50. A. Rembaum & Z. A. Tokes, Eds., "*Microspheres: Medical and Biological Applications*", CRC Press, Boca Raton, 1988.
51. J. A. Bakan, in: "*Polymers in Medicine and Surgery*", R. L. Kronenthal, Z. Oser & E. Martin, Eds., pp. 213-235, Plenum Publ., New York (1975).
52. F. Lim & A. M. Sun, Science, 210, 980 (1980).
53. T. Kondo, in: "*Surface and Colloid Science*", E. Matijevic, Ed., Vol. 10, pp. 1-43, Plenum Publ., New York (1978).
54. T. M. S. Chang, Ed., "*Artificial Kidney, Artificial Liver, and Artificial Cells*", Plenum Publ., New York (1978).
55. T. M. S. Chang, in: "*Biomedical Polymers. Polymeric Materials and Pharmaceuticals for Biomedical Use*", E. P. Goldberg & A. Nakajima, Eds., pp. 171-187, Academic Press, New York (1980).
56. A. Kato & T. Kondo in: "*Advances in Biomedical Polymers*", C. G. Gebelein, Ed., Plenum Publ., New York, 1987, pp. 299-310.
57. Anon. Polymer News, 13, 114-115 (1988)
58. C. H. Li, Ed., "*Hormonal Proteins and Peptides*", Vol. I & II, Academic Press, New York (1973).
59. M. Ghosh, Polymer News, 13, 71-77 (1988).
60. A. G. Walton, in: "*Biomedical Polymers. Polymeric Materials and Pharmaceuticals for Biomedical Use*", E. P. Goldberg & A. Nakajima, Eds., pp. 53-83, Academic Press, New York (1980).
61. J. M. Samanen in: "*Polymeric Materials in Medication*", C. G. Gebelein & C. E. Carraher, Jr., Eds., Plenum Publ., New York, 1985, pp. 227-247.
62. S. H. Snyder, Chem. Eng. News, Nov. 28, 1977, pp. 26-35.
63. J. A. Pavlisko & C. G. Overberger in: "*Biomedical and Dental Applications of Polymers*", C. G. Gebelein & F. F. Koblitz, Eds., Plenum Publ. Corp., New York, 1981, p. 257.
64. A. S. Lindsey, in: "*Reviews in Macromolecular Chemistry*", Vol. 4, G. B. Butler & K. F. O'Driscoll, Eds., pp. 1-47, Dekker, New York (1970).
65. Y. Imanishi, J. Polymer Sci., Macromol. Revs., **14**, 1 (1979).
66. Y. Imanishi in: "*Bioactive Polymeric Systems*", C. G. Gebelein & C. E. Carraher, Jr., Eds., Plenum Publ., New York, 1985, pp. 435-511.
67. M. H. Keyes & S. Saraswathi in: "*Bioactive Polymeric Systems*", C. G. Gebelein & C. E. Carraher, Jr., Eds., Plenum Publ., New York, 1985, pp. 249-278.
68. S. Saraswathi & M. S. Keyes in: "*Polymeric Materials in Medication*", C. G. Gebelein & C. E. Carraher, Jr., Eds., Plenum Publ., New York, 1985, pp. 249-264.
69. Anon., Chem. Week, July 6, 1988, p. 16.
70. H. B. Levy & T. Quinn in: "*Bioactive Polymeric Systems*", C. G. Gebelein & C. E. Carraher, Jr., Eds., Plenum Publ., New York, 1985, pp. 387-415.
71. K. Takemoto, J. Polymer Sci., Poly. Symp., **55**, 105 (1976).
72. K. Takemoto in: "*Polymeric Drugs*", L. G. Donaruma & O. Vogl, Eds., Academic Press, New York, 1978, p. 103.
73. K. Takemoto in: "*Bioactive Polymeric Systems*", C. G. Gebelein & C.

E. Carraher, Jr., Eds., Plenum Publ., New York, 1985, pp. 417-433.

74. J. Pitha, in: "*Biomedical and Dental Applications of Polymers*", C. G. Gebelein & F. F. Koblitz, Eds., pp. 203-213, Plenum Publ., New York (1981).

75 J. Pitha, M. Akashi & M. Draminski, in: "*Biomedical Polymers. Polymeric Materials and Pharmaceuticals for Biomedical Use*", E. P. Goldberg & A. Nakajima, Eds., pp. 271-297, Academic Press, New York (1980).

76. C. G. Gebelein, R. M. Morgan, R. Glowacky & W. Baig, in: "*Biomedical and Dental Applications of Polymers*", C. G. Gebelein & F. F. Koblitz, Eds., pp. 191-201, Plenum Publ., New York (1981).

77. C. G. Gebelein, in: "*Biological Activities of Polymers*", C. E. Carraher, Jr. & C. G. Gebelein, Eds., pp. 193-203, American Chemical Society, Washington, DC (1982).

78. J. L. Alderfer, R. E. Loomis, S. D. Soni, M. Sharma, R. Bernacki & R. Hughes, Jr., in: "*Polymeric Materials in Medication*", C. G. Gebelein & C. E. Carraher, Jr., Eds., Plenum Publ., New York, 1985, pp. 125-138.

79. M. Ghosh & S. Maiti in: "*Polymeric Materials in Medication*", C. G. Gebelein & C. E. Carraher, Jr., Eds., Plenum Publ., New York, 1985, pp. 103-114.

80. C. Schuerch in: "*Bioactive Polymeric Systems*", C. G. Gebelein & C. E. Carraher, Jr., Eds., Plenum Publ., New York, 1985, pp. 365-386.

81. J. F. Kennedy & N. R. Williams, Eds., "*Carbohydrate Chemistry, A Review of the Literature*", Royal Society (London).

82. L. S. Goodman & A. Gilman, Eds., "*The Pharmacological Basis of Therapeutics*", 4th, 5th & 6th Editions, Macmillan Co., New York, 1970, 1975, 1980.

83. A. Usmani & I. O. Salyer in: "*Modifications of Polymers*", C. E. Carraher, Jr. & J. Moore, Eds., Plenum Publ. Corp., New York, 1983, p. 247.

84. C. G. Gebelein, Polymer News, 4, 163-171 (1978).

85. L. G. Donaruma & O. Vogl, Eds., "*Polymeric Drugs*", Academic Press, New York (1978).

86. L. G. Donaruma, R, M. Ottenbrite & O. Vogl, eds., "*Anionic Polymeric Drugs*", Wiley-Interscience, New York (1980).

87. S. M. Samour, Chemtech, 8, 494-501 (1978).

88. H. Ringsdorf, J. Polymer Sci., Symposium No 51, 135-153 (1975).

89. H. G. Batz, in: Advances in Polymer Science, Vol. 23, H. J. Cantrow, Ed., pp. 25-53, Springer-Verlag, New York (1977).

90. D. S. Breslow, Pure & Appl. Chem., 46, 103-113 (1976).

91. V. A. Kropachev, Pure & Appl. Chem., 355-361 (1976).

92. R. M. Ottenbrite in: "*Bioactive Polymeric Systems*", C. G. Gebelein & C. E. Carraher, Jr., Eds., Plenum Publ., New York, 1985, pp. 513-529.

93. K. Dorn, G. Hoerpel & H. Ringsdorf in: "*Bioactive Polymeric Systems*", C. G. Gebelein & C. E. Carraher, Jr., Eds., Plenum Publ., New York, 1985, pp. 531-585.

94. G.B. Butler, in: "*Anionic Polymeric Drugs*", L. G. Donaruma, R. M. Ottenbrite & O. Vogl, Eds., Wiley-Interscience, New York (1980), pp. 49-141.

95. L. G. Baird & A. M. Kaplan, in: "*Anionic Polymeric Drugs*", L. G. Donaruma, R. M. Ottenbrite & O. Vogl, Eds., Wiley-Interscience, New York (1980), pp. 185-210.

96. M. C. Breinig, A. E. Munson & P. S. Morahan, in: "*Anionic Polymeric Drugs*", L. G. Donaruma, R. M. Ottenbrite & O. Vogl, Eds., Wiley-Interscience, New York (1980), pp. 211-226.

97. E. M. Hodnett in: "*Polymeric Materials in Medication*", C. G. Gebelein & C. E. Carraher, Jr., Eds., Plenum Publ., New York, 1985, pp. 211-226.

13

98. C. E. Carraher, Jr., W. S. Scott & D. J. Giron in: "*Bioactive Polymeric Systems*", C. G. Gebelein & C. E. Carraher, Jr., Eds., Plenum Publ., New York, 1985, pp. 587-620.
99. M. J. Ostro, Ed., "*Liposomes From Biophysics to Therapeutics*", Marcel Dekker, New York, 1987.
100. M. J. Ostro, Ed., "*Liposomes*", Marcel Dekker, New York, 1983.
101. J. D. Rodwell, Ed., "*Antibody-Mediated Delivery Systems*", Marcel Dekker, New York, 1988.
102. S. Ferrone & M. P. Dierich, Eds., "*Handbook of Monoclonal Antibodies. Applications in Biology and Medicine*", Noyes Data Corp., Park Ridge, NJ, 1985.
103. C. E. Carraher in: "*Bioactive Polymeric Systems*", C. G. Gebelein & C. E. Carraher, Jr., Eds., Plenum Publ. Corp., New York, 1985, Chapters 20, 22.
104. A. Phillip, Prog. Org. Coatings, 2, 159 (1973/74).
105. T. Hof, J. Inst. Wood Sci., 4, 19 (1969).
106. M. P. Levi, J. Inst. Wood Sci., 4, 45 (1969).
107. R. Cockroft, J. Inst. Wood Sci., 6, 2 (1974).
108. R. V. Subramanian, B. Gard, J. Jakubowski, J. Corredor, J. Montemarano & E. C. Fisher, Org. Coatings & Plastics Chem., 36 (2), 660 (1976).
109. R. V. Subramanian & M. Anand in: "*Chemistry and Properties of Crosslinked Polymers*", S. S. Labana, Ed., Academic Press, New York, 1977, p. 1.
110. R. V. Subramanian, B. K. Garg & J. Corredor, J. Macromol. Sci.-Chem., **A11**, 1567 (1977).
111. R. V. Subramanian, B. K. Garg & J. Corredor in: "*Organometallic Polymers*", C. E. Carraher, Jr., J. Sheats & C. Pittman, Eds., Academic Press, New York, 1978, p. 181.
112. K. N. Somasekharan & R. V. Subramanian in: "*Modification of Polymers*", C. E. Carraher, Jr. & M. Tsuda, Eds., American Chemical Society, Washington, DC, 1980, p. 165.
113. A. W. Sheldon, J. Paint Technol., **47** (600), 54 (1975).
114. E. J. Dyckman & J. A. Montemarano, "*Antifouling Organometallic Polymers: Environmentally Compatible Materials*", NSRDC Report 4136, Feb. 1974.
115. H. B. Scher, "*Controlled Release Pesticides*", American Chemical Society, Washington, DC, 1977.
116. D. L. Gustafson in: "*Bioactive Polymeric Systems*", C. G. Gebelein & C. E. Carraher, Jr., Eds., Plenum Publ., New York, 1985, pp. 179-201.
117. J. M. Miller & A. Yahiaoui in: "*Bioactive Polymeric Systems*", C. G. Gebelein & C. E. Carraher, Jr., Eds., Plenum Publ., New York, 1985, pp. 121-141.
118. D. L. Wise, "*Biopolymeric Controlled Release Systems*", Vol. II, CRC Press, Boca Raton, FL, 1984.
119. S. B. H. Kent in: "*Biomedical Polymers*", E. Goldberg & A. Nakajima, Eds., Academic Press, New York, 1980, p. 213.
120. I. Chibati, "*Immobilized Enzymes*", John Wiley & Sons, New York, 1978.
121. P. W. Carr & L. Bowers, "*Immobilized Enzymes in Analytical and Clinical Chemistry*", John Wiley & Sons, New York, 1980.
122. A. I. Laskin, "*Enzymes and Immobilized Cells in Biotechnology*", Butterworth Publ., Stonehan, MA, 1985.
123. R. A. Messing, Ed., "*Immobilized Enzymes for Industrial Reactors*", Academic Press, New York, 1975.
124. H. H. Weetal, ed., "*Immobilized Enzymes, Antigens, Antibodies and Peptides*", Dekker, New York (1975).
125. T. M. S. Chang, ed., "*Biomedical Applications of Immobilized Enzymes and Proteins*", Vol. 1 & 2, Plenum Publ., New York (1977).
126. M. D. Trevan, "*Immobilized Enzymes*", Wiley, New York (1980).

127. M. H. Keyes, in: *"Kirk-Othmer, Encyclopedia of Chemical Technology"*, 3rd. ed., Vol. 9, pp. 148-172, Wiley, New York (1980).
128. S. P. O'Neill, Rev. Pure & Appl. Chem., 22, 133-143 (1972).
129. T. Fujimura, F. Yoshii, I. Kaetsu, Y. Inoue & K. Shibata, Z. Naturforsch., 35c, 477-482 (1980).

PESTICIDE-POLYMER RESEARCH: A REVIEW OF 1976-87

David A. Kurtz and Kevin Hassett

Department of Entomology
Pesticide Research Laboratory
The Pennsylvania State University
University Park, PA 16802

The usefulness and effectiveness of polymers in pesticide applications is shown in this literature review covering from 1976 to 1987. Pesticides have been physically incorporated in the polymer matrix; release has been by desorption, by true solution movement through the polymer matrix, by leaching, by breaking of microencapsulated droplets, by flow through hollow fiber tubes, and by chemically breaking the polymer bonds. Pesticides have also been chemically bonded in a polymer formulation either before or after polymerization; their release has been accommodated through breakup of cross-linking bonds, through breakup of the main polymer backbone, and by hydrolysis of the pendant chain. Sometimes pesticidal action is effective without polymer degradation. Polymer interaction with pesticide formulations has also been shown in flocculation control, spray-drift control, and in devices utilizing this concept (leg bands, ear tags, plastic strips and mulches). References have been cited showing either practical or theoretical use. Some tables and figures have been presented to show this usefulness and efficacy.

INTRODUCTION

Pesticides have been applied in a variety of formulations onto soils and crops for the control of insects, noxious weeds, fungi, and other bioagents that interfere in the production of food and fiber. Examples of such formulations are dusts, suspensions prepared from solid powders, and suspensions prepared from concentrated liquid formulations. The formulations, however, can have some undesired effects in that the active ingredient in these preparations can easily move about to a non-target area. Dusts can easily be carried for long distances away from the field even in the slightest winds. Evaporation to the atmosphere can take place with both dusts and liquid suspensions sprayed onto fields.

In recent times polymeric materials have been used to improve the application and effectiveness of pesticides and to remove at least some of the disadvantages described above. Incorporation of a pesticide within a polymer has allowed a lower concentration of pesticide to be applied.

This results from a retention of the agent within the polymer body obviating its spread into the environment. It has also prevented degradation from taking place either from contact with water, ultraviolet radiation, or atmospheric oxygen. Hence, polymers have been used to modify the concentration of a pesticide by containing and protecting it as well as slowing down its release as a free agent to the environment. Polymers have thus controlled undesired movement in the environment. Supplementary uses have been to control the flocculation in pesticide suspensions and to control the drifting of the spray.

Gebelein suggests that there are five methods of immobilizing enzymes, but three are actually physical methods and only two are chemical binding.[1] These can be applied to a description of immobilizing pesticides. The three physical methods are: (1) adsorption, (2) matrix entrapment and (3) encapsulation. The methods by which these physical binding methods release the pesticide are: (1) desorption, (2) diffusion and (3) polymer degradation or destruction. Physical desorption from such strong adsorbents as silica gel, mica, and activated charcoal were the first to appear in use.[1] Later diffusion-based processes were employed. The physical processes of release were the primary processes studied at the time of the 1976 ACS symposium.[1]

The two chemical methods are: (1) bonding in chain and (2) bonding through crosslinking. A number of these methods will be reported here. They are the most interesting, of course, to the polymer chemist. The pesticide is chemically bonded to a monomer or polymer. Its usefulness depends on inherent activity of the pesticide-polymer itself or on the chemical release of the pesticide through chemical degradation. The active material is degraded through action of air, sunlight, water, or microorganisms. Equation 1 illustrates this approach, where synthesis and environment (water, air, sunlight, microorganisms) operate in opposing directions.[1]

POLYMER + PESTICIDE $\longrightarrow$ POLYMERIC PESTICIDE   (Equation 1)

The most common linkages are esters, anhydrides and acetals.[1] Most likely the chemical degradation will take place through an hydrolysis reaction, the anhydride being the easiest to hydrolyze. A crosslinked polymer will afford more resistance to degradation than linear polymers. Also, a crystalline polymer is less reactive than an amorphous or atactic polymer.

In the following discussion, pesticides that have been dispersed within the polymer in some way or encapsulated as a solution within a polymeric "skin" will be discussed under the "Physically Bonded" topics. These systems are those that physically hold the pesticide within the polymeric matrix. On the other hand, the "Chemically Bonded" systems bind the pesticide or pesticidal ligand to part of the molecule of the polymer itself. Their action is due to either the action of the polymer itself or to the gradual breakdown of the molecule leaving a smaller molecule having pesticidal action. Specialized uses will be found in the sections on "Flocculation Control" and "Spray Drift Control". References that emphasize the incorporation of pesticide-polymers as "Polymeric Devices" and those that control insects and weeds through "Plastic Mulches" will be discussed last.

Polymeric materials originally were used as a control mechanism in agriculture twenty years ago in simplistic ways. Largely as sheeting materials, these uses were either to keep crops dry, such as the outside storage of hay, or to keep them wet to conserve soil moisture. However as much as fifteen years ago, fertilizers and insecticides were used in conjunction with polymeric concepts or materials to alter the release or activity of the product.[2,3] The classic example of such an application was the physical incorporation of dichlorvos in poly(vinyl chloride) coated on paper or pressed into blocks.[4,5] Such uses have found favor in reducing costs by using less pesticide and in reducing the release of toxic compounds to the environment. Recent advances in the utilization of polymeric materials for the control of insects, noxious weeds, and the like will be listed.

The scope of this paper is to update a previous symposium on this topic which was also held in New Orleans, in March 1977.[6] Papers published in 1976 and later will generally be discussed here. The reader is referred to several earlier references on this topic.[1,7,8] Two additional texts have been published since 1976.[9,10]

PESTICIDE POLYMERS - PHYSICALLY BONDED

1. Preparation of Physically Bonded Formulations

A. Adsorption. The physical adsorption of the nonionic, nonpolar chlorinated pesticides, lindane and toxaphene, were measured in two types of polymers: ionic exchange resins and nonionic styrene:divinylbenzene polymers.[11] The following results were obtained:

a. Lindane was adsorbed best in the strongly basic hydroxyl form of the exchange resin Wofatit SBW[TM]. This resin, from W. Germany, is a quaternary trimethylammonium exchanger. When 1 g/L solution, dissolved in 60% aqueous methanol, was allowed to be in contact for only 2 hours, 70 mg/g of lindane was adsorbed. This amount was much larger than when other salt forms of the exchanger were used.

b. Toxaphene was adsorbed from 50% acetone solution to the extent of 36 mg/g of Wofatit SBU[TM], hydroxyl form, after 24 hours. Similar quantities were adsorbed, 36 and 41 mg/g, from resin that contained primary and secondary amino groups as anchor groups from solutions of 60% methanol and 50% acetone, containing the toxaphene. These latter data were also determined from 24 hours contact time.

c. The best adsorption of lindane and toxaphene was from macroporous styrene:divinylbenzene copolymer. At a 2 hour adsorption time, 100 mg/g of lindane and 117 mg/g of toxaphene was adsorbed from the respective solutions.

B. Matrix Incorporation. Matrix incorporation is probably the most common method for the preparation of physically bonded pesticides. Five methods illustrate the wide variety available for the preparation of incorporated aldicarb[12] and diflubenzuron (Dimilin[TM])[13]. Both are carbamate insecticides. Selected methods were used for the matrix adsorption of the following organic insecticides: Abate[TM], Dursban[TM], malathion, and naled[14]:

a. Polymerization of a solution of monomers and a pesticide. An example of this is the addition of aldicarb to the monomeric precursors of urea-formaldehyde polymer. Treatment of the solution with trace quantities of phosphoric acid afforded the polymerization.

Formaldehyde and urea with plasticizers and Dimilin[TM] were allowed to react together and then harden in a circular pan. The dimilin™ was incorporated within the urea-formaldehyde polymer at the time of polymerization. The plasticizers used were glycerol and granular gelatin. The organophosphorus compounds were also incorporated with polyurethane foam but at the completion of foaming.[14]

b. Polymers and pesticides are mutually dissolved in a solvent. Aldicarb[12] and Dimilin™,[13] were stirred with a turbid solution of the polyamide Elvamide™, in methanol. When dried, the sheets of white opaque resin were ground to granules. The polymer formulations with the organophosphorus compounds were also made in this manner.[14]

In a similar manner, cellulose acetate, along with aldicarb and plasticizers, were dissolved in acetone and refluxed. The hot solution was poured into glass containers, allowing the acetone to evaporate. Other solvents can be used, as necessary.

Methoprene is a non-persistent systemic insect growth regulator effective against the horn fly, *Haemotobia irritans* (L.) and the common cattle grub, *Hypodermia lineatum* (de Villers). Methoprene, [isopropyl (E,E)-11-methoxy-3,7,11-trimethyl-2,4-dodecadienoate], was physically enclosed in poly(dl-lactic acid) by dissolving the starting materials in methylene chloride and then evaporating the solvent.[15] When pressed into pellets, a useful form of the insecticide was formed. The pellets were found to release the methoprene at a relatively constant rate from *in vitro* laboratory experiments. When implanted in Black Angus steer ears, however, the release became less uniform although the active ingredient was still present in the pellets.

c. Precipitation by solvent changes. Carbopol resin formulations were mixed with Dimilin™. Granules were formed by the careful addition of small amounts of water. When the water was allowed to evaporate, the granules could be blended and sieved for later use.

d. Solid mixing of polymer and pesticide. Aldicarb was incorporated in Isofoam PE-20™ as an example of this method.

Poly(vinyl chloride), as a plastisol, was used with Dimilin™ for incorporation by heating to moderate temperatures to afford mixing. In the earliest work,[14] the temperature was 150°C and the pesticides successfully incorporated were naled, Abate™, Dursban™, and malathion. Later, aldicarb was successfully incorporated.[12]

e. Melting polymer and pesticide together. Poly(vinyl chloride) plastisol and aldicarb were melted together at 260°C for 1 min in small metal planchets. Little aldicarb decomposition was found.

A matrix incorporation of organophosphorus and carbamate pesticides into a polyamide polymer was found to have good use under tropical conditions (see Figure 1). The best combination of carbofuran with the polymer was found to suppress attacks of the mahogany shootborer, *Hypsipyla grandella Zeller*, for almost a year.[16]

The older preparation of the plastic devices was made by melting Versamid 940™ (General Mills Chemicals) at about 110°C. This polymer had an average molecular weight of 6000 and was prepared from ethylenediamine and dilinoleic acid.[17] The respective pesticide was added and mixed until it was homogeneously dissolved. The solution was then poured into molds and cut as cylinders, 1 cm in diameter by 2 cm long (carbofuran cylinders were 8 cm long). These cylinders, 12 in number, were buried under the soil 15 cm from the tree seedling.

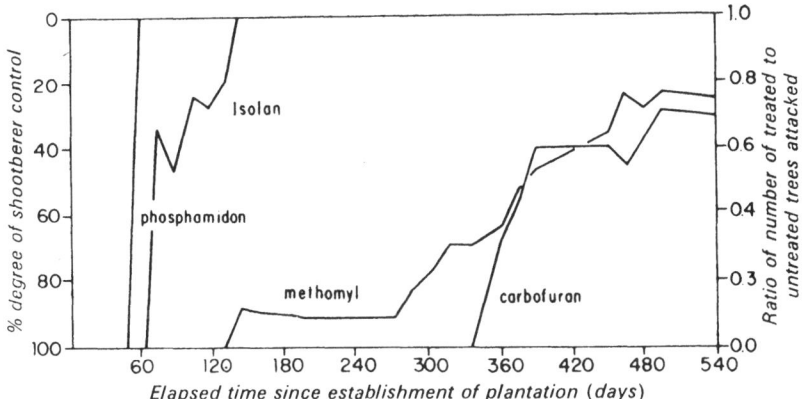

Figure 1. The control of the mahogany shootborer by polyamide polymer combinations with organophosphorus and carbaryl insecticides. Reproduced from *International Pest Control* by permission of McDonald Publications of London.[16]

All insecticides were found to have an effect for 60 days. The control by Isolan™ and phosphamidon quickly was reduced at this time. Methomyl gave good control up to 280 days and then slowly fell off after that. Since the area was sprayed at the beginning of the experiments with normal formulations of the same material, the 60 day control period may have resulted from that application. Hence only methomyl and carbofuran plastic-impregnated cylinders provided control.

The effectiveness of two of the formulations of Dimilin™ against face fly larval development are shown in Figure 2.[13] While the percentage inhibition of adult emergence with technical Dimilin™ drops off precipitously after 20 days, reaching zero at 60 days, the effectiveness of two of the polymer formulations increased during this time. The Polyurethane foam and the polyamide formulations containing 5% Dimilin™ active ingredient increased in effectiveness from zero at the start to 100% after 30 to 50 days. The total effectiveness was held for at least 110 days with the polyurethane foam maintaining a high effectiveness for at least 150 days.

2. Release of Physically Bonded Pesticides

An example of the variety available for controlled release of pesticides from physically bonded polymer materials is found in incorporating aldicarb and dimethoate.[3] The pesticides were generally mixed with preformed polymers and additional additives and the solvents were allowed to evaporate. The efficacy from the release of these two pesticides from such a combination is shown in Table 1. It is clear that various polymer formulations give quite a large range of release times. Release of these two pesticides from plastic formulations into soil have given similar percentages when compared over a 28 day period.

An additional example of physically held controlled release pesticide is the release of tri-n-butyltin fluoride in polyethylene.[18] After 24 days, the release of tributyltin fluoride is fairly constant at about 0.03% per day when placed in water. The formulation has a molluscicidal role in ship bottom application and can be used also as a mosquito larvicide.

21

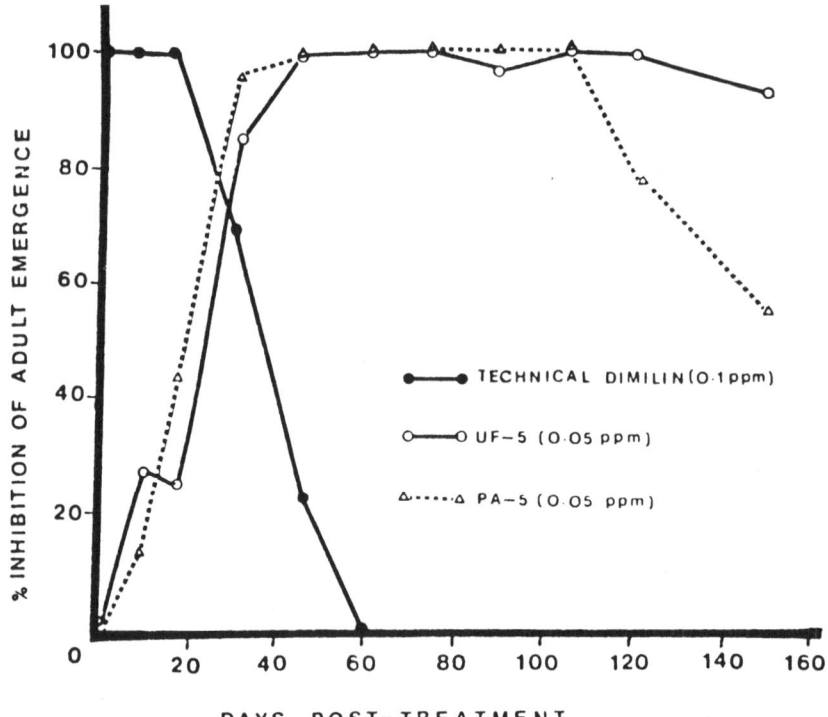

Figure 2. The effectiveness of Dimilin™ formulations on the
percentage inhibition of adult emergence of face
Fly larva. Reproduced from *Controlled Release of
Bioactive Materials* by permission of Academic
Press.[13]

Table 1. Release of Aldicarb and Dimethoate from polymer
formulations into water.[3]

Formulation	Percentage pesticide found in water at the indicated hour of immersion			
	Aldicarb		Dimethoate	
	2 Hr.	24 Hr.	2 Hr.	24 Hr.
Corn Cobs (a)	100	100	84	100
Urea-formaldehyde	74	100		
Poly(vinyl chloride) #4	72	91	60	100
Polyurethane	43	67		
Petroleum charcoal with 20% binder (b)	32	48	60	74
Cellulose acetate	8	23	9	30
Polyester	1	3		
(a) Fast release standard (b) Slow release standard				

A. Desorption. Historically, the first method that was developed was desorption. No current work has been found in this area in the current literature. Unbonded Sn has now been outlawed in paint applications.

B. True Solution Release. The next method was the release of solutions of pesticides incorporated in polymers. These were true solutions. In these cases the polymers were usually elastomers and they were homogeneous. Examples were the herbicide 2,4-D dissolved in natural rubber[50] and the molluscicides tributyl tin fluoride and tributyl tin oxide dissolved in elastomers.

The physically bonded solution preparations rely on diffusion for the most part for release from the polymer. Also possible is a chemical or biological erosion of the matrix to release the agent. The biocide is trapped in a hard plastic, such as nylon, polyethylene, or poly(vinyl chloride); a rubber; or in a natural polymer, such as cellulose or starch.

The diffusion-dissolution process occurs when pesticides and other compounds are evenly distributed in a polymer. An example of this is the preparation of the antifouling agent, tributyl tin oxide, in an elastomer, butyl rubber. The process by which the active agent moves to the surface of the polymer to become effective in its intended purpose has been termed diffusion-dissolution,[19] and has been described in more detail in another publication.[20] In this process, the molecules of the added agent distribute themselves evenly throughout the polymer in what is described as a homogeneous solution process. Removal of molecules of the agent at the surfaces through formation of a true aqueous solution, for example, produces a momentary state of nonsolution. Other active agent molecules move in or diffuse to again set up a condition of equal distribution. The rate of release can be controlled either by the diffusion process or by the boundary release process.

One example: The use of the pinolene polymer (β-Pinene) with carbaryl allows an increased deposition and decreased rate of decay of the carbaryl on tomato leaves. There is a three-fold period of release that the carbaryl remains on the leaf. This residual extension of the pesticide by the use of pinolene results from the occlusion and dissolution of the pesticide within the pliant film that pinolene forms on the leaf.[21]

A three-layer plastic flake has been prepared as one form of a matrix entrapped polymer relying on a physical diffusion of the active agent.[22] The outside layers were a vinyl plastic. The inside layer was any one of several pheromones of the pink bollworm, *Pectinophora gossypiella* (Saunders) including gossyplure, TF, virelure, or Z-9 TDF pheromones. Gossyplure is a 1:1 mixture of the Z,Z and Z,E isomers of 7,11-hexadecadienyl acetate. TF is 1-tetradecenal formate. Virelure is a 16:1 mixture of (Z)-11-hexadecenal and (Z)-9-tetradecenal. Z-9-TDF is (Z)-9-tetradecen-1-ol formate.

In another work, the pheromone treatment reduced catches of the male pink bollworm moths in pheromone-baited traps, boll infestations, and female mating. The effect was compared to both the use of insecticide control and an untreated check plot.[22] These flakes, alone or in combination, were sprayed and dispensed by air either in flake form or in a liquid formulation. The effectiveness of the gossyplure-treated flakes is seen in Figure 3.

The rate of release can be controlled by incorporation of various amounts of the pesticide. Molten polyamides have been shown to possess "remarkable solvent powers for pesticides in general".[23] Solid solutions

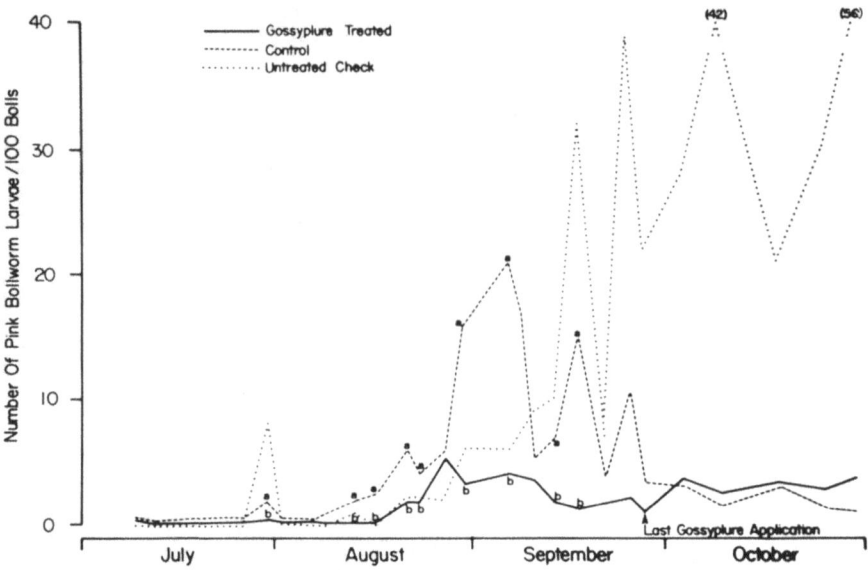

Figure 3. Mean pink bollworm larva found from gossyplure-
treated and check plots. Reprinted with permission
from *Journal of Economic Entomology*, c. 1981,
Entomological Society of America.[22]

of pesticide greater than 25% (w/w) in polyamides (M_n 2,000-15,000) were
possible. The data shown in Figure 4 indicates the wide variety of
release amounts of the house fly chemosterilant, hexamethylphosphoric
triamide (HMPT) that can be obtained.[24,25] The released amounts can be
varied simply by mixing together any desired amounts of the pesticide at
the time of the polymer preparation. This compound is an example of an
organophosphorus pesticide. The polymer in this case (M_n = 15,000) was
prepared from ethylenediamine and dimerized linoleic acid.[25]

Considerable effort has been made in the area of snail control in
utilizing slow-release incorporated tri-n-butyl fluoride within elastomeric substrates.[26] Using mostly rubber-type substrates, at least five
different formulations are cited in controlling seven species of snails
under a variety of conditions. Although all of these are physically
entrapped, a variety of shapes and densities are now available to allow
quite a range of use in the field. The citations in reference 26 showed
complete control under a variety of conditions for periods up to 19
months long.

The efficacy pathway of chemical pesticides physically incorporated
within a polymer medium and acting on mollusks is much more complicated
than a simple release of an active chemical. Tributyl tin oxide (TBTO)
and tributyl tin fluoride (TBTF) have been dispersed within a natural
rubber, an elastomer, because of the latter's natural biodegradability.[27]
"Upon immersion in water the tributyl tin molecules are slowly emitted
from the dispenser surface through a diffusion-dissolution mechanism."
The dispensing medium may take the form of pellets, granules, powders,
strips, sheets, cords, or tubes, etc. The release rate can be moderated
by various additives as described below. Figure 5 shows the loss of C^{14}
labeled TBTO released from BioMet™ SRM over a period up to 60 days. This
agent release can be stretched up to 20 years or even longer, yielding
levels from 1 to 7 ppm per day.[28] When TBTF is dissolved in a plastic, on
the other hand, it is released through a leaching mechanism.

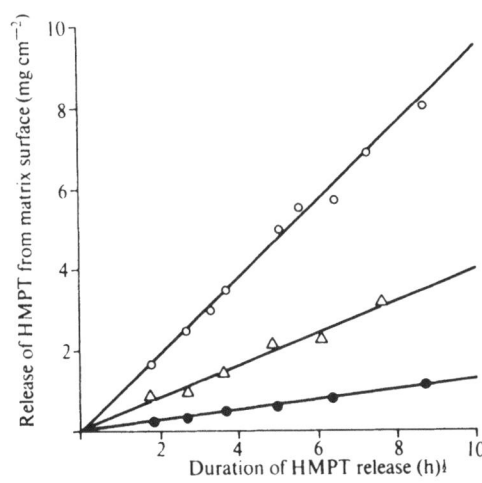

Figure 4. Rate of release of hexamethylphosphoric triamide
(HMPT) from a polyamide matrix. O, 21.48% HMPT; <,
14.00% HMPT; ●, 6.9% HMPT. Reprinted from *Nature*,
234, 349-351. Copyright 1971, Macmillan Magazines,
Ltd.[25]

Carrier Systems have improved performance over desorption and true
solution methods. These systems consist of three components. The pesticide is soluble in an additive, which is the carrier. The carrier solution is then soluble in the polymer. As the components are mutually
soluble, they are homogeneous preparations. Examples of carriers are soya
oil and lecithin. Useful examples have been in the DDVP containing No-
Pest™ strips, the roach-type traps, and baits.

The technology for bait insecticides has already been well developed
by the late 70's. An advance from this occurred when a dual purpose
additive was devised.[29] This material served as both a carrier and an
attractant. Two formulations are shown in Table 2 that illustrate this
process. Soya oil and lecithin serve both as a carrier and an attractant.

Table 2. Bait contact insecticides for German Cockroach Control.

Ingredient	Parts by weight	
	A	B
Ethylene-propylene copolymer	–	84.0
Ethylene-vinyl acetate copolymer	68.8	–
Zinc stearate	1.0	1.0
Diazinon	–	10.0
Baygon™	15.2	–
Soya Oil	10.0	–
Lecithin	–	5.0

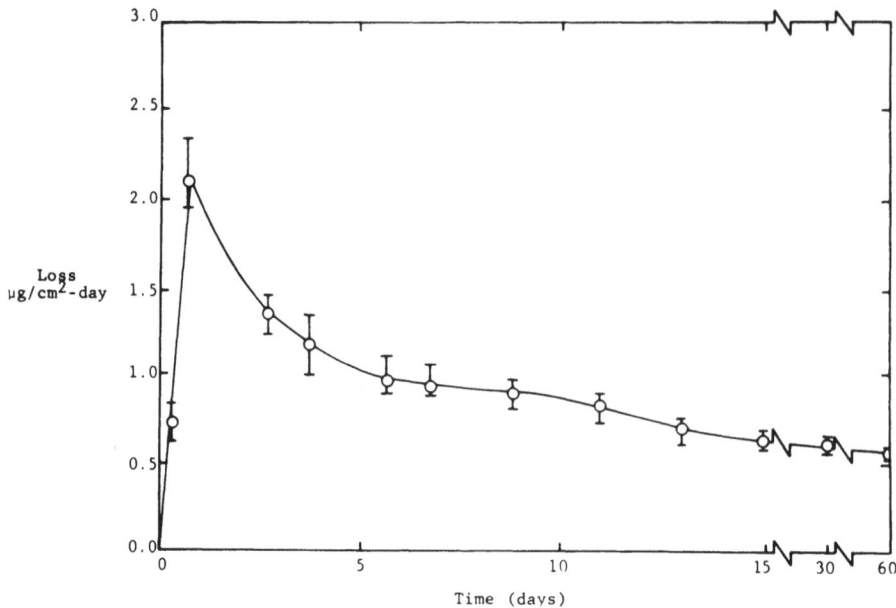

Figure 5. Emission of C-14 Tri-n-butyltin oxide (TBTO) from BioMet™ SRM. Reproduced from *Controlled Release of Bioactive Materials* by permission of Academic Press.[27]

Other bait attractant-carrier material was useful in snail abatement. Wheat germ, beef-heart infusion agar, powdered lettuce (for freshwater snails) and fish flour (for marine snails) are examples in this use.[30]

C. Leaching. A third release method has been the leaching type. The pesticide is prepared in high concentration. The materials produced, however, have a short term and are of low efficiency. The preparations containing copper sulfate are of this type. (See Table 3.)

The elastomers utilize a diffusion-dissolution mechanism because true solutions of the pesticide in the elastomer solvent are obtained. When true solutions are not possible, as in thermoplastic polymers, a leaching mechanism would be used. Large loadings were required to create the proper porosity that would allow the pesticide to escape to the sur-rounding medium. Other additives have other functions. An example is given in Table 3.[31,32] Unfortunately, copper sulfate does not provide the proper release for mollusk control and is less effective than the various tin compounds discussed.[31]

Carrier systems, however, suffer from poor efficiency due to their inability to produce complete agent release. A better method of deve-loping release from thermoplastics was found in the porosity generated systems, or porosigens.[33] For these, a co-leachate included in the mix-ture allows a controlled pore size. These types have long term and high efficiency. Examples of porosigens have been calcium carbonate, copper sulfate, in the right concentrations, and ammonium sulfate.

Low solubility agents, such as, tributyltin fluoride (TBTF), had very low solubility in such thermoplastics as polyethylene and low solubility in its acting environment as well. For this porosigen system, water soluble salts and oxides were added to the thermoplastic. As this soluble portion was leached out of the plastic, a porosity system was developed

Table 3. A formulation of the leaching type.

	Parts by weight
Epcar 5465[TM] monomer	100.0
Sulfur (curative agent)	1.0
Mercaptobenzothiazole	0.2
Zinc Oxide	3.0
Tetramethylthiuram Disulfide	1.0
HAF Carbon Black	0.0
Ammonium Sulfate (pH control)	2.0
Copper Sulfate Monohydrate	157.2

to allow incoming water to have better contact with the TBTF. Such soluble agents used were calcium carbonate and ammonium sulfate.[34]

The following herbicides have been used in porosigen containing mono-liths: diuron, diquat, Fenac[TM], simazine, bromacil, dichlobenil, 2,4-D acid, the dimethylamine salt of 2,4-D, and the isooctyl ester of 2,4-D. Thermoplastic polymers prepared included polyethylene, polypropylene, polystyrene, polyurethane, and polyamide. Thermosetting plastics prepared included polyesters and epoxies. Hence it is seen that the choice of the porosity preparing agent is perhaps the more important ingredient in such a polymer rather than the precise binding matrix.[35]

Later research has improved devices to be more effective. One method has been to include more than one active agent to be disseminated. An example is the inclusion of a liquid agent, dimethyl-1,2-dibromo-2,2-

Table 4. Successful microencapsulated systems.

Pesticide	Target	Polymer	Reference
INSECTICIDES			
Temephos	Mosquito Larvae	Polyethylene	37
Sumithion[TM]	Cockroaches	Polyurethane	38
Famphur	Tick Control	Poly(lactic acid)	39
Diflubenzuron	Fly Larvae		40
HERBICIDES			
2-(2,4,5-trichlorophenoxy) propionic acid	Broadleafs	Silicone	41
OTHER PESTICIDES			
Dimilin[TM]	Chitin Inhibitor		42
Diamphenetide	Parasitic Infections		43

dichloroethyl phosphate, and a non-volatile solid carbamate.[36] In this particular example a plasticizer, such as di-2-ethylhexylphthalate, and a porosity control additive are also added to the formulation.

D. Microencapsulation. Microencapsulation is also an effective release mechanism where small central pockets of active agents are formed within a polymeric outer coating or skin. The effect depends on the relative polarities of the core and skin as well as the relative amounts of the two. Polymers used as encapsulated skins include gelatin gum arabic, starch, sugar, ethyl cellulose, carboxymethylcellulose, and paraffin. Examples of successful systems include but are not limited to those shown in Table 4.

The classical case of a physically encapsulated pesticide has been the preparation of Penncap M™.[44] Methyl parathion is encapsulated in a water polycondensation reaction. The oil soluble ingredients for the condensation are dissolved in the oil phase (methyl parathion) and the water soluble components in water. The two phases are brought together and allowed to form the polymer. Operating conditions allow various wall thicknesses, degrees of capsule wall crosslinking, and microcapsule size. The polymerization process encapsulates the pesticide oil. Dosages in this type of pesticide formulation were set up at similar amounts of active ingredient per acre of crop compared to the emulsifiable concentrate. The polymerized formulation dosages were found to last considerably longer than the EC formulation. The data in Table 5 shows the comparison of the 25% crosslinked encapsulated product with the EC formulation. The crosslinked product lasted seven days at a 100% mortality level for bollworms on cotton (greenhouse tests) whereas the EC formulation lasted less than one day. Other results in this early work are shown in Table 6.

No phytotoxicity with Penncap M was found even at concentrations as high as 5.6 kg/ha. Mammalian toxicity was found also to be much lower with the encapsulated formulation - 500 times less toxic to rabbits by skin absorption, 80-100 times less toxic to white mice, and 40-50 times less toxic to rats by ingestion. The encapsulated product was thus found to be more effective, less costly, less phytotoxic and less hazardous an insecticide.

Penncap M was also found to give good control of grasshoppers in Montana rangeland at levels of 4 and 8 oz./acre. Similar control was obtained when compared with 8 fl. oz./acre of 95% technical malathion.

Table 5. Effectiveness of encapsulated insecticide with respect to crosslinking percentage.

Treatment	% Cross linked	Kg/ha	\% Mortality of bollworm by days				
			0	3	5	7	11
Penncap M	0	1.12	100	96	76	25	0
	10	1.12	100	100	96	60	24
	25	1.12	100	100	100	100	72
	50	1.12	100	100	100	84	56
Me Parathion EC	–	1.12	94	60	16	4	0

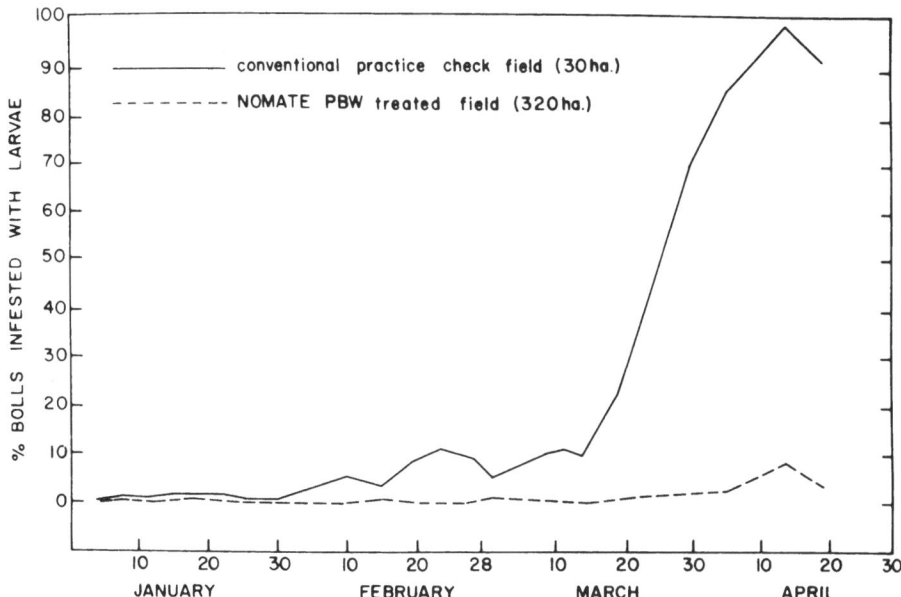

Figure 6. *P. gossypiella* larval infestations in cotton bolls
from eight fields permeated with gossyplure-Nomate
PBW™ and a conventional practice field. 1978-79,
near Saluta Cruz, Bolivia. Reproduced from
Controlled Release of Bioactive Materials by
permission of Academic Press.[47]

Initially the two Penncap M concentrations gave 85 and 89% control
compared to 87% for the malathion. Later at 3, 7, and 14 days, the
control was found to continue at 81, 89, and 90%.[45]

Matrix bound coumaphos and trichlorfon and encapsulated toxicants
containing ethyl and methyl pirimiphos, permethrin, and diazinon were
found to be ineffective against the fire ant.[46] However, the ineffective-
ness was not due to the controlled release mechanism but rather the
ability of the ant to filter particles in its infrabuccal pocket in its
head. Particles as small as 0.88 microns can be filtered and never come
in contact with internal parts.

E. Hollow Fiber Tubes. The use of hollow fiber types of physically
incorporated pesticides have been the last to be invented and developed.
Insect pheromones, contained in hollow fiber tubes that were closed at
one end,[47] were broadcast on the cotton fields to be protected. The
effectiveness of the slow release is shown in Figure 6.

F. Destruction of polymer bonds. The release of physically bound
pesticides by chemical destruction of polymer bonds affords the effectiveness of some physically bonded pesticide polymer mixtures. This can
be done in two ways: First, by breaking crosslinking bonds that hold the
polymer in a tight matrix. Second, by breaking the backbone polymer
chains themselves.

An example is the preparation of a starch xanthate:sludge polymer
with herbicides, such as thiocarbamates.[49] The starch xanthate was formed
by using oxidatively crosslinked aqueous starch xanthate in the presence
of active agents to produce a granular matrix that entraps the agent. The
sludge is formed by a heterogeneous mix of polysaccharides, crosslinked

Table 6. Penncap M use parameters for encapsulated formulation.

Formulation	Insect controlled	Applied concentration kg/ha	Effective time in days
Penncap M	2-Spot Spider Mite	0.56	13
EC		0.56	ineffective
Penncap M	Japanese beetles	0.56	8
EC		0.56	3
Penncap M	Gypsie moth larva	1.12	32 (87%)
EC			4 (48%)

in the presence of the active agent by dialdehyde starch, thus entrapping the agent. Starch xanthate mixtures with trifluralin showed increased activity over the emulsifiable concentrate. Those with alachlor, metalochlor, or several thiocarbamates did not greatly increase the residual activity. Formulations with EPTC were found to provide less protection to corn than the emulsifiable concentrate.

Polymers derived from lactic acid and glycolic acid allow matrix entrapment and subsequent release by destruction of the polymer structure.[50] These materials are inexpensive and easy to polymerize. They will degrade to the respective acids, CO_2, and water, all harmless in the environment. The monomer for lactic acid, for example, is d,l-lactide which can be polymerized to a high molecular weight. 2,4-D can be mixed with the powdered polymer and compressed into pellets at low heat. These pellets will degrade very slowly by reaction with moisture when applied to outdoor areas. The resulting hydrolysis allows the 2,4-D to become free. The half life of this system in wet sand was found to be about 6-8 days. (See Figure 7.)

G. An unusual case. A polymer-based spray was found to control powdery mildew on Zinnea elegans. In this case the active agent, Acti-Dione [(3)-2-(3,5-dimethyl-2-oxocyclo-hexyl)-2-hydroxyethyl]-glutarimide acted as a polymer based anti-transpirant. The hydrophobic film causes enough changes in the surface to disorient the pathogen germ tubes.[51]

CHEMICALLY BONDED PESTICIDE-POLYMERS

1. Preparation

A. Introduction. A variety of chemically bonded schemes are possible. In general, however, the schemes involve either covalent or ionic bonding to a preformed polymer,[52,53] or the pesticide becomes a part of the polymerization process itself,[54-56] as shown in Equations 2 and 3, respectively. The mode of pesticidal action is dependent on either in situ activity or a gradual degradation of the polymer itself.

The bonding to preformed polymer requires macromolecules with pendant functional groups capable of reaction with herbicides or their derivatives. The nature of the bond can vary with different rates of cleavage

$$[-CH_2-CH-]_n \quad + \quad A-PEST \quad \longrightarrow \quad [-CH_2-CH-]_n \quad + \quad A-Z \qquad \text{(Equation 2)}$$
$$\Big|\Big|$$
$$ZPEST$$

$$X-CH_2CH_2-Y \quad + \quad A-PEST-B \quad \longrightarrow \quad [-CH_2CH_2-(PEST)-]_n \quad + \quad A-Y \quad \text{(Equation 3)}$$

in the environment. The advantage of this type is the availability of relatively inexpensive, biodegradable polymers like chitin, starch, and cellulose.

The preparation of polymers from monomeric pesticides, on the other hand, has the advantage in the ability to control both the molecular design and the pesticide-polymer weight ratio. This preparation type offers the most interesting concepts for the polymer chemist to consider. The problem is to take proven pesticides and create a polymer from them without losing their pesticidal action. On the other hand the reactive part of a pesticide molecule can be joined with a polymer functional group to create a molecule that has both functions. This monomer is then polymerized to get the longer lasting material.

B. Chemical Bonding with Polymerization. Two examples of this type are pesticide-isocyanate adducts with PVA and pentachlorophenyl acrylate with vinyl acetate (or ethyl acrylate).

For the first, diisocyanates, such as 4,4'-diphenyl methane diisocyanate, 1,6-hexamethylene diisocyanate and toluene diisocyanate were allowed, as an example, to react with metribuzin to yield a pesticide-isocyanate adduct.[57] This was then allowed to react with poly(vinyl alcohol) to form a copolymer with controlled release properties. (See Equation 4.) Crosslinked systems were also made by using an excess of the diisocyanate prior to the reaction with polyvinyl alcohol. The metribuzin was released faster from the linear preparation than the crosslinked due to its ability to swell with the hydrophilic polymer; hydrolysis and diffusion of the herbicide occurred more easily. Only the hydrolyzed or released metribuzin moved; the polymer remained immobile. The commercial formulation of metribuzin was found to be non-toxic after 78 days, but the linear polymer version was found to retain activity even after 112 days. Polymer crosslinking can be varied to provide even longer activity times.

The other example, a polymer-bound fungicide, is found in the copolymerization of pentachlorophenyl acrylate with vinyl acetate and ethyl acrylate.[58] This pentachlorophenol-based product could have use as an anti-fouling agent in marine coatings. In this case it was necessary to copolymerize with ethyl acrylate. The homopolymer was found to be too hydrophobic to allow decomposition of the polymer and allow release of the active agent in sufficiently high concentrations to have the appropriate biocide effect.

Poly(ethylenimine S-alkyldithiocarbamate) polymers were prepared from respective poly(ethylenimine sodium dithiocarbamate) and alkyl chlorides, aralkyl chlorides, substituted alkyl esters of chloroacetic acid, β-chloroethyl esters of carbamic and carboxylic acids, and N-substituted chlorocarboxamides. The derivatives thus obtained were decomposed both physically and chemically to release sulfur and sulfur-containing substances which acted as controlled-release herbicides or fungicides.[59] One author has proposed reactions of the pesticide 2,6-dichlorobenzaldehyde with diols and amines to form polyamide polycondensation products.[60]

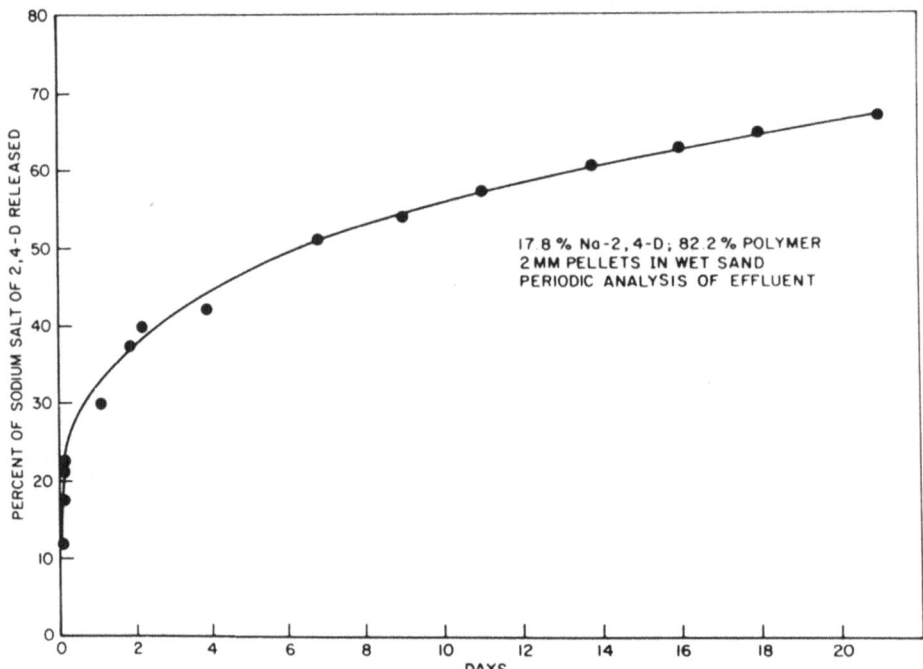

Figure 7. Release time of polylactic acid-encapsulated sodium
salt of 2,4-D. Reprinted with permission from
Environmental Science and Technology, 7(10), 955-6,
copyright 1973, American Chemical Society.[50]

$$(CH_3)_3C-C \underset{N}{\overset{C}{\underset{\diagdown}{\overset{O}{\underset{\diagup}{\parallel}}}}} N-NH_2 \quad + \quad OCN-R-NCO \quad \longrightarrow \quad (CH_3)_3C-C \underset{N}{\overset{C}{\underset{\diagdown}{\overset{O}{\underset{\diagup}{\parallel}}}}} N-NH-C-NH-R-NCO$$

(Metribuzin)   (Equation 4)

$$[-CH_2-CH-]_n \quad \xrightarrow{\hspace{2cm}} \quad [-CH_2-CH-]_x-[-CH_2-CH-]_{n-x}$$

$$(CH_3)_3C-C \quad N-NH-C-NH$$

C. Chemical Bonding after Polymerization. A convenient example of a chemically bonded slow release pesticide is found when herbicidal phenoxyacetic acid is to be bound. This type of compound is easy to attach to a polymer moiety containing an labile hydrogen, as found in polymers containing an amine, alcohol, or mercaptan side chain group. Equation 5 illustrates this reaction.[25] The carboxyl group is only one of many possible reactive groups.[61,62]

$$\text{Polymer-X-H} \ + \ \text{HOOCR} \ \longrightarrow \ \text{Polymer-X-COR} \ + \ \text{HOH} \qquad \text{(Equation 5)}$$

where $X = N, O,$ or S

Phosphorylation of 1,2,3,4-tetra-o-acetyl-β-d-glycopyranose with diethyl phosphorochloridothiolate gave the corresponding phosphorothioate.[63] Cellulose-6-(diethyl phosphorothioate) was prepared by treating sodium cellulose with the diethyl compound above in benzene in the presence of pyridine. Periodate oxidation of the cellulose compound above showed that the phosphorylation took place at the C-6 position of anhydroglucose units.

2. Release of Chemically Bonded Pesticides from Polymers

Efficacy in the field depends on the nature of the pesticide-polymer bond, the chemical character of the pesticide and polymer, and the dimensions and structure of the system. Most pesticidal action will result from a degradation of the polymer to free the bonded pesticide.[60] In a few cases, effective action will result from the effect of the bonded material as a whole.

An excellent review[48] of the theory of diffusion for pesticide release (48) discusses three mechanisms: (1) Solubilization by crosslink cleavage that is readily destroyed by the aqueous environment. Release is dependent on the matrix erosion rate. (2) Solubilization by hydrolysis, ionization, or protonation of pendant groups. In this case there is no change of molecular weight. (3) Solubilization by backbone cleavage. If the process occurs on the surface, it is termed heterogeneous; if it occurs throughout the polymer, it is termed homogeneous.

A. Solubilization via Cross-linking Cleavage. Tributyl tin oxide, often used as a dispersion in a paint or rubber, has also been effectively used when chemically bonded within a polymer chain or network.[28,64] The tin compound is allowed to react with pendant carboxyl or anhydride groups to form an ester. This polymer is then crosslinked by allowing unreacted carboxyl groups to react with diepoxides. Curing is then accomplished at 150°C. Room temperature cured polyesters, urethanes and aziridines have also been used to incorporate organo-tin groups in other studies.[65]

B. Solubilization via Pendant Chain Degradation. "In the biological environment, side chain degradation occurs so that the chemical bonds holding the pesticide within its polymeric prison are sequentially broken to provide a sustained release of the pesticide over an extended period of time. The rate of release will clearly be determined by the nature of the pesticide-polymer bonds, the chemical characteristics of the pesticide and polymer, as well as the dimensions and structure of the resultant macromolecular combination".[25]

Polyvinyl alcohol related polymers provide solubilization of a pesticide bound as a side chain. Polyacetals, polyketals, and poly-o-esters also provide for side chain degradation. In addition, cleavage of the main chain with these latter compounds also provides for pesticide activity.

Whether the polymeric backbone is water soluble or insoluble will determine the expected release function. Equations for either case have been written and show that the amount of release over time can be controlled by the amount of pesticide-polymer combination used. Figure 8 shows the relationship between the herbicide level of 2,4-D and the achieved level of application over time.[23] In this case, water is needed for the degradation. The polymer combination can be made less water soluble by preparing a longer chain length in the polymer, by using low molecular weight oligomers, or by lowering the percentage of hydrophilic monomers. Figure 8 also shows that the use of the polymer combination allows a much smaller application of 2,4-D at a given period of time or for an extended period of time.

In a brush application instead of an aquatic one, the results were found to be different. 2,4-D (2,4-dichloro-phenoxyacetic acid), 2,4,5-T (2,4,5-trichlorophenoxyacetic acid), dicamba (3,6-dichloro-o-anisic acid), and picloram (4-amino-3,5,6-trichloropicolinic acid) were prepared in this same way and applied to brush control alone and in combinations. Generally there was no difference in effectiveness between conventional and polymerized herbicides. Picloram, however, was more effective when applied conventionally.[66]

A controlled release herbicide was prepared from poly(vinyl chloride) and thiourea.[67] The resulting polymer, poly(S-vinylisothiourea-vinylene-vinyl thiocyanate) was allowed to decompose under both aqueous alkaline and acidic conditions to give thiocyanate and other compounds. The use of the polymer was not effective to retard germination but was effective for inhibiting the growth of seedlings of barnyard grass on the treated soil for 28 days. When treated with acid or base, the herbicidal effect was more effective on the germination and the growth of the plant.

C. Solubilization via Hydrolysis Cleavage of the Polymer Chain or Backbone. A number of chemical reactions are available to provide for solubilization of polymer backbone to yield an active pesticide. Some of these reactions are illustrated in Equations 6-9.[99]

$$[-CH_2-O-\overset{\overset{\displaystyle O}{\|}}{C}-CH_2-]_n \xrightarrow{HOH} HO-CH_2-\overset{\overset{\displaystyle O}{\|}}{C}-OH \qquad \text{(Equation 6)}$$

$$[-CH_2-NH-\overset{\overset{\displaystyle O}{\|}}{C}-CH_2-]_n \xrightarrow{HOH} H_2N-CH_2-\overset{\overset{\displaystyle O}{\|}}{C}-COH \qquad \text{(Equation 7)}$$

$$\underset{\underset{\displaystyle (O-R)_2}{|}}{[-P=N-]_n} \xrightarrow{HOH} ROH + NH_3 + H_2PO_4 \qquad \text{(Equation 8)}$$

$$[-CH_2-C(CN)_2-]_n \xrightarrow{HOH} H_2C=O + CH_2(CN)_2 \qquad \text{(Equation 9)}$$

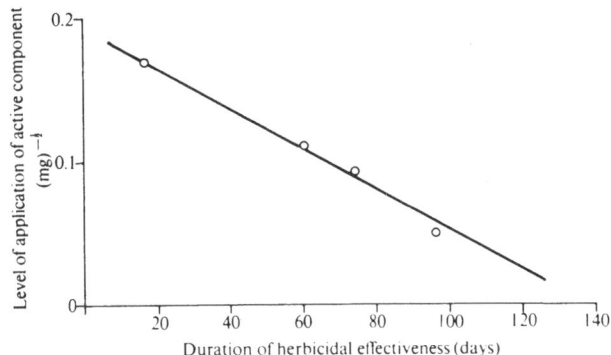

Figure 8. Relationship of the duration of herbicidal effectiveness to the level of application for 2,4-D acid
chemically combined with a water soluble polymer.
Reprinted from *Nature*, **234**, 349-351. Copyright
1971, Macmillan Magazines, Ltd.[25]

D. Solubilization via Enzymatic Action. Although enzymatic action
should be an important consideration for the decomposition of a pesticide
polymer combination, no references were found describing work in this
important area.

E. Action of Chemically Bonded Pesticides as a Whole, Non-degraded
Polymer. Preparations of biologically active polymers depending on the
slow release of the active agent are quite common. On the other hand the
preparation of a biologically active polymer that depends on activity of
parts of the polymer itself without degradation have offered challenges
to the polymer chemist. Such a system could use specific isocyanates that
would be polymerized with polyvinyl alcohol.[61] In this example propham,
chlorpropham, and swep are all similar carbamate herbicides. The isopropyl group on the one end of the molecule could become the backbone of
the polymer. Such polymers have a structure similar to that of the
original herbicide, suggesting that the biocidal properties could be
retained in the polymer. The preparation of such material would proceed
by allowing polyvinyl alcohol to react with chlorophenyl isocyanates in
dimethylsulfoxide in the presence of triethyl amine. A host of other
possibilities exist.

In situ pesticides have limited uses since the polymer is generally
not free to move. One area of use, however, is in marine antifouling. In
this case a copolymer with ethyl acrylate was found to be necessary to
impart some hydrophilicity to the polymer. It would increase the release
so as to get concentrations high enough to be effective.

Nine poly(S-vinyl alkyldithiocarbamates were tested for activity on
barnyard grass, *Panicum crusgalli*.[68] After 19, 27, and 32 days post
application, the most effective polymer was one having the following
formula: $(CH_2CHSCSNR_1R_2)_{138}$ where R_1 was butyl and R_2 was H. Other forms
tested varied R_1 as C_1-C_4 alkyl and R_2 as H or C_1-C_3 alkyl. None of these
compounds showed antifungal activity against *Aspergillus niger*, *Tricho-
derma viride*, and *Pythium debaryanum*. Two polymers were found to have
fungicidal activity against these fungi.[69] These two were poly(ethylenimine) and poly(vinyl sodium xanthate). The most active decomposition
product against the same fungi was found to result from the decomposition
of copoly(vinyl sodium dithiocarbamate-vinyl isothiocyanate).

APPLICATION FUNCTIONS

1. Flocculation Control

Polymer uses other than polymeric or slow-release pesticides have also been developed. Polymers have been used for the control of flocculation of traditional pesticide suspension formulations. This is particularly true in the preparation of concentrated suspensions, those in excess of 0.4 volume fractions of the solid.[70] Surface active agents, of the ionic or nonionic types, can be used, but they suffer for various reasons and are not able to prevent flocculation under all conditions.

Good results can be obtained, however, with the use of block and graft polymers, where two main types of monomers make up the chain. One type of monomer should have a strong affinity for the suspended particles, and the other one will provide steric stabilization. For example, the first or anchoring group can be strongly hydrophobic, such as polystyrene or poly(methyl methacrylate) which will have a strong affinity to the hydrophobic pesticide particle. The second portion can be a water soluble chain, such as poly(ethylene oxide). An example where this combination polymer has been successfully used was in the preparation of a dispersion with ethirimol, a fungicide.[70]

2. Polymers in Spray Drift Control

Utilizing a pesticide-polymer combination can also increase the safety in spraying by controlling the drift following spraying. To do this the pesticide is prepared as a methanol-treated activated sludge polymer (MAS polymer). It is a heterogeneous polysaccharide that has film-forming properties, and it will hydrate but not redissolve in water once dried. MAS can be mixed with dialdehyde starch (DAS) and a pesticide. When diluted with water for the proper dosage, it can be applied using ordinary spray nozzles. The drift can be controlled by varying the viscosity and the concentration of MAS.[71]

Another example of drift control is through the addition of a poly(vinyl chloride) polymer. The polymer is very shear resistant without increasing the viscosity in relation to increased droplet size. Addition of the polymer causes a "viscoelastic" effect that reduces the number of droplets less than 100 microns in size.[72] At higher concentrations the polymers appear to encapsulate the herbicide and bond it to the plant allowing longer contact times. The proprietary product, Nalco-trol™, was found to have 5-10 times less drift with an increased spray deposition of 25% above standards. Half of the spray with Nalco-trol™ was found on-target as compared to 28% without.[73] When used with Diquat and Komeen™ it gave 95% submerged weed control and 75% open lake control after 4 weeks.[72]

Another use of anti-drift additions to sprays is in the controlled direction of the spraying. In the control of johnson grass, redroot, pigweed, and hemp sesbania in soybeans sprays were directed across the rows to catch the higher weeds in June, July, and August. The anti-drift polymer at 0.1% in the spray balanced the increased effectiveness through the use of surfactants in the formulation.[74] The Nalco-trol™ polymer consisted of a long chain polymer that thickened water and eliminated the production of spray droplets smaller than 200 microns.

36

3. Devices Using Bioactive Pesticide Polymers

Bioactive polymeric material can be used in applications other than formulations which are broadcast or applied to a target surface. Devices such as bands or food wrap prepared from biocide-impregnated polymers or can be used. These devices are often used on animals where a low, constant dose is useful which does not harm the animal. In these cases, much lower doses can be used than that found in sprays or dips because of their long term presence.

A. Leg Bands. One example of the impregnated device is used in protecting leg horn chickens from northern foul mites. Permethrin was impregnated into polyvinyl chloride plastic leg bands at the 10% level.[75,76] These bands were also effective when banded to the floor of the chicken cages. These bands have been more productive than dusting because the latter upsets egg production.

Poultry cages have been treated in either of two ways to control fowl mites at an almost 100% success rate. One method involved the hanging of pesticide-impregnated strips in the cages and the other method involved circulating the insecticide through plastic tubes.[77]

Dichlorvos, Dursban[TM], and naled were used separately in a slow release plastic formulation to control the house fly (Musca domestica) in Florida poultry houses containing caged layers. The dichlorvos formulation (20% Shell Vapona[TM] resin strip resin) controlled the larvae and adults for 7 weeks with 3 applications of 2 g toxicant per square meter of breeding area.[78]

B. Ear Tags. Plastic ear tags impregnated with tetrachlorvinphos have been used for fly control on pastured cattle.[79] Placed on the ears, these tags are transferred to other parts of the body by the cows bumping or rubbing together. This method has been particularly effective against horn flies (94% control over an entire season) and face flies (37% control in 4-5 weeks).

Chlorpyrifos and its metabolite, 3,5,6-trichloro-2-pyridinol, were determined at various intervals from ear tag use. The pesticide was used at a level of 10% in the tags (3.3 g per ear, 6.6 g total exposure to each cow) to control for Gulf coast ticks, Amblyomma maculatum Kooh. Chlorpyrifos was found at 0.09 ppm only in fatty tissue after a two-week biopsy. The metabolite was found in fat, liver, and kidney tissues at a maximum of 0.037 ppm after 5 weeks and in two heart samples at 0.01 ppm. The ear tags provided 88-100% protection for 10 weeks from the ticks. The tags, however, caused severe necrosis of either one or both ears of each animal.[80] At a level of 1.2 g chlorpyrifos in each ear tag, residues of chlorpyrifos were found in fatty tissues only (0.030 ppm, at 5 weeks). Residues of pyridinol were found only in fat, liver, and kidney tissues (maximum of 0.032 ppm in the kidney at 5 weeks). The application was given to control not only the ticks but also Cochliomyia hominivorax (Coquerel). In this case no adverse effects resulted from the attachment of the tags to the ears.[81]

C. Military Wraps. Military ready-to-eat diets (MRE's) have overwraps of pesticide treated plastic to protect against insects in storage.[82] Chlorpyrifos-methyl was applied to polyethylene film and permethrin was applied to polypropylene. The permethrin film was placed as an outer layer of a triple film consisting of polypropylene and polybutylene middle adhesive layer and a polypropylene inner layer. When cartons wrapped with these films were placed in a test room containing 11 species of stored-product insects, the chlorpyrifos treated area was insect-free until 18 months and the permethrin treated area was free even longer.

D. Plastic Strips. Impregnation of deltamethrin on cerulean blue strips has afforded effective control of tsetse flies (*Glossina fuscipes quanzenzis*) when used in a trap device. The trap is protected by a plastic cone during the rainy season. It may prove to be effective for trypanosomiasis control in Africa.[83]

Control of corn rootworm was obtained in a unique way by the spraying of tiny plastic tubes dropped by plane or helicopter. The tubes were coated by a three-part mixture consisting of a synthetic sex pheromone to lure the male beetles, compounds from the squash and cucumber family to encourage feeding, and a minute amount of an appropriate insecticide.[84]

In a different type of use, the sex attractant of the pink bollworm operating in cotton fields of Arizona and California impregnated into plastic strips confused mating enough to reduce crop damage 40%.[85] Effective control was maintained for two months. This is a particularly encouraging in view of the fact that many insects are developing resistance to pesticides. The use of the sex attractant reduced applications of chemical pesticides from an average of 11.4 for conventionally treated fields to 6.6 applications for pheromone treated fields over the growing season. This method was also successful in controlling the tea tortrix moth in Japan.

E. Plastic Mulch. The use of plain plastic sheeting, with and without a separate application of a pesticide, has many gardening uses. Black plastic mulch has effectively controlled weeds in the vicinity of musk melons and has also served as a barrier for additional herbicide applications to spread to the areas protected by the plastic.[86,87] Clear plastic mulch raised the soil temperature and when the soil was moist served to kill weed seeds without chemical treatment.[88] The clear plastic also increased growth earliness.[89]

Chemical weed control was better with the pineapple-ananas-comosus cultivar curola crop than was the plastic mulch associated with either hoe weeding or weedicide between the rows.[90]

The use of black plastic mulching of strawberries (*Fragaria ananassa Duch.* 'Midway') gave similar results to the use of applications of either glyphosate applied at the rate of 2.2, 4.5, and 5.6 kg/ha or paraquat applied at the rate of 0.6, 1.1, and 2.2 kg/ha.

Polyethylene plastic tarpaulins covering 14 year old (Frost Valencia) orange stumps controlled sprouts as well as did chemical treatment.[91] The chemicals applied in the test were ammonium sulfamate, 2,4-D, and ammonium ethyl carbamoylphosphonate.

Plastic mulching combined with a foliar spray gave control of the stem blight disease of asparagus, *Asparagus officialis* caused by *Phoma asparagi*. The pesticides found effective were Topsin[TM], applied at 154 g active ingredient, and Difolatan[TM], at 220 g a.i., per 10 acres. These were applied at 10-day intervals during the growing season. In addition to the reduction of the disease, the mulching gave good moisture retention for asparagus growth when the soil moisture was about 10 cm below the soil surface in July-August.[92]

White and blue plastic mulches were compared with various other agents in controlling mosaic virus, nematodes, and fungi. Both mulches reduced the watermelon mosaic virus (WMV) in both fruits and plants. All significantly reduced infestations of serpentine leaf miners, *Liriomyza munda Frick*. However, the film mulches did not significantly alter the populations of plant parasitic nematodes and plant pathogenic fungi. The film mulch did significantly increase the yellow squash yield 70-610% over the unmulched control. Also, white mulches with no fumigation control produced significantly greater yields than did the blue film.[93]

4. Miscellaneous Examples

An unusual application of a physically bound pesticide is the incorporation of a fungicidal agent in an epoxy to prevent fungicidal breakdown of the epoxy polymer over time.[94]

Thiolignin was treated with sodium hydride in dimethyl formamide (DMF) and the derivative obtained reacted with a dialkyl phosphorochloridothioate to give the corresponding thiolignin (dialkyl phosphorothioate).[95] Phosphorylation of the thiolignin occurred at both phenolic and aliphatic OH groups. The possibility exists for this polymer to have an *in situ* pesticidal effect.

Synthesis was accomplished of the s-triazine derivatives from uronic and polyuronic acids.[96] 5(R)-(2-Amino-4-di-methylamino-1,3,5-triazin-6-yl)-L-arabinopyranose and its methyl glucoside were prepared from galacturonic acid. 5(R)-(2-amino-4-dimethylamino-1,3,5-triazin-6-yl)-β-d-xylopyranose was prepared from glucuronolactone. Methyl 5(R)-(2-Amino-4-dimethyl-amino-1,3,5-triazin-6-yl)-α-D-lyxopyranoside was prepared from mannuronolactone by ring closure with N,N-disubstituted biguanide. s-Triazine derivatives of polyuronic acids, such as pectin and alginic acid, were prepared similarly.

In the early 70s it was announced that organotin compounds had been bonded to such plastics as polystyrene, polymethacrylate, polyester, polyvinyl chloride, and cellulose polymer backbones.[97] These have been termed organometallic polymers (OMP). Triethyltin hydroxide was allowed to react with a copolymer of styrene-maleic anhydride. These polymers can be incorporated in a marine paint which, when applied, would retain an anti-fouling activity through hydrolytic cleavage of the metal-oxygen-polymer bond.

The herbicide 2,4-D was bound to functionalized polystyrene through the ester and anhydride groups. The release of the 2,4-D by hydrolysis was measured by the effect on the growth of duckweed (*Lemna minor*) under laboratory conditions. The anhydride form released the herbicide at a faster rate than from the ester, but it was much slower than the release from a mechanical mixture of 2,4-D and polystyrene.[98]

ACKNOWLEDGMENT

This paper is published as Journal Series paper No. 7872 of the Pennsylvania Agricultural Experiment Station.

REFERENCES

1. H. B. Scher, ed., "*Controlled Release Pesticides*", ACS Symposium Series, No. 53., American Chemical Society, Washington, DC, 1977.
2. J. T. Hayes, & W. B. Hewson, J. Ag. Food Chem., 21(3), 498-499 (1973).

3. R. A. Stokes, J. R. Coppage, D. L. Bull & R. L. Ridgway, J. Ag. Food Chem., **21**(1), 103-108 (1973).
4. B. J. Smittle & G. S. Burden, Pest Control., **33**, 10 (1965).
5. T. L. Harvey & D. G. Ely, J. Econ. Entomol., **61**, 1128 (1968).
6. C. G. Gebelein, Ed., "Symposium on the Controlled Release of Bioactive Materials", American Chemical Society 174th National Meeting, New Orleans, LA, 1977.
7. N. F. Cardarelli, Ed., *"Controlled Release Pesticides Formulations"*, CRC Press, Cleveland, OH, 1976.
8. D. R. Paul & F. W. Harris, Eds., *"Controlled Release Polymeric Formulations"*, ACS Symposium Series No. 33, American Chemical Society, Washington, DC, 1976.
9. R. Baker, *"Controlled Release of Bioactive Materials"*, Academic Press, New York, 1980.
10. D. Lewis, *"Controlled Release of Pesticides and Pharmaceuticals"*, Plenum Publishers, New York, 1981.
11. F. Wolf & S. Lindau, Acta Hydrochim. Hydrobiol., 5(3), 251-258 (1977).
12. R. A. Stokes, J. R. Coppedge, D. L. Bull & R. L. Ridgway, J. Agr. Food Chem., **21**(1), 103-108 (1973).
13. F. W. Knapp & C. Nontapan in: *"Controlled Release of Bioactive Materials"*, R. Baker, Ed., Academic Press, New York, 1980, pp. 267.
14. J. T. Whitlaw, Jr., & E. S. Evans, Jr., J. Econ. Entomol., **61**(4), 889-892 (1968).
15. H. Jaffe, J. A. Miller, P. A. Giang & D. K. Hayes in: *"Controlled Release of Bioactive Materials"*, R. Baker, Ed., Academic Press, New York, 1980, pp. 237-250.
16. G. G. Allan, R. I. Gara & R. M. Wilkins, Int. Pest Control, **16**(4), 4-11 (1974).
17. G. G. Allan & A. N. Neogi, Int. Pest. Control, **14**(4), 21 (1972).
18. L. R. Sherman, J. Appl. Polymer Sci., **28**, 2823-2829 (1983).
19. N. F. Cardarelli & B. M. Cardarelli in: *"Bioactive Polymeric Systems"*, C. G. Gebelein & C. E. Carraher, Jr., Eds., Plenum Press, New York, 1985, p. 34.
20. E. H. Bollinger, *"Proceedings of the Controlled Release Pesticide Symposium"*, University of Akron, OH, 1974, p. 19.1.
21. C. H. Blasquez, A. D. Vidyarth, T. D. Sheehan, M. J. Bennett & G. T. McGrew, J. Agr. Food Chem., **18**(4), 681-684 (1970).
22. T. J. Henneberry, J. M. Gillespie, L. A. Bariola, H. M. Flint, P. D. Lingren & A. F. Kydonieus, J. Econ. Entomol., **74**(4), 376-381 (1981).
23. A. N. Neogi, Thesis, University of Washington, Seattle (1970).
24. P. H. Terry, & A. B. Borkovec, J. Med. Chem., **11**, 958 (1983).
25. G. G. Allan, C. S. Chopra, A. N. Neogi & R. M. Wilkins, Nature, **234**, 349-351 (1971).
26. E. S. Upathan, M. Koura, M. A. Dagal, A. H. Awad & M. D. Ahmed in: *"Controlled Release of Bioactive Materials"*, R. Baker, Ed., Academic Press, New York, 1980, p. 449-459.
27. N. F. Cardarelli & W. Evans in: *"Controlled Release of Bioactive Materials"*, R. Baker, Ed., Academic Press, New York, 1980, pp. 357-385.
28. A. J. Allen, B. M. Quitter & C. M. Radick in: *"Controlled Release of Bioactive Materials"*, R. Baker, Ed., Academic Press, New York, 1980, pp. 399-413.
29. N. F. Cardarelli "Biologically Active Insecticide Containing Polymeric Formulation", U. S. Patent 4,237,113, Dec. 2, 1980.
30. N. F. Cardarelli & B. M. Cardarelli in: *"Bioactive Polymeric Systems"*, C. G. Gebelein & C. E. Carraher, Jr., Eds., Plenum Press, New York, 1985, p. 48.
31. N. F. Cardarelli & B. M. Cardarelli in: *"Bioactive Polymeric Systems"*, C. G. Gebelein & C. E. Carraher, Jr., Eds., Plenum Press, New York, 1985, p. 46-47.

32. N. F. Cardarelli & K. E. Walker, "Slow Release Copper Toxicant Composition", U. S. Patent 4,012,221, 1977.
33. N. F. Cardarelli & B. M. Cardarelli in: "*Bioactive Polymeric Systems*", C. G. Gebelein & C. E. Carraher, Jr., Eds., Plenum Press, New York, 1985, p. 59.
34. N. F. Cardarelli "Method and Composition for the Long Term Controlled Release of a Non-Persistent Organotin Pesticide from an Inert Monolithic Thermoplastic Material", U. S. Patent 4,166,111, August 28, 1979.
35. N. F. Cardarelli & B. M. Cardarelli in: "*Bioactive Polymeric Systems*", C. G. Gebelein & C. E. Carraher, Jr., Eds., Plenum Press, New York, 1985, p. 69.
36. J. Greenberg & G. D. Lloyd, "Pet Collar", U. S. Patent 4,150,109, June 12, 1979.
37. K. G. Das & V. B. Tungikar, "*Proceedings of the Controlled Release Bioactive Materials Symposium*", New Orleans, LA, p. IV. 37, 1979.
38. H. Fuyama, G. Shinjo, & K. Tsuji, "*Proceedings of the Controlled Release of Bioactive Materials Symposium*" (Abstracts), Fort Lauderdale, FL, p. 145, 1982.
39. H. Jaffe, D. K. Hayes, P. A. Giang, R. O. Drummond, & T. M. Wetsone, "*Proceedings of the Controlled Release Pesticide Symposium*", Corvallis, OR, p. 272, 1977.
40. R. W. Miller & C. Corley, "*Proceedings of the Controlled Release Pesticide Symposium*", Corvallis, OR, p. 264, 1977.
41. R. Helfner, "*Proceedings of the Controlled Release Bioactive Materials Symposium*", New Orleans, LA, p. III. 16, 1979.
42. R. D. Sjogren, "*Proceedings of the Controlled Release Bioactive Materials Symposium*", Wright State University, Dayton, OH, p. 217, 1975.
43. R. S. Rew & R. H. Fetter, "*Proceedings of the Controlled Release of Bioactive Materials Symposium*", Fort Lauderdale, FL, p. 209, 1982.
44. E. E. Ivy, J. Econ. Entomol., 65(2), 473-4 (1972).
45. J. A. Onsager & P. C. Mazuranich, J. Econ. Entomol., 69(6), 747-748 (1976).
46. R. K. Vander Meer & D. H. Lewis in: "*Controlled Release of Bioactive Materials*", R. Baker, Ed., Academic Press, New York, 1980, pp. 251.
47. T. W. Brooks, C. C. Doane, D. G. Osborn & J. K. Haworth in: "*Controlled Release of Bioactive Materials*", R. Baker, Ed., Academic Press, New York, 1980, pp. 227-236.
48. J. Heller, & R. W. Baker in: "*Controlled Release of Bioactive Materials*", R. Baker, Ed., Academic Press, New York, 1980, pp. 1-18.
49. M. E. Foley & L. M. Wax, Weed Science, 28, 626-632 (1980).
50. R. G. Sinclair, Environ. Sci. Technol., 7(10), 955-6 (1973).
51. M. Kamp, Hort. Science, 20, 879-881 (1985).
52. C. E. Carraher, Ed., "Modification of Polymers," Am. Chem. Soc., Washington, DC, 1980.
53. J. A. Moore, Ed., "Reactions on Polymers," Reidel Publ., Dordrecht, Holland, 1973.
54. C. G. Gebelein & F. F. Koblitz, Eds., "*Biomedical and Dental Applications of Polymers*", Plenum Press, New York, NY, 1982.
55. C. G. Gebelein, Polymer News 4, 163, 1978.
56. C. G. Gebelein, R. M. Morgan, R. Glowacky & W. Baig in: "*Biomedical and Dental Applications of Polymers*", C. G. Gebelein & F. F. Koblitz, Eds., Plenum Press, New York, 1981, p. 191.
57. C. L. McCormick & D. K. Lichatowich, J. Miss. Acad. Sci., 23, 6-10 (1978).
58. C. U. Pittman, Jr., & G. A. Stahl, J. Appl. Polymer Sci., 26, 2403-2413 (1981).
59. H. Naruse & K. Maekawa, J. Fac. Agric. Kyushu Univ., 21(2-3), 107-16 (1977); CA, 87,63924w.

60. E. Schacht, G. Desmarets & Y. Bogaert, Makromol. Chem., **179**, 837-840 (1978).
61. C. G. Gebelein and C. E. Carraher, Eds., "*Biological Activities of Polymers*", ACS Symposium Series, No. 186, American Chemical Society, Washington, DC, 1982, pp. 75-82.
62. G. G. Allan, Belgian Patent, 706,507 (1967).
63. C. S. Lee & K. Maekawa, J. Fac. Agric. Kyushu Univ., **19**(1), 1-9 (1974); CA, **82**, 113365j.
64. K. N. Somasekharan & R. V. Subramanian in: "*Controlled Release of Bioactive Materials*", R. Baker, Ed., Academic Press, New York, 1980, pp. 415-431.
65. R. V. Subramanian, B. K. Garg & K. N. Somasekharan, Org. Coatings and Plastics Chem., **39**, 572 (1978) and in: "*Controlled Release of Bioactive Materials*", R. Baker, Ed., Academic Press, New York, 1980, p. 415.
66. R. W. Bovey, R. E. Meyer, R. D. Baker & J. R. Baur, Weed Sci., **20**(4), 332-335 (1972).
67. H. Naruse & K. Maekawa, J. Fac. Agric. Kyushu Univ., **21**(4), 167-72 (1977); CA, 87, 178869z.
68. H. Naruse & K. Maekawa J. Fac. Agric. Kyushu Univ., **21**(4), 173-9 (1977); CA, 87, 146932y.
69 H. Naruse & K. Maekawa, J. Fac. Agric. Kyushu Univ., **21**(4), 153-9 (1977); CA, 87, 178833h.
70. D. Heath, Th. F. Tadros, R. D. Knott, and D. A. Knowles, ACS Symposium Series, No. 254, American Chemical Society, Washington, DC, 1984, pp. 11-28.
71. L. E. Bode, M. E. Foley, B. J. Butler & L. M. Wax, Proceedings of the Annual Meeting North Central Weed Control Conf., **32**, 141-144 (1977).
72. G. E. Wortley, Jr., Proc. South Weed Sci. Soc., **30**, 345-351 (1977).
73. K. I. Rash, Proc. South Weed Sci. Soc., 30, 423-427 (1977).
74. C. G. McWhorter, Weed Sci., **25**(2), 135-141 (1977).
75. E. M. Jones & J. B. Kissam, Poultry Sci., **62**, 1113-1116 (1983).
76. R. D. Hall, J. M. Vandepopuliere, F. J., Fischer, J. J. Lyons & K. E. Doisy, Poultry Sci., **62**, 612-615 (1983).
77. Anon., The Furrow, **90**(3), 26 (1985).
78. D. L. Bailey, G. C. LaBrecque & T. L. Whitfield, J. Econ. Entomol., **64**(1), 138-140 (1971).
79. S. Moore, III & G. F. Cmarik, Bulletin No. 8, Dixon Springs Agricultural Center, 11-20 (1980).
80. M. C. Ivey, J. S. Palmer & E. C. Hooten, J. Econ. Entomol., **71**(4), 697-700 (1978).
81. M. C. Ivey, J. Econ. Entomol., **72**(6), 909-911 (1979).
82. H. A. Highland, L. D. Cline & R. A. Simonaitis, J. Econ. Entomol., **79**, 775-778 (1986).
83. J. Lancien, Cah. O R S T O M, Ser. Med. Parasitol., **19**(4), 235-238 (1981).
84. J. J. Reagon, The Furrow **90**(4), 4 (1985).
85. USDA Press Release, USDA, May 14 (1986).
86. J. R. Teasdale, Hort. Sci., **20**, 871-872 (1985).
87. S. F. Gorske, Proc. Northeast Weed Sci. Soc., **34**, 284 (1980).
88. C. E. Bell, A. Durazo, III, & C. L. Elmore, Calif. Agric. Experi. Station, **39** (11-12), 17-18 (1985).
89. S. F. Gorske, Acta Horticulturea, **1983**(136), 35-39 (1983).
90. D. H. R. C. Reinhardt, N. F. Sanches & G. A. P. D. Cunha, Pesqui. Agropeco. Bras., **16**(5), 719-724 (1981).
91. S. B. Boswell, D. R. Atkin & K. W. Hench, Hortic. Science, **13** (section 1), 49-50 (1978).
92. J. K. Choi, Y. S. Kwon & Y. H. Yu, Korean J. Plant Prot., **20**(2), 83-86 (1981).
93. R. B. Chalfant, C. A. Jaworski, A. W. Johnson & D. R. Sumner, J. Am. Soc. Hortic. Sci., **102**(1), 11-15 (1977).

94. V. F. Smirnov, A., A. Anisimov & A. S. Semicheva, Appl. Biochem. Microbiol., **13**(1), 102-105 (transl.) (1977).

95. C. S. Lee & K. Maekawa, J. Fac. Agric. Kyushu Univ., **19**(1), 65-72 (1974); CA, **82**, 100427f.

96. C. S. Lee & K. Maekawa, Agric. Biol. Chem., **40**(4), 785-790 (1976); CA, 85, 21745s.

97. N. F. Cardarelli & B. M. Cardarelli in: "*Bioactive Polymeric Systems*", C. G. Gebelein & C. E. Carraher, Jr., Eds., Plenum Press, New York, 1985, p. 37.

98. M. B. Shambhu, G. A. Digenis, D. K. Gulati, K. Bowman & P. S. Sabharwal, J. Agric. Food Chem., **24**(3), 666-668 (1976).

99. C. G. Pitt, T. A. Marks & A. Schindler in: "*Controlled Release of Bioactive Materials*", R. Baker, Ed., Academic Press, New York, 1980, pp. 19-44.

CHITOSAN AND DERIVATIVES AS ACTIVATORS OF PLANT CELLS IN TISSUES AND SEEDS

Shigehiro Hirano, Masahiko Hayashi, Kakuko Murae, Hisaya
Tsuchida and Takeshi Nishida

Department of Agricultural Biochemistry
Tottori University
Tottori 680, Japan

Chitosan and its derivatives (O-carboxymethylchitosan, O-glycolchitosan, chitosan oligosaccharides, and low molecular weight chitosan) were tested for inducing plant chitinase and chitosanase activities and for increasing plant growth. Chitinase and chitosanase activities were widely distributed in plants, and especially high in their exo-tissues. These enzymes activities were increased up to 3.5-fold in the presence of low molecular weight chitosan (0.05%) in the callus formation of cabbage leaves on the Murashige-Skoog medium, and up to 3.0-fold in the germination stage of soybean and Japanese radish seeds coated with a thin membrane of low molecular weight chitosan. These coated Japanese radish seeds were cultivated in the field, and the yield of the radish plants was 7-13% higher than that of the uncoated seeds.

INTRODUCTION

Chitin is a $(1\rightarrow4)$-linked 2-acetoamido-2-deoxy-β-D-glucan, and chitosan is its N-deacetylated product. These polysaccharides are naturally abundant and are present in the cuticles of insects and in the cell walls of plant pathogens,[1,2] but absent in the higher plant kingdom. Chitin and chitosan are (a) natural, (b) biocompatible, (c) almost nontoxic, (d) biodegradable, and (e) bioactive polymers. Our interest in these polymers is two-fold. (1): the molecular design of chitin and chitosan by chemical modification (Figure 1) in view of (a) the inversion of their molecular conformation,[3] (b) the development of their potential molecular functions[4] and (c) the addition of novel functions to these polymers.[5] (2): The effective uses of these functions in connection with their related enzymes.[6] Chitin and chitosan are known as novel materials utilizable in the biomedical,[7] pharmacology,[8] agricultural,[9] and biotechnological[10] fields. These polysaccharides are now commercially available for medical, cosmetic, food additive, agricultural and flocculent uses. It is well known that chitinase (EC 3.2.1.14) and lysozyme (EC 3.2.1.17) hydrolyze chitin into chitin oligosaccharides,[11] and chitosanase hydrolyzes chitosan into chitosan oligosaccharides.[12] Chitin and chitosan are not found as a structural constituent in higher plants, but their hydrolyzing enzyme (chitinase and chitosanase) activities are present in

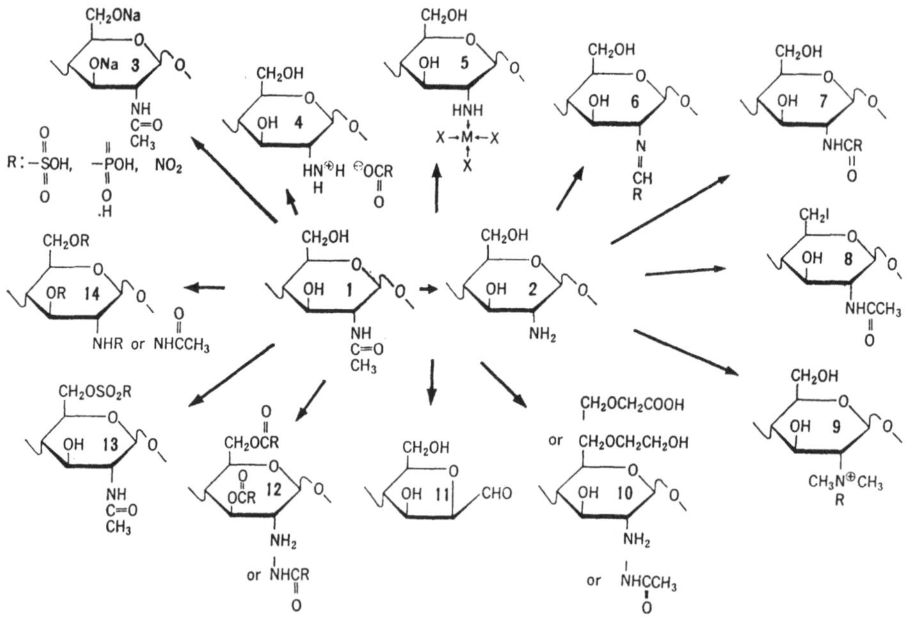

Figure 1. Some chemical reactions for the molecular design of chitin and chitosan. [1], chitin; [2], chitosan; [3], alkoxide (alkali chitin); [4] salt (carboxylate); [5], chelation; [6] Schiff's base; [7], N-acylation; [8], halogenation; [9], N-alkylation; [10], O-alkylation; [11], oxido-deaminative cleavage; [12], O-acylation; [13], sulfonation; [14], sulfation, phosphorylation and nitration.

higher plant tissues and seeds. In fact, several plant chitinases have been purified,[13-23] and attention has been focused on the biological function of these enzymes in the plant kingdom.

We now report crab shell chitosan and its derivatives can have a novel function as an activator of plant cells in (a) the callus formation of cabbage leaves, (b) the germination of soybean and Japanese radish seeds, and (c) the field cultivation of Japanese radish seeds. In addition, we will discuss a possible function of plant chitinase and chitosanase in connection with the wide distribution of these enzymes in plants.

EXPERIMENTAL

Materials

Chitosan, $[\alpha]_D^{24}$ = -8° (1% in aqueous 10% acetic acid) was prepared from commercial crab shell chitosan (Flonac-N, Kyowa Yushi Co., Ltd.) by treating with 45% NaOH solution at 120°C for 4 hrs. under a stream of nitrogen. The product had a negligible signal for NAc at about 2 ppm in the ^{1}H NMR spectrm (9:1, D_2O:DCOOD). The observed C/N ratio from the elemental analyses was 6.11 (calcd. = 6.00). N-Acetylchitosan xerogel (a regenerated chitin, d.s. = 1.0 for NAc) was prepared by selective N-acetylation of chitosan.[24] Low molecular weight chitosan ($[\alpha]_D^{20}$ = +26°,

1% in water, mol. wt. ca. 3,000) was prepared by partial chlorolysis of chitosan.[25] Chitosan oligosaccharide mixture (degree of polymerization = 2-8) was supplied by Katakura Chikkarin Co., Ltd.[26] O- Carboxylmethylchitosan Na salt {CM-chitosan $[\alpha]_D^{18}$ = -7°, 0.5%, aqueous 5% NaOH, d.s. = 0.9 for CM, mol. wt. ca. 250,000} and O-glycolchitosan {$[\alpha]_D^{14}$ = -6°, 1% aqueous 10% acetic acid, d.s. = 0.8 for glycol} were prepared from CM-chitin and glycolchitin {$[\alpha]_D^{18}$ = +8°, 0.7% in water, d.s. = 0.9 for glycol}, respectively, in our laboratory.

Methods

Specific rotations were recorded with a JASCO DIP-181 digital polarimeter, and absorption spectra were recorded with a Hitachi 100-50 spectrophotometer. ^{1}H-NMR were recorded with a Hitachi R-24NMR spectrometer (60 MHz) and the ^{13}C-NMR spectra were recorded with a single contact 75.46 MHz ^{13}C-CP/MAS NMR method on a Bruker CXP-300 spectrometer equipted with a CP/MAS accessory.

1. Preparation of a Crude Enzyme Solution. All the following treatments were performed at 4°C. Each of the plant tissues (100-200 g), the soybean (30 grains) and Japanese radish seeds (100-200 grains), the calluse (3-11 g) of cabbage leaves, and the germinated seeds (30 or 100 grains) was homogenized in an appropiate volume (usually 2-10 volumes) of 0.05 M potassium phosphate buffer solution (pH = 6.8). After centrifuging at 15,000 x g for 45 min., the supernatant solution was adjusted to 20% and 80% saturation with ammonium sulfate. The precipitates produced between 20% and 80% saturations were collected by centrifugation at 15,000 x g, and redissolved in a small volume of 0.1 M potassium phosphate buffer solution (pH = 6.8). The solution was then dialyzed against about 2L of 0.02 M potassium phosphate buffer solution (pH = 6.8) overnight. A small amount of precipitate was removed by centrifugation at 15,000 x g for 20 min. to give a crude enzyme solution.

2. Chitinase and Chitosanase Assays. A standard assay mixture for chitinase and chitosanase consisted of the enzyme solution (1.0 mL), 0.05 M citric acid-0.1 M Na₂HPO₄ buffer solution (pH = 6.8, 2.0 mL), and a substrate (each 30 mg of N-acetylchitosan xerogel and chitosan for the analysis of the enzymes from plants and seeds, or each 5 mg of glycolchitin and glycolchitosan for the analysis of the enzymes from the calluse). Blank tests were also performed in the absence of these substrates. The suspended mixture was incubated in test tubes with constant shaking at 30°C at pH = 6.8 for exactly 2 hr, and the reaction was stopped by treating in a boiling water bath for 5 min. Aliquots (0.5 mL) were withdrawn from the supernatant solution, and the release of the reducing sugar value was measured by a modified Schales method,[27] and by the Morgan-Elson method[28] or the Elson-Morgan method.[29] The reducing sugar was expressed as U/100 g seeds, mU/mg protein or U/g protein using an average value from three to five experiments. One unit (U) of enzyme activity was defined as the release of 1 μmol of reducing sugar value as N-acetyl-D-glucosamine for chitinase and as D-glucosamine for chitosanase per min. at 30°C. Protein was determined by the method of Lowry, et al.,[30] using crystalline bovine serum albumin (Wako Pure Chemical Industries, Ltd.) as a standard.

3. Callus Formation of Cabbage Leaves. Each sample (0.01, 0.05 and 0.10%) of CM-chitosan, low molecular weight chitosan, and chitosan oligosaccharides was added to the Murashige Skoog (M-S) medium,[31] and the pH of the medium was adjusted to 5.7 with 1.0 M NaOH, and the medium (20 mL) was poured into 50 mL Erlenmeyer flasks with silicon stoppers. The flasks were autoclaved at 120°C for 15 min. A piece of cabbage leaf was washed

with distilled water and cut into small pieces (ca. 0.5 x 1.5 cm, 0.75-1.20 g). The leaf pieces were sterilized by soaking in 70% ethanol for a few seconds, followed by soaking in 5% sodium hypochlorite solution containing 5% Tween 20 for 15 min., and the leaf pieces were washed five times with sterilized water. Each of the pieces was planted on the corresponding medium, and it was incubated in the dark at 25°C for 25 days. Chitinase and chitosanase activities in the callus and the weights of the callus were analyzed.

4. Coating Procedures for the Seeds. Each sample (60 g) of soybean and Japanese radish seeds was gently stirred in 10-15 mL aqueous 1% lactic acid for chitosan (0.1 g) or in distilled water for low molecular weight chitosan and chitosan oligosaccharides (0.1 g). The seeds were air-dried and used in the present study. A portion (30 or 100 grains) of the seeds was placed on an absorbent cotton sheet, wetted with distilled water, in a Petri dish (9 cm diameter), and was allowed to germinate in the dark at 25°C.

5. The Field Cultivation of Japanese Radish Seeds. The radish seeds coated with low molecular weight chitosan were cultivated in the field of the Tottori University farm in two autumn seasons (84 and 109 days, respectively) and one spring season (69 days) in 1984-1986. The results were compared with those of the uncoated seeds. Each experimental plot size was 0.75 x 3.5 m (2.6 m²).

RESULTS

Figure 2 shows the ^{13}C-NMR spectra of chitosan (d.s. = 0.05 for NAc) and N-acetylchitosan (d.s. = 1.0 for NAc/GlcN). N-Acetyl signals were detected at 23 (CH_3) and 174 ppm (C=O) in the spectrum of N-acetylchitosan, but were almost absent in that of chitosan, in spite of the presence of one acetyl group per about 20 monosaccharide units. The signal of $^{13}C_1$ at 1.07 ppm and that of $^{13}C_4$ at 86 ppm were multiplets in the spectrum of chitosan, but the signals in that of N-acetylchitosan (d.s. = 1.0 for NAc) were singlet, indicating a polymorph for the chitosan molecule.[32]

1. Distribution of Chitinase and Chitosanase Activities in Plant Tissues

Chitinase and chitosanase activities were found in all the plants and seeds examined (Table 1), and their activities varied not only with the species of the plants, but also with the morphological parts of their tissues. These enzyme activities were generally higher in the exo-tissues than in the endo-tissues. Chitinase activity in the skin of radish roots was about 2 times (U/100 g tissue) and 1.5 times (mU/mg protein) the values in the core. The chitinase activity in the chaff of rice seeds was 2.5 times (U/100 g tissue) and 12 times (mU/mg protein) the values in the hulled rice. Chitinase activity was found in the cuticle of soybean seeds, but only traces were in their embryo and albumen parts. Chitinase activity was up to 15 times higher than chitosanase activity in these tissues, except carrot roots and spinach leaves. Plant pathogens and insects, whose cuticles consist of chitin and chitosan, may attack plant tissues externally, and the localization of chitinase activity in the plant exo-tissues may have a function to prevent their external invasion. Furthermore, chitinase, which was immobilized in the plant tisues, was relatively stable against the heat treatment as shown in the parentheses in Table 1. Up to 34% of the original enzyme activity remained, and the specific activity increased up to 3.3 times that of the originals even after treatment in a boiling water bath for 10 min. in the cases of sweet pepper, Japanese radish leaves, and spinach leaves. However, chitinase

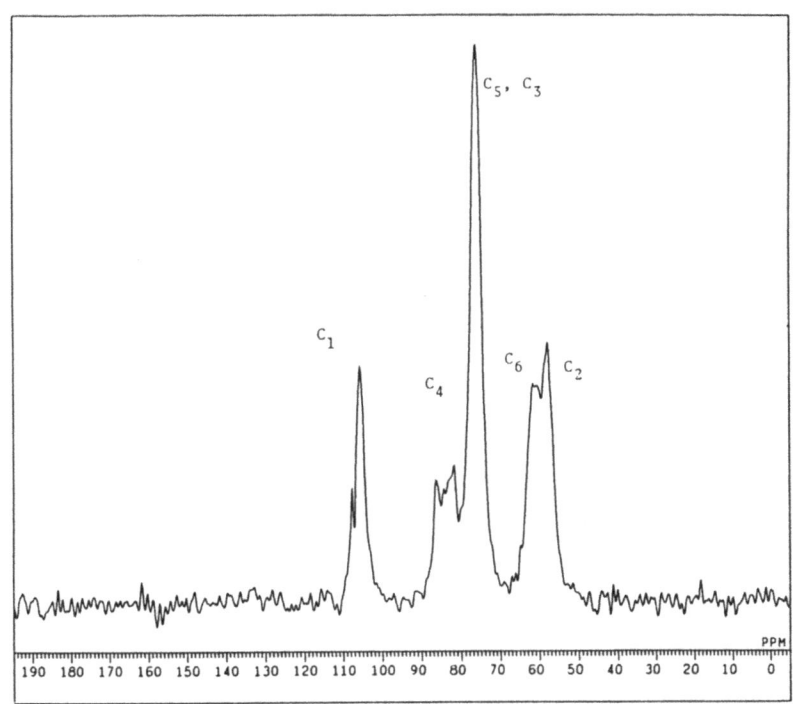

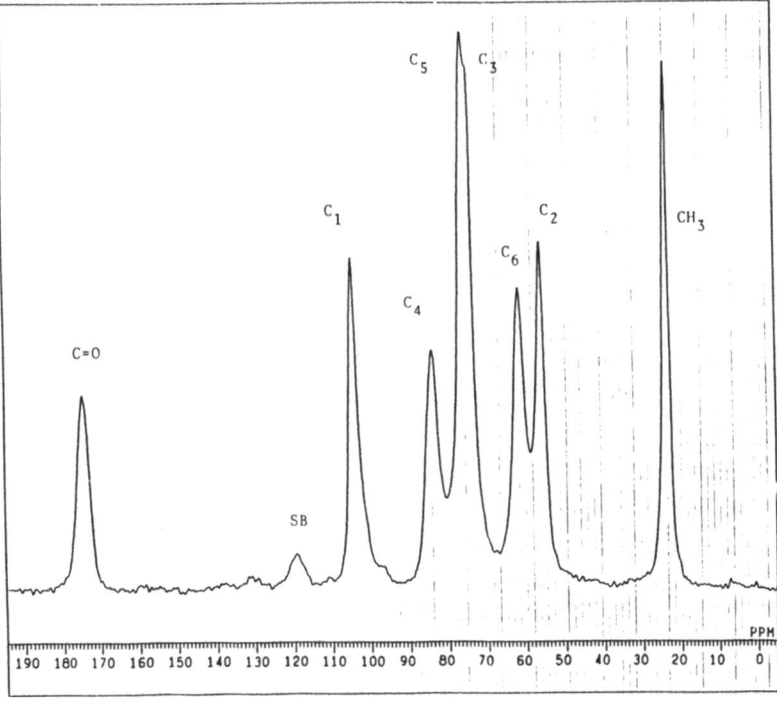

Figure 2. ^{13}C-CP/MAS nmr spectra of chitosan (above) and N-acetylchitosan (below). Chitosan (d.s. = 0.05 for NAc): C_1 = 107-105, C_2 = 58, C_3 = 76, C_4 = 86-82, C_5 = 76 ppm; N-acetylchitosan (d.s. = 1.0 for NAc): C_1 = 104, C_2 = 56, C_3 = 76, C_4 = 84, C_5 = 76, C_6 = 61, CH_3 = 23, C=O = 174 ppm.

Table 1. Distribution of chitinase and chitosanase activities
by fresh weight in some plants and seeds (a).

Plants	Chitinase		Chitosanase	
	(b)	(c)	(b)	(c)
Allium cepa L. (onion)				
Whole fruit	978	4.9	n.d.	n.d.
Apium graveolens L. var. *dulce* DC. (celery)				
Stem with leaves	140(10)	0.69(0.21)	40(4.0)	0.19(0.09)
Brassica oleracea L. var. *capitala* L. (Cabbage)				
Leaves	596(11)	10(1.8)	68(0.9)	1.1(0.14)
Stem (core)	527	4.0	n.d.	n.d.
Capsicum annum L. (Red pepper)				
Whole fruit	290(15)	1.7(0.39)	38(10)	0.22(0.26)
Citrus unshiu MARCOV. (Mandarin)				
Whole fruit	260	0.48	n.d.	n.d.
Fruit endocarp	1150	0.61	n.d.	n.d.
Fruit exocarp	2220	1.0	n.d.	n.d.
Citrullus vulgaris SCHRAD. (Water melon)				
Fruit cortex	1100	n.d.	n.d.	n.d.
Sarcocarp	280	n.d.	n.d.	n.d.
Cucurbita moschata DUCHESNE. (Pumpkin)				
Whole fruit	540	1.8	37	0.07
Cucumis stativus L. (Cucumber)				
Whole fruit	810	3.2	n.d.	n.d.
Dioscorea japonica THUNB. (Yam)				
Root cortex	2650	0.16	n.d.	n.d.
Diospyros kaki THUNB. (Persimmon)				
Whole fruit	230	0.50	n.d.	n.d.
Fruit cortex	500	1.3	n.d.	n.d.
Ducus carota L. var. *sative* DC. (Carrot)	trace	trace	158	0.82
Glycine hispida MAX. (Soybeans)				
Whole beans	20	0.1	n.d.	n.d.
Bean embryo	trace	trace	n.d.	n.d.
Bean albumen	trace	trace	n.d.	n.d.
Bean cortex	320	22	n.d.	n.d.
Sprouted beans	1000	2.2	n.d.	n.d.

Table 1. Continued

Plants	Chitinase		Chitosanase	
	(b)	(c)	(b)	(c)
Ipomoea batatas LAM. (Sweet potato)				
Whole potato	286	0.26	n.d.	n.d.
Potato cortex	2180	1.6	n.d.	n.d.
Stem and leaves	1333	22	n.d.	n.d.
Oryza sativa L. (Rice)				
Whole seeds	340	1.4	n.d.	n.d.
Hulled rice	330	1.4	n.d.	n.d.
Sed chaff	840	17	n.d.	n.d.
Paphanus sativas L. var. *macropodus*				
MAKINO (Japanese radish)				
Leaves	130	0.32(0.11)	67	0.17(0.56)
Whole root	660	5.1	81	0.63
Root skin	1900	5.1	n.d.	n.d.
Root core	500	7.4	n.d.	n.d.
Whole seeds	18000	6.5	n.d.	n.d.
Solanum melomgena L.				
(Eggplant)				
Whole fruit	1220	2.7	n.d.	n.d.
Solanum tuberosum L. (Potato)				
Whole potato	270	0.69	n.d.	n.d.
Fruit cortex	1470	27	n.d.	n.d.
Spinacia oleracea L. (Spinach)				
Leaves	20(210)	0.01(2.9)	107(35)	0.09(0.49)
Taraxacum ceratolepis KITAM				
(Dandelion)				
Leaves	230	0.31	n.d.	n.d.
Tulipa gesneriana L. (Tulip)				
Bulb	3270	0.50	n.d.	n.d.
Vicia faba L. (Broad bean)				
Bean sheath	1200	0.40	n.d.	n.dn

(a) Activity after treating the fresh tissues in a boiling water bath at 110°C for 10 min. is shown in the parentheses.
(b) mU/100g.
(c) mU/mg protein.

purified from cabbage leaves was completely inactivated under the present conditions.

2. Induction of Chitinase and Chitosanase Activities

A. In the Callus Formation of Cabbage Leaves. As shown in Figure 3, chitinase activity (nU/mg protein) was induced in the sequence: CM-chitosan (2.68 ± 0.05) > low molecular weight chitosan (2.11 ± 0.07) > chito-

san oligosaccharides (1.64 ± 0.04) > control (1.4 ± 0.03), with respect
to U/g protein, and in the sequence low molecular weight chitosan (1.81 ±
0.04) > chitosan oligosaccharides (1.54 ± 0.0) > CM-chitosan (0.90 ±
0.03) > control (0.60 ± 0.04) with respect to U/100 g tissue. Chitinase
and chitosanase activities were 1.4 and 2.5 mU/mg protein (control),
respectively, in the callus formed on the M-S medium for 25 days. The
induction rates of chitinase and chitosanase activities, in the presence
of 0.1% CM-chitosan, was 1.9 and 3.5 times those of the control, respectively, but the induction rate in the presence of 0.05% CM-chitosan was
low. Almost no induction was observed in the presence of 0.01% CM-chitosan. Chitinase and chitosanase activities in the presence of 0.05% low
molecular weight chitosan were 1.5 and 1.8 times, respectively, those of
the control. Chitosanase activity in the presence of 0.01 and 0.10% low
molecular weight chitosan was 1.6 times that of the control. However,
these enzyme activities were only slightly induced in the presence of
0.01-0.10% chitosan oligosaccharides. These data indicate that low molecular weight chitosan induced chitinase and chitosanase activities in
plant tissues and is a good activator for plant cells.

B. In the Germination of Soybean and Japanese Radish Seeds. Chitinase
and chitosanase activities increase in the course of the natural germination of the uncoated soybean seeds (Figure 4). The maximum activities

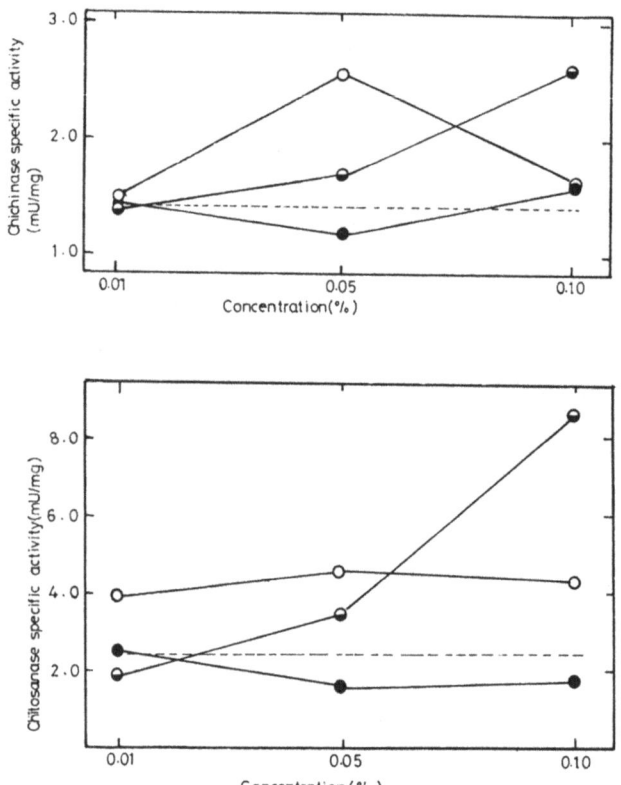

Figure 3. Induction of chitinase and chitosanase activities
in the callus formation of cabbage leaves on the
Murashige-Skoog medium. The following compounds
were added to the medium: low molecular weight
chitosan, -o-; CM-chitosan, -●-; chitosan oligosaccharides, -●-.

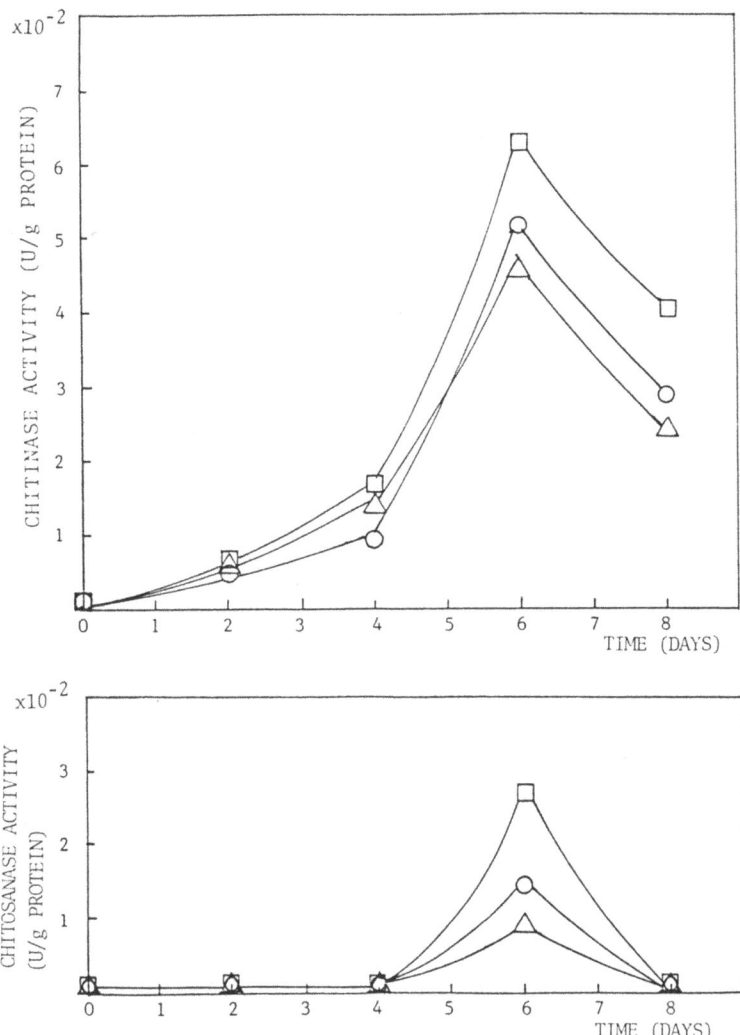

Figure 4. Induction of chitinase and chitosanase activities
in the germination of soybean seeds (each 30
grains) coated with a thin membrane of chitosan and
low molecular weight chitosan. Chitinase activity
(U/mg protein): uncoated, -△- ; coated with chitosan, -o- ; coated with low molecular weight chitosan, -■- . The fresh and dry weights (g) of each 30
grains during the germination process were 16 and
6.0 (2nd day), 18 and 5.5 (4th day), 27 and 5.4
(6th day), and 32 and 5.1 (8th day), respectively.

achieved by coating seeds with low molecular weight chitosan were 6U/100
g protein for chitinase and 3U/100 g protein for chitosanase, which were
about 1.4 and 3.0 times those of the uncoated seeds. Chitosanase was more
induced than that of chitinase by this treatment. Both the enzyme activities were slightly induced by coating with chitosan.

A similar induction of chitinase was observed with the germination
stage of radish seeds by coating with chitinase and its derivatives

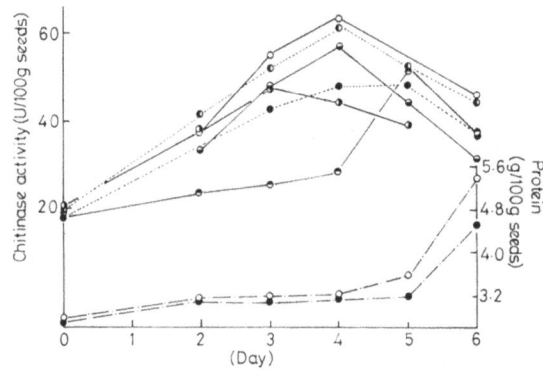

Figure 5. Induction of chitinase activity in the germination
of Japanese radish seeds (each 100 g) coated with a
thin membrane of chitosan and its derivatives.
Chitinase activity: uncoated (control) -•-; coated
with chitosan, -⊖-; coated with CM-chitosan, -⊕-
coated with chitosan oligosaccharides, -⊙-; coated
with glycolchitosan, -⊙-; coated with low molecular
weight chitosan, -o-; Protein: uncoated, ··-•-;
coated with low molecular weight chitosan, ··-o-. The
fresh and dry weights (g) of each 100 grains
during the germination process were 240 and 98 (2nd
day), 562 and 83 (3rd day), 823 and 81 (4th day),
843 and 80 (5th day), and 883 and 78 (6th day),
respectively.

(Figure 5). The maximum activity of chitinase by coating with low molecular weight chitosan was 64U/100 g seeds on the 4th day, which was 1.3
times that of the uncoated seeds. The maximum activity of chitinase by
coating with each of CM-chitosan and chitosan oligosaccharides was 1.2
and 1.1 times, respectively, that of the uncoated seeds. However, the
enzyme activity was only slightly induced by coating with each of chitosan and glycolchitosan.

3. Growth Increase in the Callus Formation From Cabbage Leaves in the Presence of Chitosan and Its Derivatives

As shown in Table 2, the growth rate (times) relative to the original
weight of cabbage leaves in the presence of 0.1% concentration was in the
sequence chitosan oligosaccharides (10.8 ± 0.9) > low molecular weight
chitosan (8.3 ± 0.7) > control (7.2 ± 0.6) > CM-chitosan (3.3 ± 0.5). The
growth rate of the callus was 7.2 times that of the original cabbage
leaves (control). An average value of three to five experiments is shown.
The growth rate in the presence of 0.1% chitosan oligosaccharides was 1.5
times that of the control, and the growth rate in the presence of 0.1%
low molecular weight chitosan was 1.2 times that of the control. Figure 6
shows a view of the callus formed after incubation for 25 days in the
presence of low molecular weight chitosan (0.01, 0.05 and 0.10%). However, the growth rate was inhibited in the presence of CM-chitosan.

4. Field Cultivation of Japanese Radish Seeds

Japanese radish seeds coated with a thin membrane of chitosan or low
molecular weight chitosan were cultured in the farm field of the Tottori

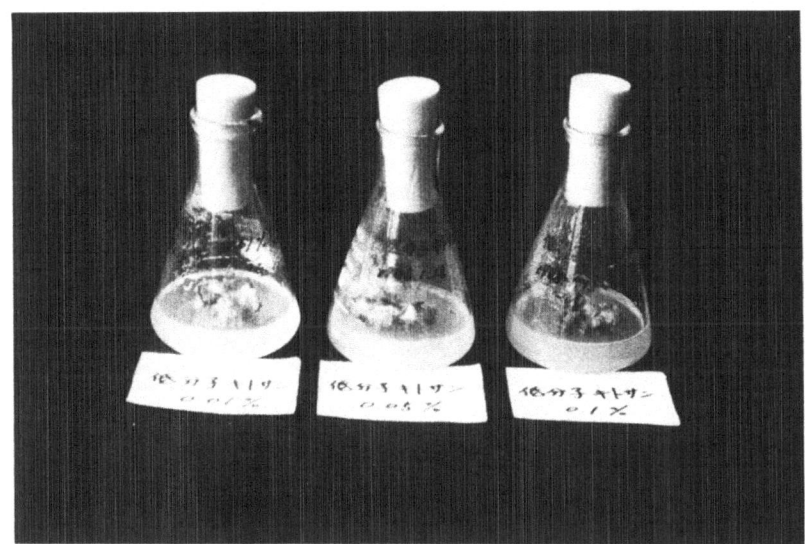

Figure 6. A view of the callus of cabbage leaves after incubation at 25°C for 25 days in the presence of low
molecular weight chitosan (0.01, 0.05 and 0.10%
from the right to the left).

Table 2. Callus formation from cabbage leaves (a)

Derivatives	% Added	Growth Rate(b)	% Relative to control
CM-Chitosan	0.01	6.0 ± 0.4	84
	0.05	6.5 ± 0.5	90
	0.10	3.3 ± 0.5	46
Low molecular weight chitosan	0.01	7.0 ± 0.3	98
	0.05	7.3 ± 0.7	100
	0.10	8.3 ± 0.7	120
Chitosan oligosaccharides	0.01	7.0 ± 0.3	98
	0.05	7.7 ± 0.4	110
	0.10	10.8 ± 0.8	150
None (control)	-	7.2 ± 0.6	100

(a) An average of three to five experiments is shown. Pieces
of cabbage leaves were planted on the Murashige-Skoog
medium (control) and on the three media containing the
corresponding chitosan derivative. They were incubated
in the dark at 25°C for 25 days, and their weights were
measured.

(b) Times relative to the weight of the original leaves.

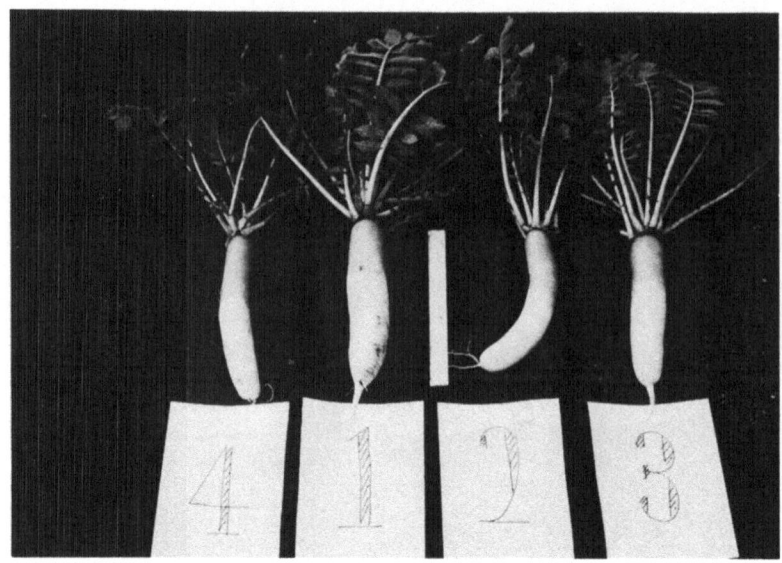

Figure 7. A view of Japanese radish plants after field cultivation. [1], from the seeds coated with low molecular weight chitosan; [2], from the uncoated seeds
by spraying an aqueous 2% solution of the low molecular weight chitosan over the young leaves twice a
week for the first two weeks after germination;
[3], from the seeds coated with high molecular
weight chitosan; [4], from the uncoated seeds
(control).

University. Figure 7 is a typical of the harvested radish plants: 4
(control) is from the uncoated seeds; 1 is from the seeds coated with low
molecular weight chitosan; 2 is from the uncoated seeds by spraying an
aqueous 2% solution of low molecular weight chitosan over the young
leaves twice a week for the first two weeks after germination; 3 is from
the coated seeds with chitosan. Their weights were in the sequence 1 > 3>
4 > 2. The plant growth was slightly inhibited by spraying over young
leaves.

Based on these results, Japanese radish seeds coated with low molecular weight chitosan were cultivated in the farm field of the Tottori
University. Total weight yields of radish plants and radish roots are
shown in Table 3, and the parentheses indicates an average weight/radish
plant or radish root. Coating the seeds with low molecular weight
chitosan increased the weight yields of radish plant (7-13%) and radish
root (15%). It is of interest to note that the weight increase of radish
roots was higher than that of the leaves. The present results is in
agreement with the data reported by Hadwiger, et al[39] for 8-21% increases
of the yield in the field cultivation of the wheat seeds coated with
chitosan.

DISCUSSION

The activation of plant cells with chitosan and its derivatives may
relate to (a) the induction of chitinase and chitosanase, (b) an increase
of the callus growth of cabbage leaves, and (c) a yield increase in the
field cultivation of Japanese radish plants. The growth and chitinase
activity of the callus increased in the presence of low molecular weight

Table 3. Effect of coating Japanese radish seeds with a thin
membrane of low molecular weight chitosan on the
weight yield of the plants and roots (a).

Radish	Treatment	Total Weight Yield(a)		
		1984 Autumn(b)	1985 Spring(c)	1986 Autumn(d)
Plants (leaves and roots)	Coated(e)	15,800 (605 ± 126)	12,500 (636 ± 108)	9,850 (704 ± 195)
	Control(f)	14,800 (568 ± 145)	11,100 (614 ± 193)	9,000 (643 ± 256)
% Increase over control:		7	13	9
Roots	Coated	n.d(g)	n.d.	5,290 (388 ± 137)
	Control	n.d.	n.d.	4,610 (338 ± 134)
% Increase over control:		13(h)	19(h)	15

(a) One plot size for the cultivation was 0.75 m x 3.5 m. The
parenthesis indicates the average weight/plant or root.

(b) Seeded on September 15, 1984 and harvested on January 1,
1985.

(c) Seeded on April 29 and harvested on July 6, 1985.

(d) Seeded on September 15 and harvested on December 7, 1986.

(e) Coated with a thin membrane of low molecular weight
chitosan (see experimental section for details).

(f) Uncoated.

(g) Not determined.

(h) Estimated from the value of 1986.

chitosan and chitosan oligosaccharides, and the specific activity of
chitinase also increased. This strongly suggests an increase in the protein synthesis in the presence of chitosan and its derivatives. Several
investigators reported the induction of chitinase and chitosanase activities in entomopathogenic fungi with the degradation products of chitin
and chitosan,[40] in bean leaves with ethylene,[15,35] in pea pods with
chitosan,[16] pathogens and elicitors,[36,37] and in melon leaves and seedlings with pathogens.[38]

Recently we found that chitinase has a relatively broad substrate
specificity not only for the structure of N-acyl groups,[33] but also for
the degree of substitution for N-acyl groups. Chitinase from *Streptomyces
griseus* digests partially N-acetylated chitosans, having a d.s. = 0.5-0.9
for N-acetyl, at a slightly higher rate than those having a d.s. = 1.0
for N-acetyl.[34] Plant chitinase also hydrolyzes not only chitin, but also
partially N-deacetylated chitin.[34] Chitosan (cell walls of pathogens and
cuticles of insects) adheres to plant tissues, and plant chitinase and

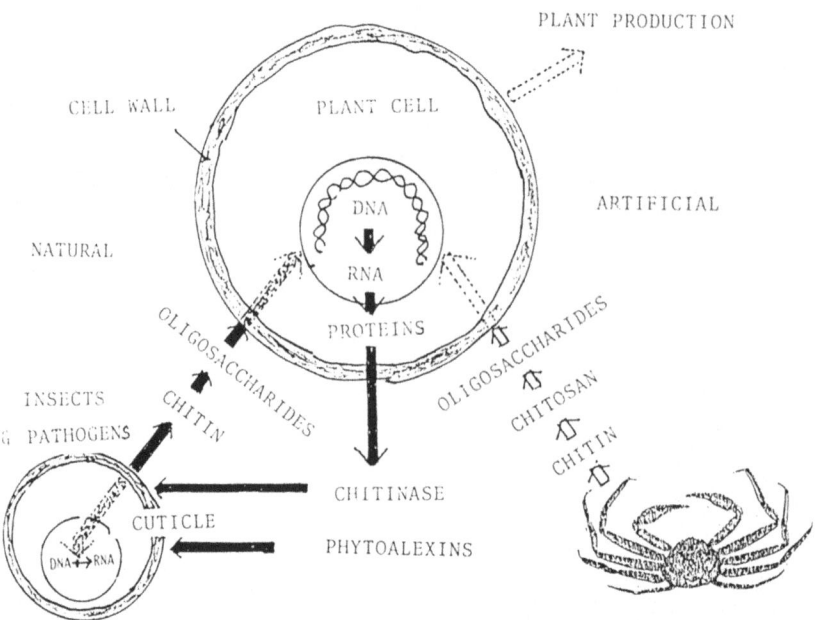

Figure 8. A proposed model for the molecular interaction of the plant cells with a pathogen or an insect in nature, and artificial activation of plant cells with crab shell chitosan to enhance the plant production. See the text for details.

chitosanase hydrolyzes it to low molecular weight chitosans and chitosan oligosaccharides, which bind to both the specific regions on the cell walls of plant cells and on the cuticle of pathogens. Chitosan oligosaccharides activate plant cells, which induce chitinase, chitosanase, β-D-glucanase, phytoalexin-synthetic enzymes, etc.,[41,42] as indicated with a black arrow in Figure 8. Chitosan oligosaccharides also inhibits the transcription of DNA to mRNA,[42] and chitinase inhibits the growth of pathogens.[43] As demonstrated in the present study, chitinase and chitosanase activities increased in the early germination stage of soybean and radish seeds. The soft young tissues of germinating seeds are possibly attacked by pathogens and insects more easily than that of the matured tissues, but these young tissues are generally resistant to their invasion. This is probably owing to chitinase and chitosanase activities present in the surface of plant tissues. These plant pathogens and plant insect contacts are essential for the natural growth of plants. As shown in the white arrows, Figure 8, we may artificially activate plant cells and enhance the plant production by coating with chitosan, or spraying chitosan over plant leaves, and by fertilizing chitosan for plant roots in soil.

REFERENCES

1. B. R. Johnson & G. C. Chen, Holzforshung, 37, 255 (1983).
2. H. Tanaka, S. Kamiyama, T. Miki & M. Kominato, Agric. Biol. Chem., 49, 1393 (1985).
3. S. Hirano & R. Yamaguchi, Biopolymers, 15, 1685 (1976).
4. S. Hirano& J. Kinugawa, Carbohydrate Res., 159, 295 (1986).
5. S. Hirano & Y. Che, Carbohydrate Polym., 4, 15 (1984).
6. S. Hirano & T. Matsumura, Carbohydrate Res., 165, 120 (1987).

7. S. Hirano & Y. Noishiki, J. Biomed. Mater. Res., **19**, 413 (1985).
8. K. Suzuki, T. Mecum, Y. Ohkawa, A. Tokoro, S. Suzuki & M. Suzuki, Carbohydrate Res., **151**, 403 (1986).
9. S. Hirano, H. Senda, Y. Yamamoto & A. Watanabe in: *"Chitin, Chitosan and Related Enzymes"*, J. P. Zikakis, Ed., Academic Press, Orlando, 1984, p. 77.
10. S. Hirano & O. Miura, Biotechnol. Bioeng., **21**, 711 (1979).
11. K. Amano & E. Ito, Eur. J. Biochem., **85**, 97(1987).
12. A. Ohtakara, H. Ogata, Y. Tamketomi & M. Mitsutomi in: *"Chitin, Chitosan and Related Enzymes"*, J. P. Zikakis, Ed., Academic Press, Orlando, 1984, p. 147.
13. R. F. Powning & H. Irzykiewicz, Comp. Biochem. Physiol., **14**, 127 (1965).
14. F. B. Abeles, R. P. Bosshart, L. E. Forrence & W. H. Habig, Plant Physiol., **47**,129 (1970).
15. T. Boller, A. Gehric, F. Mauch & U. Vogeli, Planta, **157**, 22(1983).
16. E. J. Nichols, J. M. Beckman & L. A. Hadwiger, Plant Physiol., **66**, 199 (1980).
17. A. Toppan & D. Roby, Agronomie, **2**, 829 (1982).
18. G. F. Pegg & D. H. Young, Physiol. Plant Pathol., **21**, 389 (1982).
19. J. Molano, I. Polacheck, A. Duran & E. Cabib, J. Biol. Chem., **254**, 4901 (1979).
20. T. Tsukamoto, D. Koga, A. Ide, T. Ishibashi, M. Horino-Matsushige, K. Yagishita & T. Imoto, Agric. Biol. Chem., **48**, 931 (1984).
21. S. A. Wadsworth & P. Zikakis, J. Agric. Food Chem., **32**, 1284 (1984).
22. L. A. Hadwiger & J. M. Beckman, Plant Physiol., **66**, 205 (1980).
23. L. A. Hadwiger & D. C. Loschke, Phytopathol., **71**, 756 (1981).
24. S. Hirano, Y. Ohe & H. Ono, Carbohydrate Res., **47**, 315 (1976).
25. S. Hirano, Y. Kondo, M. Fuketa & A. Yamashita in:*"Chitin and Chitosan"*, S. Hirano & S. Tokura, Eds., Japanese Society of Chitin & Chitosan, Tottori, Japan, 1982, p. 54.
26. M. Izume & A. Ohtakara, Agric. Biol. Chem., **51**, 1189 (1987).
27. O. Schales & S. Schales, Arch. Biochem., **8**, 285 (1945).
28. J. L. Ressig, J. L. Strominger & L. F. Leioir, J. Biol. Chem., **217**, 959 (1955).
29. G. Blix, Acta Chim. Scand., **2**, 467 (1948).
30. O. H. Lowry, N. J. Rosebrough, A. L. Farr & R. J. Randall, J. Biol. Chem., **193**, 265 (1951).
31. T. Murashige & F. Skoog, Physiol. Plant, **15**, 473 (1962).
32. K. Ogawa, S. Hirano, T. Miyanishi, T. Yui & T. Watanabe, Macromolecules, **17**, 973 (1984).
33. S. Hirano & Y. Yagi, Carbohydrate Res., **83**, 103 (1980).
34. S. Hirano & H. Tsuchida, Seikagaku, **59**, 898 (1987).
35. T. Boller & U. Vogeli, Plant. Physiol., **74**, 412 (1984).
36. M. Walker-Simmons, L. Hadwiger & C. A. Ryan, Biochem. Biophys. Res. Comm., **110**, 194 (1983).
37. F. Mauch, L. A. Hadwiger & T. Boller, Plant Physiol., **76**, 607 (1984).
38. D. Roby, A. Toppan & M. T. Esquerre-Tugaye, Plant Physiol., **81**, 228 (1986).
39. L. A. Hadwiger, R. Fristensky & R. C. Riggleman in: *"Chitin, Chitosan and Related Enzymes"*, J. P. Zikakis, Ed., Academic Press, Orlando, 1984, p. 291.
40. R. J. St. Leger, R. M. Cooper & A. K. Charnley, J. Gen. Microbiol., **132**, 1509 (1986).
41. C. R. Alan & L. A. Hadwiger, Exp. Mycology, **1979**, 285.
42. L. A. Hadwiger, D. F. Kandra, B. W. Fristensky & W. Wagoner in: *"Chitin in Nature and Technology"*, R. Muzzarelli, C. Jeuniaux & G. W. Gooday, Eds., Plenum, New York, 1986, p. 209.
43. A. Schlumbaum, F. Mauch, U. Vogeli & T. Boller, Nature, **324**, 365 (1986).

BIODEGRADATION OF HYDROXYLATED POLYMERS

Laura J. DiBenedetto, J. A. Cameron, and Samuel J. Huang*

Institute of Materials Science
University of Connecticut
Storrs, Connecticut 06268

Both qualitative and quantitative microbial methods have been used to investigate the biodegradability of two hydroxylated polyesters and their polyurethane derivatives. Bitritto and Huang reported that poly(hexamethylene tartrate) and poly(octamethylene tartrate), synthesized using para-toluene sulfonic acid as a catalyst, were good substrates for fungal growth.[1] In this study it was found that tin chloride could also be used as a catalyst for the polyesterification reactions with no apparent effect on the biodegradability of the polymers. Both polymers, as well as polyurethanes synthesized from the polyesters, supported the growth of *Aspergillus niger* on film surfaces. On the other hand, when zinc chloride was either used as a catalyst or incorporated into the polymer matrices, fungal growth was inhibited. Based on these results, further experiments were conducted to test the feasibility of using these biodegradable polymers as controlled release matrices for fungicidal agents. In these experiments, zinc chloride was incorporated into polymer tablets, the release profile examined, and the effect on fungal growth observed.

INTRODUCTION

A biodegradable polymer is a polymer which is capable of being enzymatically degraded by microorganisms.[2] The study of biodegradable polymers has become increasingly important over recent years. There are many reasons for this but perhaps the most obvious is that biodegradable synthetic materials eventually decompose, thus alleviating current waste disposal problems by diminishing the accumulation of waste products in the environment. There are many uses for biodegradable polymers, including applications in the packaging industry as well as in the field of medicine. For example, there are many advantages to using biodegradable polymers as surgical implants, as bioabsorbable sutures, and as controlled release devices for biologically active agents.[3]

Polymer biodegradation may be studied by exposing the polymer to an enzymatic source such as fungi, bacteria, or purified enzyme preparations.[3] One method by which the degree of biodegradation can be determined is by the examination of the extent of microbial growth on polymer surfaces according to the ASTM Standard Practice for Determining Resistance of Synthetic Polymeric Materials to Fungi and Bacteria.[4] In this procedure, the polymer and certain test microbes are placed in a system such that the polymer is the only source of carbon available to the microbes. The extent of microbial growth after a given period of time is used as a semi-quantitative measure of the ability of the microbes to degrade the polymer.

Changes in the physical characteristics of the polymer can also be detected using the ASTM protocol. For example, a change in the color or morphology of the polymer can be used as an indicator of polymer degradation. Scanning Electron Microscopy has been used to examine polymer samples for morphological changes resulting from degradation.[3,5,6] The use of the SEM is in addition to the ASTM recommended procedure of direct visual examination of the polymer sample.

The ASTM Testing Procedures are a semi-quantitative measure of polymer degradation. On the other hand, the methods of Huang and coworkers can be used to quantitatively determine the extent of polymer biodegradation.[3,7] These methods involve the use of GPC to examine the changes in the molecular weight and molecular weight distribution of the polymer following degradation by either microorganisms or purified enzyme preparations.

The structure and morphology of polymers affects their biodegradability. For example, biodegradable polymers tend to contain hydrolyzable linkages such as ester, amide, urethane, or urea bonds.[3] This is not surprising since in biological systems, natural polymers are degraded first by hydrolysis and then by oxidation. In addition, substituents such as benzyl, hydroxyl, carboxyl, methyl, and phenyl groups, adjacent to hydrolyzable bonds, tend to increase polymer biodegradability as long as the chiral specificities of the enzymes are maintained. For example, the L-isomers of poly(ester ureas) derived from phenylalanine are more readily degraded than the D,L-isomers.[3]

Morphological factors, such as the flexibility of polymer chains, tend to have an effect on the rate of polymer degradation. Flexible aliphatic polymers are more readily degraded than the rigid aromatic ring-containing polymers.[3] Flexibility is important since in order to hydrolyze the substrate, the enzymes must be able to fit into active sites along the polymer chains. Jarrett, using polycaprolactone (PCL) as the polymer substrate, did an extensive quantitative study of the effects of crystallinity and crosslinking on rates of biodegradation by microorganisms and purified enzyme preparations.[5] He found that increasing the extent of crystallinity or increasing the degree of crosslinking tended to decrease the rate of polymer biodegradation. Both the crystalline lattice structure and the crosslinked chains limit polymer flexibility and therefore limit enzyme accessibility to the active site.

The hydrophilic/hydrophobic character of polymers has also been found to influence their biodegradability. This was studied by Bitritto and Huang in 1979.[1] They synthesized poly(alkylene tartrates) by reacting a series of alkylene diols with tartaric acid. Polymer films were cast in glass vials, the samples were inoculated with a suspension of *Aspergillus niger* spores in a buffered solution, and then incubated for two weeks at 37°C. The extent of fungal growth was then rated on a scale of 0-4 according to the ASTM recommended rating system. The results are shown in Table 1. The hexamethylene diol and octamethylene diol derivatives were found to support fungal growth to a greater extent than either the more hydrophilic polymers (ethylene diol or butylene diol derivatives), or the more hydrophobic polymers (decamethylene diol and dodecamethylene diol derivatives). The addition of isocyanates to the dodecamethylene derivative did not affect its biodegradability. These data indicated that a balance of hydrophilicity and hydrophobicity was optimal for fungal degradation.

The poly(alkylene tartrates) are synthesized by melt polymerization. Both Bronsted-Lowry acids and Lewis acids can be used to catalyze the reaction. Bitritto used para-toluene sulfonic acid (pTSA). The resulting polymers were, in general, colored brown, indicating that the alpha-hydroxyls of the tartaric acid may have been oxidized. When tin chloride was used as the catalyst a lightly colored polymer was formed, indicating that some oxidation probably occurred. Upon purification of the product however, the yellow color was removed.[8] It appears that more favorable reaction conditions exist when tin chloride is used as the catalyst and thus it has become the catalyst of choice for future syntheses.

Because tin chloride is a heavy metal, it may have fungicidal activity. It is clear that the biodegradability of the polymer may be affected by the use of this catalyst. Therefore, the primary objective of this research was to evaluate the effect of using tin chloride as a catalyst on the biodegradation of the polyesters and their respective polyurethane derivatives. Both qualitative and quantitative microbial assays were used in these studies. In addition, experiments were conducted to test the feasibility of the use of poly(alkylene tartrates) and their polyurethane derivatives as biodegradable controlled release matrices for fungicidal agents. In these studies, zinc chloride was incorporated into polymer matrices, the release profile studied, and the effect on fungal growth observed. Zinc chloride was chosen as a model fungicide since since zinc is a component in many antifungal pharmaceutical preparations.

EXPERIMENTAL

1. Polyester Synthesis

Into a three neck 250 mL flask equipped with a mechanical stirrer and a vacuum distillation head was added 0.11 m of 1,6-hexanediol (or 1,8-octanediol), 0.10 m L-tartaric acid, and 2% (w/w) $SnCl_2 \cdot 2H_2O$ as catalyst. The mixture was heated under argon atmosphere to 120°C. After two hours, the pressure was reduced to 5-10 mm Hg. When the distillation of water was complete, the mixture was heated to 130°C and allowed to react for two more hours. The resulting crude polymer was dissolved in dioxane, precipitated from cold anhydrous ethyl ether, and dried *in vacuo* 48-72 hours. Poly(hexamethylene tartrate) was isolated as a clear elastomeric gum, while poly(octamethylene tartrate) was isolated as a dry white powder. Poly(caprolactone diol) or PCL was obtained commercially.

2. Polyurethane Synthesis

Into a three-neck 250 mL flask was added 30 g of polymer dissolved in a minimum of THF. Ninety eight percent hexamethylenediisocyanate (0.3 g, 0.002 m) in 10 mL THF was added dropwise with stirring into the flask. The mixture was allowed to react for 24 hours at room temperature. The reaction was terminated by the addition of excess ethanol. The polyurethane was precipitated from solution with cold anhydrous ethyl ether and then dried *in vacuo* 48-72 hours. The resulting product was, in the case of the poly(hexamethylene tartrate) derivative, a clear sticky solid, and in the case of the poly(octamethylene tartrate) derivative and

Table 1. Extent of growth of *A. niger* on poly(alkylene-d-tartrates) after 14 days at 37°C.

n	Extent of Growth
2	1
4	1
6	4
8	4
10	3
12	3
12 + 2% HDI	3-4
12 + 7% HDI	4
12 + 7% TDI	3

*ASTM rating: % surface covered: 4 = 60 - 130%, 3 = 30 - 60%, 2 = 10 - 30%, 1 = <10%m, 0 = no growth. Reproduced from Reference 1.

the PCL derivative, a dry white powder. In some cases 50 mol% HDI was used. In these cases, a hard, white, insoluble solid was formed.

3. Characterization

The polymer structures were verified by infrared and proton NMR analysis. Films for infrared (IR) analysis were cast onto KBr discs from THF/CHCl₃ solutions. IR spectra were recorded on a Nicolet FT-IR. Proton NMR were recorded on an EM 360 60 MHz spectrometer.

4. Biodegradation Studies

The preparation of the *Aspergillus niger* spore suspension and the non-nutritive growth medium (basal mineral salts, agar) was as described previously.[7] Briefly, the *A. niger* spores were washed from several nutrient agar slants with a solution of 0.1% Triton X-100 in sterile distilled water. The number of spores were counted under an optical microscope and then diluted with the Triton X-100 solution to a concentration of 1 x 10⁶ spores/mL. The buffer (BMS) was prepared by combining 500 mL of sterilized Solution A (K₂HPO₄, 0.7 g/L; KH₂PO₄, 0.7 g/L in distilled water) with 500 mL of sterilized Solution B (MgSO₄·7H₂O, 0.7 g/L; NH₄Cl, 1.0 g/L; NaNO₃, 1.0 g/L in distilled water). Sterile trace salts (1.0 mL) containing NaCl, 0.005 g/mL: FeSO₄·7H₂O, 0.002 g/mL; ZnSO₄·7H₂O, 0.002 g/mL; and MnSO₄·H₂O, 0.0007 g/mL were added to the buffer. For the solid surface studies, 14 g of Noble Agar (Difco, Detroit, MI) was added to the BMS buffer.

A. Qualitative Study. The purpose of the following preliminary study was to examine the effect of using different catalysts on the biodegradability of the poly(alkylene tartrates). Poly(hexamethylene tartrate) was synthesized according to the above procedure using either tin chloride (5% w/w), zinc chloride (10% w/w), or pTSA (5% w/w) as catalysts. Films were cast from a THF/CHCl₃ solution (30 mg/mL) onto the bottom of Erlenmeyer flasks. Mud and water from a local pond were poured over the

films. The flasks were loosely capped and then incubated at room temperature for four weeks. After four weeks, liquid and mud from each flask
were transferred to fresh polymer films that had been cast in clean
Erlenmeyer flasks. After two weeks this procedure was repeated. At the
end of the study, microbial growth in each flask was rated on a scale of
0-4 according to the ASTM recommended rating system.

B. Semi-Quantitative Solid Surface Studies. The qualitative tests
were next supplemented using the ASTM semi-quantitative solid surface
tests. For these experiments, polymer films were cast on the agar surface
by spreading 2.0 mL of a polymer solution (30 mg/mL) over the agar. When
the solvent evaporated, the plates were inoculated with 0.1 mL of the
spore suspension. After a two week incubation at room temperature the
extent of fungal growth was rated according to the ASTM recommended
rating system. All plates were done in triplicate.

C. Quantitative Studies. Quantitative studies were initiated in order
to quantify the extent of microbial growth on polymer surfaces. In the
first set of quantitative studies, turbidity was used as an indicator of
microbial growth. Polymer films were cast in the base of sterile 150 mL
bottles. Sterile buffer (100 mL) and an *A. niger* spore suspension
(1 x 10^6 spores) were poured over the films. Turbidity was monitored each
day for two weeks by removing a small sample (3 mL) from each bottle and
measuring its change in optical density (580 nm) on a Bausch and Lomb
Spectronic 21. Controls were included to correct for the contribution of
buffer and polymer to turbidity. All experiments were done at room
temperature.

In the second set of quantitative experiments, the extent of polymer
biodegradation by *A. niger* was quantified by measuring the increase in
the number of live spore colonies with time. Sterile scintillation vials
(20 mL) were coated with polymer films. In some cases, zinc chloride (10%
w/w) was dissolved in acetone and added to the polymer solution prior to
casting into films. Sterile buffer (15 mL) and an *A. niger* spore suspension (2 X 10^{13} spores) were added to each vial. After two weeks, nutrient
agar plates were inoculated with 1 mL of solution from each vial. After
four days the spore colonies on each plate were counted. Triplicates of
each sample were done at each step of the procedure resulting in a total
of 9 culture plates for each polymer sample.

D. Modified Semi-Quantitative Solid Surface Studies. The ASTM protocol for polymer biodegradation by fungus was modified for the studies
involving the zinc chloride-containing polymer matrices. Zinc chloride
(10% w/w) was dissolved in 2 mL acetone and added to the polymer solutions. Films were cast on the bottom of sterile petri dishes and the
solvent allowed to evaporate. Warm glucose supplemented (1% w/w) BMS-agar
(20 mL) was inoculated with 0.1 mL of the spore suspension and then
poured over the surface of each polymer film. The plates were incubated
at room temperature for two to four weeks after which the effect of the
zinc on microbial growth was visually observed.

E. Zinc Release Experiments. The purpose of these experiments was to
examine the release profile of zinc from polymer tablets. Poly(octamethylene tartrate) (500 mg) and zinc chloride (10% w/w) were thoroughly mixed
with a mortar and pestle. The mixture was placed in a mold and then
pressed in a Carver Press at 10,000 psi for 10 minutes. Coated tablets
could also be prepared by this method by sandwiching the drug-laden polymer between pure polymer layers. The uncoated edges of the tablets were
covered with wax so that diffusion of the zinc could occur only via the
top and bottom surfaces of the tablets.

The *A. niger* spore suspension was incorporated into glucose supplemented agar. The warm mixture was poured into sterile petri dishes. When the agar was almost gelled, the polymer tablets were placed into the center of the plates. As the zinc diffused out of the tablet and into the agar a precipitate formed. The release profile of zinc could be examined by measuring at various time points the distance from the center of the tablets to the outside edges of the precipitate.

RESULTS AND DISCUSSION

The effect on microbial growth of using various catalysts for polymer synthesis are shown in Table 2. In this experiment, the polymers were exposed to pond water and mud containing a mixture of bacteria and fungi. Regardless of which catalyst was used, microbial growth was very heavy during the first four weeks. When p-toluene sulfonic acid was used as a catalyst, growth was heavy in each flask even after successive periodic transfers to fresh polymer films. When tin chloride was used as a catalyst, growth dropped off somewhat when a small amount of the mixture was transferred to a fresh film. After the next transfer two weeks later, growth picked back up although the extent of growth was not as heavy as that for the pTSA-catalyzed films. When zinc chloride was used as a catalyst, growth dropped off following each successive transfer. In the final incubation flask, there was no apparent microbial growth. These results indicate that that, while the use of 5% tin chloride as a catalyst did inhibit microbial growth, the inhibition was not very dramatic. On the other hand, the use of 10% zinc chloride as a catalyst did dramatically inhibit microbial growth.

These experiments were refined by using the ASTM Standard Practice for Determining Resistance of Synthetic Polymer Material to Fungi.[4] The results of this study are shown in Table 3. The results indicate that the tin chloride catalyzed poly(alkylene tartrates) and their polyurethane derivatives are biodegradable. Each of the polymers supported the growth of *Aspergillus niger* on film surfaces to approximately the same extent. Figures 1-4 are photographs of the plates after the 14 day incubation period. Figure 1 shows a control plate. The background represents the agar base. On the surface of the plate, a few isolated fungal colonies

Table 2. Effect of catalyst Used for polyester synthesis on microbial growth.

Catalyst	Growth		
	Flask 1	Flask 2	Flask 3
p-toluene sulfonic acid	4	4	4
5% tin chloride	4	2	3
10% zinc chloride	4	2	0

*Extent on growth where 4 means heavy growth, 0 means no growth.

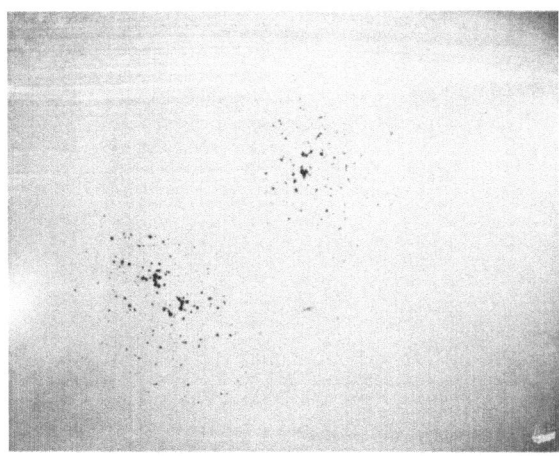

Figure 1 *A. niger* growth on a non-nutritive agar plate.

are visible. Figure 2 shows an agar plate over which a PCI film has been cast. *A. niger* growth is heavy and extensive hyphal development is apparent. PCL was included as a positive control for fungal growth since it is known to be readily biodegradable.[7] Growth was in fact heavier on the PCL films than it was on either the poly(alkylene tartrate) films or the films of their respective polyurethane derivatives (Figures 3 and 4 respectively). When 50 mol% HDI was used for polyurethane synthesis from the poly(octamethylene tartrate), a crosslinked polymer was formed. The extent of fungal growth on this sample was minimal. It is thought that with time (greater than the time course of this experiment), degradation would occur.

Next, an attempt was made to quantify the extent of microbial growth on polymer films. In the first set of experiments, turbidity was used as an indicator of microbial growth. As the fungus multiplies, it increases in mass and thus the turbidity of its solutions increase. In this experiment, extreme fluctuations in turbidity readings on a day to day basis made it impossible to make a quantitative statement. These fluctuations were the result of two major factors. The first is that as the fungus multiplied, it clumped together, decreasing the overall turbidity. In

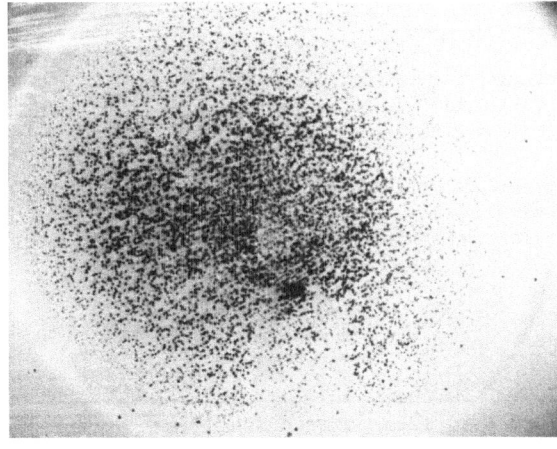

Figure 2. *A. niger* growth on the surface of a PCL film.

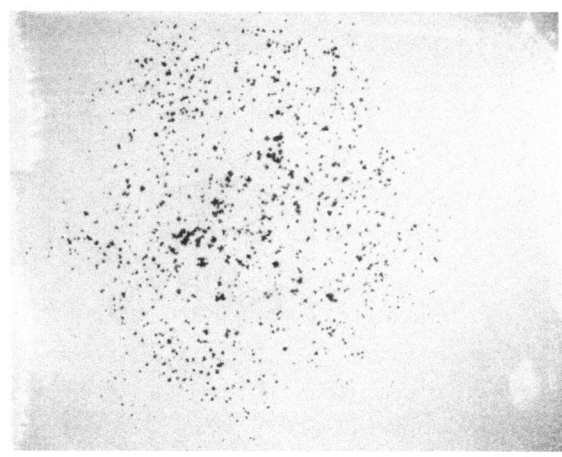

Figure 3. *A. niger* growth on the surface of a poly(alkylene tartrate) film.

addition, as the polymer films dissolved or flaked off the bottle surfaces, large unreproducible contributions to turbidity were made. Although a quantitative statement could not be made, several qualitative observations which supported the previous data were made. It was observed that both PCL and PCL + HDI were very good substrates for *A. niger*, with peak growth occurring after only 5 days. Very high optical density readings were obtained. The poly(alkylene tartrates) and the uncrosslinked polyurethane derivatives had, on the other hand, much lower optical density readings (approximately four times less) with no peak in growth even after fourteen days. The crosslinked polyurethane sample

Table 3. Extent of growth of *A. niger* on polymer films after 14 days at 37°C.

Substrate	Extent of Growth
Control	1
Poly(hexamethylene tartrate)	2-3
Poly(hexamethylene tartrate) + 3% HDI	2-3
Poly(octamethylene tartrate)	2-3
Poly(octamethylene tartrate) + 3% HDI	2-3
Poly(octamethylene tartrate) + 50% HDI	1-2
PCL	4
PCL + 3% HDI	4
PCL + 50% HDI	4

*ASTM rating: % surface covered 4 = 100 - 60, 3 = 60 - 30, 2 = 30 - 10, 1 = <10, 0 = no growth.

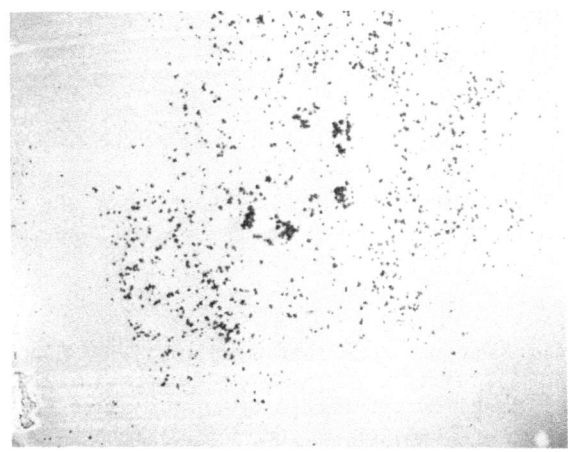

Figure 4. *A. niger* growth on the surface of a polyurethane
derivative of a poly(alkylene tartrate).

showed only a very minimal increase in optical density after fourteen
days.

A second quantitative study was attempted. In this study, the number
of live spore colonies (over time) was used as a measure of fungal growth
and polymer biodegradation. An increase in number of colonies would be
expected if the fungus could utilize the polymer as a carbon source. In
some cases, zinc chloride was incorporated in the polymer matrix. A
decrease in the number of colonies was expected in these cases. The
results of this experiment are shown in Table 4. There was no difference
between the polyester and the polyurethane in the number of spore
colonies present after fourteen days incubation in solution. In addition,
zinc chloride seemed to have no effect on fungal growth. It was possible
that any polymer-polymer differences as well as the effects of the zinc
on fungal growth had occurred prior to sampling at 14 days. Therefore,

Table 4. Effect of incorporation of zinc into poly(octamethylene tartrate) films on *A. niger* growth.

Sample	Number of Colonies
Control	103 ± 18
Poly(octamethylene tartrate)	85 ± 16
Poly(octamethylene tartrate) + 10% Zn	85 ± 21
Poly(octamethylene tartrate) + 3% HDI	81 ± 17
Poly(octamethylene tartrate) + 3% HDI + 10% Zn	103 ± 20

*   After 14 days incubation in solution.
**   ± standard deviation of 9 plates.

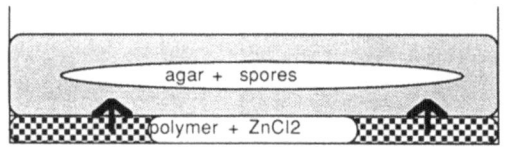

Figure 5. Experimental design for the study of the effect of
zinc on fungal growth.

the experiment was repeated such that sampling from the vials was done
daily. Again, no differences in colony counts between vials were
observed. However, based on the turbidity of the solutions, it was clear
that growth was in fact heavier in the vials without any zinc. It was
thus concluded that the test was not sensitive enough for our needs.
Clearly, polymer degradation is difficult to monitor via changes in the
microbial population. In the future, quantitative studies will be done by
monitoring changes in the physical properties of the polymer. That is,
changes in the mass, molecular weight, and molecular weight distribution
will be followed over time.

Although a quantitative statement of the effect of zinc on fungal
growth could not be made, it was still possible to perform semi-quantitative tests. A modification of the ASTM procedures was used for this purpose. The experimental design is shown in Figure 5. In this case the agar
and spores were poured over a polymer film that had been cast in the
bottom of a petri dish. As the zinc was released from the matrix it diffused into the spore-laden agar. The effect on fungal growth was quite
dramatic. The surface of a control plate that had been inoculated with
spores four days previously is shown in Figure 6. There is no zinc present in the polymer film beneath the agar surface. The agar surface is
completely coated with spores. Hyphal development is extensive. In
Figure 7 the effect of zinc chloride on *Aspergillus niger* growth is
shown. Dried hyphae indicate where colony growth was initiated but subsequently inhibited. It appears that as zinc chloride diffused from the
polymer film and became available to the fungus, it acted as a fungistat.
Polymer-polymer differences could not be discerned in this experiment
since an alternate carbon source, glucose, was added to the system.

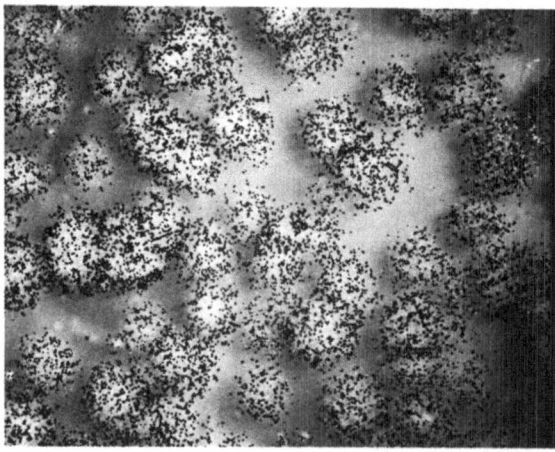

Figure 6. *A. niger* growth on the surface of a nutritive agar
plate. A polymer film was cast below the surface.

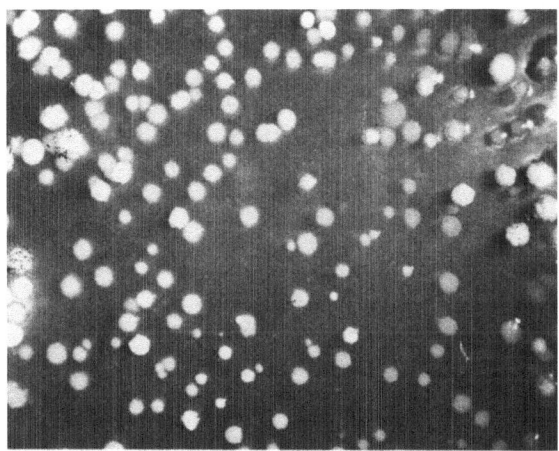

Figure 7. The effect of zinc on on *A. niger* growth. A polymer
film containing zinc was cast below the surface of
the agar.

During these experiments it was observed that a precipitate formed as
the zinc diffused out of the polymer matrix and into the agar. This is
demonstrated in Figure 8. It was postulated that the free zinc was reacting with phosphates that were present in the buffered agar to form
insoluble zinc phosphate salts. It was decided to use this phenomenon to
study the rate of release of zinc from polymer tablets. Therefore, zinc
laden polymer tablets were prepared and then placed in the center of
spore-laden agar. As the zinc diffused out of the tablets, a ring formed
around the tablet (Figure 9). With time this ring moved steadily outward,
the driving force being the release of zinc from the tablet. The
distance (r) from the center of the tablet to the outside edge of the
ring of diffusion was measured at various time intervals. The results are
shown in Figure 10. The release of zinc from poly(octamethylene tartrate)
tablets into agar at room temperature was linear with the square root of
time. This is consistent with Ficks Law for release from a matrix device.

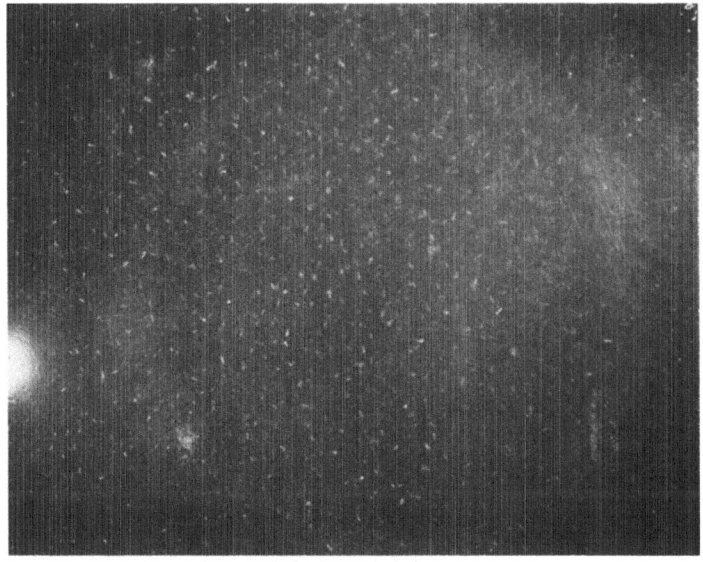

Figure 8. Precipitated zinc salts within the agar.

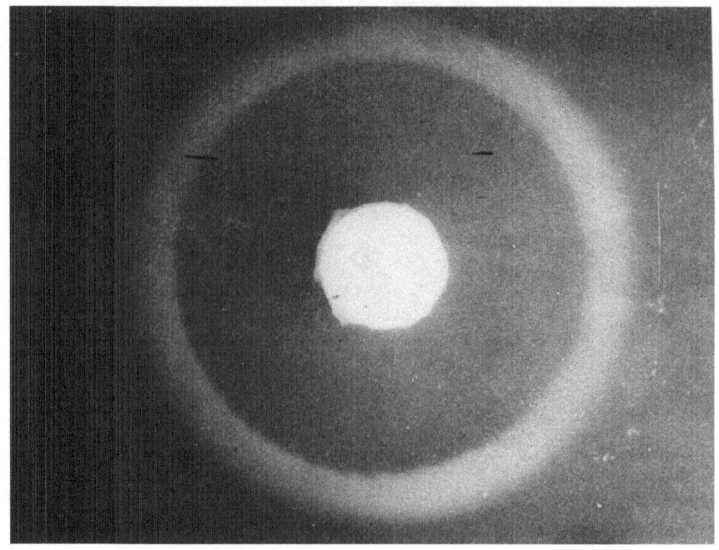

Figure 9. Ring formation following diffusion of zinc from a polymer tablet.

When a polymer coat was applied to the zinc-laden tablets, the rate of release was decreased. Release lagged approximately two hours behind that of the uncoated tablets. This result was expected since the rate of diffusion of zinc through the polymer coating is slower than its rate of diffusion through the agar, a medium composed of 1.4% solids and 98.6% water.

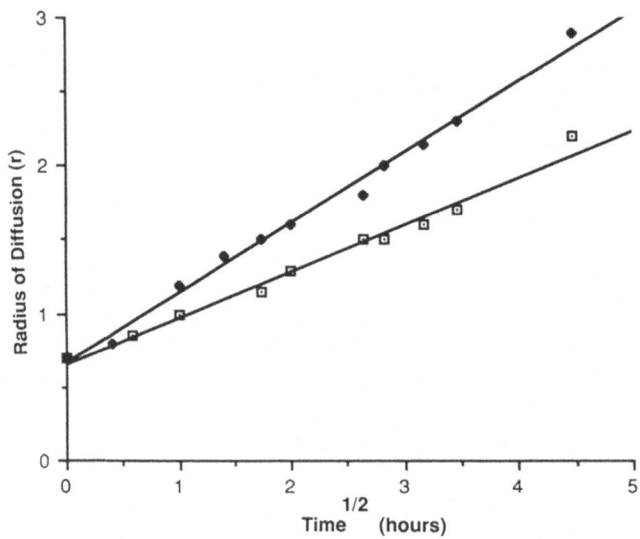

Figure 10. Release of zinc from poly(octamethylene tartrate) tablets into agar at room temperature. Diamonds: 10% zinc, uncoated tablets; squares: 10% zinc, coated tablet.

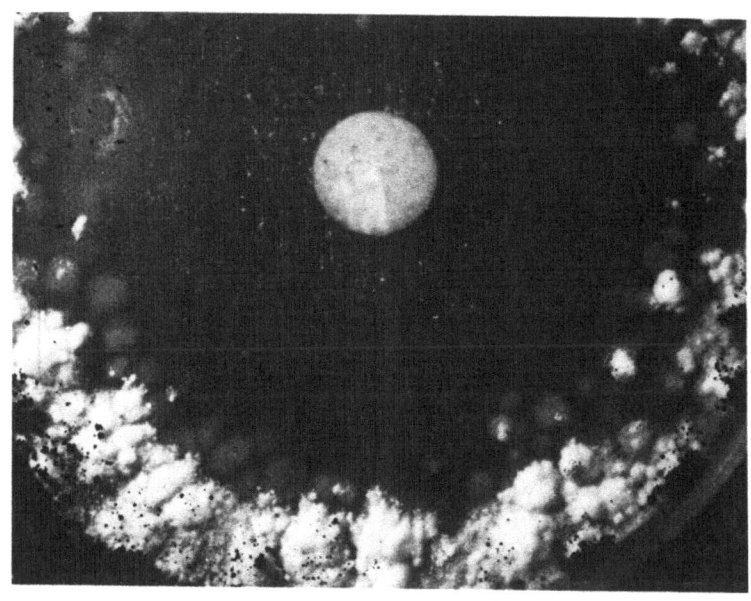

Figure 11. Effect of zinc on *A. niger* growth.

The effect of zinc chloride on fungal growth was again clearly demonstrated. Figure 11 shows the inhibition of growth within the zone of diffusion. A few colonies, both living and dead, are seen only at the edges of the plate where the concentration of zinc is minimal or not present at all. The data from this experiment has demonstrated the potential that these biodegradable polymers have for use as controlled release matrices for fungicidal agents.

Release into a stationary medium is by no means an ideal substitute for *in vitro* release studies. Clearly, future experiments must be conducted in stirred solutions. Diffusion coefficients, as well as the rate-limiting mechanisms for diffusion could then be more readily determined.

CONCLUSIONS

In this study it was found that tin chloride could be used as a catalyst for the polyesterification of alkylene diols with tartaric acid with no apparent effect on the biodegradability of the polymers. Both poly-(hexamethylene tartrate) and poly(octamethylene tartrate), as well as their respective polyurethane derivatives, supported the growth of *Aspergillus niger* on film surfaces. On the other hand, when zinc chloride was used as a catalyst or incorporated into polymer matrices, fungal growth was inhibited. Apparently, as the zinc was released from the polymer matrix into the agar, it became available to the fungus and acted as a fungistat or a fungicide. The release of zinc into the agar was found to be linear with the square root of time. Coating the drug-laden polymer tablet with a pure polymer coat decreased the rate of release. These preliminary studies have illustrated the potential use of these bio-degradable polymers as controlled release matrices for fungicidal agents.

A quantitative statement regarding polymer biodegradation could not be made. In the future, rather than looking at changes in the microbial population as indicators of polymer degradation, methods which examine changes in the polymer itself will be used. For example, changes in the mass, the molecular weight, and the molecular weight distribution can be monitored over time.

ACKNOWLEDGMENTS

Support of our research by U.S. Army (DAAG-29-85-K-0222) and NSF (DMR 80-13689) are gratefully acknowledged.

REFERENCES

1. M. M. Bitritto, J. P. Bell, G. M. Brenckle, S. J. Huang & J. R. Knox, J. Appl. Polymer Sci.: Applied Polymer Symp., **35**, 405 (1979).
2. T. Kelen: "*Polymer Degradation*", Van Nostrand Reinhold Co., New York, 1983, p.152.
3. S. J. Huang in: "*Encyclopedia of Polymer Science and Engineering*", Vol. 2, H. Mark, N. Bikales, C. Overberger & Q. Menges, Eds., John Wiley and Sons, Inc., 1985, p. 220.
4. ASTM Annual of ASTM Standards, G21, G23, 1987.
5. P. Jarrett, Ph.D. Thesis, University of Connecticut, 1983.
6. W. J. Cook, J. A. Cameron. J. P. Bell & S. J. Huang, J. Polymer Science: Polymer Letters Ed., **19**, 159 (1981).
7. S. J. Huang, C. Macri, M. Roby, C. Benedict & J. A. Cameron in: "*Urethane Chemistry and Applications*", K. N. Edwards, Ed., ACS Symposium Series, No. 172, 1981, p. 471.
8. L. DiBenedetto, Unpublished Results, 1987.

COMBINED MATRIX CONCEPT IN DELIVERY OF BIOACTIVE POLYPEPTIDES

Paul Y. Wang & Evelyn Kothe

Laboratory of Chemical Biology
Institute of Biomedical Engineering
University of Toronto
Toronto, Ontario, Canada M5S 1A4

Generally, a polymer implant may release a drug by diffusion at the same time with dissolution of the polymer component without depolymerization (Type A) or by erosion
involving depolymerization (Type B). The Type A material
induces immune response while the Type B polymer may lead to
toxicity problems. It is proposed that a combination of the
two types of polymer may attenuate the intensity of the biological responses, because the presence of one in an implant
of the same weight reduces the amount of the other. However,
it is important to know if sustained delivery may be achieved
by such an implant. In this study, partially hydrolyzed poly-
(vinyl acetate) (PVA) and polycaprolactone (PCL) were chosen
as the model Type A. and B polymers, respectively, to evaluate this objective first in vitro with methylene blue (MB) as
a model drug. Results show that sustained delivery can be
effected, but PCL erosion did not occur as intended. Therefore, PCL served only as a passive component of the implant.
while PVA was eroded with the release of MB. Consequently, it
was inferred that a polymer may not be required as a passive
component. Tests with insulin in a compressed solid admixture with palmitic acid showed that reduction of hyperglycemia in diabetic Wistar rat could be effected repro-
ducibly for at least 5 weeks. Thus, the present study,
originally planned to test a proposed concept, indicates that
non-polymeric materials of known biocompatibility may be
suitable for delivery of many bioactive polypeptides as well.

INTRODUCTION

The dissolution of the polymer component of an erodible implant system for drug delivery may be achieved in two ways. For the Type A polymer
matrix, the soluble hydrolytic products remain macromolecular. An
example of such a polymer is poly(vinyl acetate) which can be deacetylated to give the water-soluble poly(vinyl alcohol). In the Type B
scheme, the matrix is degraded into low molecular weight fragments like
in the ester hydrolysis of polycaprolactone.[1] Previous work in this

laboratory has shown that many soluble synthetic non-biological polymers of the Type A category are antigenic in mice.[2] With the exception of polymers of glycolic acid and lactic acid, many biodegradable Type B polymers, such as poly(alkyl-α-cyanoacrylate), release toxic fragments upon hydrolytic degradation.[3] If erodible polymers must he used, it is believed that the implant should incorporate features of both Type A and Type B designs as a compromise. The reason is because biological responses are mostly dose related. Therefore, in an admixture of the same weight, the presence of 1 type of polymer will reduce the amount required for the other. The decrease in amount of either types of polymer may also reduce the intensity of the unfavorable Biological responses aforementioned, and improve the chances of biocompatibility. However, even if the proposed concept is valid, but sustained delivery of the active component is not realized, then the implant will not be useful. This report describes some model experiments which demonstrates that drug delivery by the combined matrix approach is feasible. In addition. the results show that a polymer can be released on a sustained basis without total structural erosion of the implant. Furthermore, such an implant does not have to be made from polymers as structural components. Accordingly, even insulin can be delivered continuously from a compressed lipid admixture.

MATERIALS AND METHODS

1. Supplies

Maleic anhydride was purchased from British Drug Houses (Canada), Ltd., Toronto, Ont. The polycaprolactone (PCL), and partially hydrolyzed poly(vinyl acetate) (PVA) were obtained from Polysciences Inc., Warrington, PA. The poly(vinyl alcohol) is derived from poly(vinyl acetate) with 40%, 75%, 88% and 99% of the acetyl groups hydrolyzed. Their molecular weights are 3,000 for the first 2, and 25,000 for the other samples. Streptozotocin, palmitic acid, and bovine insulin (24 U,mg) were purchased from Sigma Chemicals Ltd., St. Louis, MD. The Coomassie blue dye solution was prepared by Bio-Rad Laboratories, Mississauga, Ont. The Glucometer[R] using Dextrostix[R] is a product of Miles Laboratories Ltd., Toronto, Ont. The 13-mm Specac pellet die, the hydraulic press, and the vibratory ball mill were obtained from Analytical Accessories Ltd., Dorval, Ont. The polycarbonate membrane filter was purchased from Nuclepore Corp., Pleasanton, CA. The Wistar rats are bred by Jackson Laboratories Ltd., Bar Harbor, ME.

2. Pellet Disc Preparation

Materials to be compressed were weighed and mixed thoroughly with the aid of a stainless steel ball in a capped tube mounted on the vibratory mill, before transferring to the pellet die. After the plunger components were in place, the die chamber was evacuated for 2.5 min, and the compression was then applied and kept at 5 tons for 3.5 min. After the compression was released, the pellet disc was pushed from the mold by gently tapping the exposed plunger stem. The pellet disc can be broken by bending under finger pressure to obtain pieces of desired sizes.

3. Release Rate Determination in Vitro

Release of MB from a pellet disc made of the synthetic polymers was measured at room temperature or 37°C as the case may be, in a volumetric flask containing 1 L PBS. The solution was stirred magnetically at about 70 cycles/min. At convenient intervals, 1 mL of the solution was taken and its absorbance was measured at 668 nm. The weight of the pellet disc before and after the release studies was also noted.

To estimate the release rate of insulin *in vitro*, a pellet made of 20% insulin in palmitic acid was broken and a quarter piece was dropped into a 250 mL Erlymer flask Containing 100 mL PBS. In another run, 250 mL of a 0.1 M orthophosphate solution at pH 2.4 was used with an 1/8-size piece. At daily or weekly intervals, depending on the rate of release, an aliquot of 0.8 mL of the stirred solution was withdrawn and mixed with 0.2 mL of Coomassie blue dye solution for protein analysis. After 30 min at room temperature, the intensity of the blue solution was read at 660 nm. The sensitivity of this method is 1 µg protein per mL. Since the solution was kept at 21°C, bacterial fouling would affect the dissolved protein. Changing the solution every 5 days was found to correct this problem, and the amount of protein entered the fresh solution was added to the total as the study continued.

4. Analysis of Pellet Disc Composition

After the MB release study, the sample was removed and air-dried to constant weight. It was then crushed to fine powder and transferred quantitatively into a flask. The volume of the suspension was adjusted to 500 mL, and 1 mL was withdrawn to determine the residual amount of MB, if any, by spectrophotometry. The flask was then warmed to 60°C to dissolve the remaining PVA derivative. The hot suspension was filtered through a Nuclepore membrane (0.2 micron porosity), and the weight of the insoluble PCL was obtained after air-Drying to constant weight. In a control experiment, pellet discs of a known PVA derivative to PCL ratio were assayed. The amount of the dissolved PVA recovered was determined by evaporating an aliquot of the filtrate to dryness.

5. Diabetes Induction in Wistar Rat

Male Wistar rats with body weight of 300 to 350 g were used in this study. Their normal blood glucose content was consistent at a range of 4-7 mM/L. Intravenous injection of streptozotocin in citrate buffer at a dosage of 50 mg/kg was given to induce hyperglycemia. All animals became diabetic in 24 hr with their blood glucose level exceeding 22 mM/L as determined by the reagent strip method.[4] They were studied after they had been observed to be diabetic for two weeks to ensure the permanence of their condition.

6. Implantation of Pellets

Under ether anesthesia, the abdominal skin of a diabetic Wistar rat was closely shaved and swabbed with a 10% Betadine solution. A midline cut was made, and a subcutaneous pocket 3 cm from the incision was created sideways by blunt dissection. An 1/8 piece of the pellet disc containing 20% insulin was inserted and the wound was closed by two Michel clips. The whole procedure required about 3 min, and the animal recovered in less than 1 min thereafter.

RESULTS

1. Release from Single Matrix Component

Initial tests were conducted at room temperature with pellet discs composed solely of PCL or 75%-acetate hydrolyzed PVA as the model component materials, with the amount of MB incorporated being 2.5% (w/w). It was found that the PVA pellet disc became swollen quickly and released most of the MB in 2 hrs. In contrast, the PCL pellet disc released very little even though the test was continued for over 5 days (Table 1). Changing the compression pressure during the preparation of the pellet disc to 2 or 10 tons did not alter the release characteristics as already observed.

2. Effect of Anhydride and Weight Loss

To facilitate the MB release by acid-catalyzed hydrolysis of PCL, the effect of maleic anhydride was tested. It was found that a small amount of the anhydride drastically increased the initial release rate of MB (Table 2) and depleted the dye in a few hours. However, analyses of the pellet disc after 1 week showed that the same amount of PCL used was left. Apparently the anhydride, if any remained therein, did not enhance the hydrolysis of PCL, as intended. The content of maleic anhydride which gave the slowest initial MB release was about 5% (w/w). Since acid catalysis did not occur, the addition of maleic anhydride was not studied further.

3. Release from Combined Matrix

With the MB content held at 2.5%, different ratios of PVA/PCL were evaluated to determine their effect on the release of MB, and throughout these tests, 75%-acetate hydrolyzed PVA was used. At room temperature, it was found that a ratio of 20 mg PVA/180 mg PCL had the slowest release

Table 1. Methylene blue dye released from pellet discs made of a single polymer.

Polymer	Time (min)	(hr)	MB Released** (% of total)
100% PVA*	25		16.0
	50		25.8
	75		53.3
	100		71.8
	125		82.6
100% PCL		25	4.0
		50	6.7
		75	7.3
		100	7.6
		125	7.9

  * 75% deacetylated.
 ** 2.5% MB in 200 mg pellet disc.

Table 2. Increased initial MR released from PCL matrix as a
function of the amount of MA added.

Maleic Anhydride	Time (hr)	MB Released* (% of total)
10	50	16.7
	100	20.0
	200	21.7
20	50	61.6
	100	69.1
	200	75.6
60	50	81.2
	100	81.4
	200	82.1

* Same as Table 1.

Table 3. Methylene blue dye released from compressed polymer
admixtures.

Polymer (%, w/w)		Time (hr)	MB Released* (% of total)
PVA	PCL		
10	90	25	2.3
		50	5.0
		75	8.1
		100	10.4
		150	15.2
20	80	25	6.0
		50	11.2
		100	15.5
		150	19.0
40	60	25	10.7
		50	11.5
		75	32.5
		100	38.8
		150	40.4
50	50	25	17.2
		50	36.6
		75	44.4
		100	56.2
		150	68.1

* Same as Table 1.

rate, as compared to other compositions (Table 3). Next, the effect of acetyl content of PVA on the MB release rate was determined also at room temperature for convenience. An intermediate ratio of 40 mg PVA/160 mg PCL was chosen, while the same MB content as before was used. The release was found to increase sharply with increasing percentage of the acetyl groups hydrolyzed in the polymer (Table 4). The 40% acetate-hydrolyzed PVA had the slowest MB release rate, but an intermediate grade of PVA with 75%-acetate hydrolyzed was used instead for further studies. This intermediate grade also caused a slow MB release rate that should he useful for sustained delivery. In addition, it may allow any upward and downward variations when other factors are changed to obtain the optimal combination of components in later experiments.

When the pellet discs were again analyzed after the experiment, it was found that the weight of PCL remaining closely approximated the weight of PCL put in the original discs. This occurred over several compositions of the PVA/PCL used, regardless of the duration of MB release.

4. Methylene Blue Loading

The effect of MB content was investigated at 37°C with pellet discs having a composition of 40 mg PVA/160 mg. The higher temperature enhanced the MB release slightly, and when the dye content was low, it allowed the study to be completed in a reasonable period of time which was selected as 30 days. At 10%, 5% and 2.5% loading, the number of days before the release of MB were 16, 21, and 26 days, respectively, but only the lowest MB content appeared to be useful for sustained release (Table 5). Thus, increased loading of the compressed polymer mixture with MB greatly increases the release rate. A high loading of MB also caused a very high initial release which was undesirable. The optimum amount of MB appears to be 5% or less.

Table 4. Effect of PVA deacetylation on MB release from pellet discs containing 80% PCL.

Deacetylation (%)	Time	MB Released* (hr) (% of total)
40	25	5.5
	50	8.6
	75	9.0
	100	10.4
75	25	10.1
	50	14.7
	75	16.2
	100	18.6
98	25	67.5
	50	81.2
	75	82.7
	100	85.1
* Same as Table 1.		

Table 5. Effect of MB content on release rate.

MB Amount (mg)	Time (hr)	MB Released* (% of total)
5	25	4.1
	50	6.2
	75	7.6
	100	10.1
10	25	7.5
	50	11.0
	75	13.1
	100	16.7
20	25	11.9
	50	19.6
	75	25.4
	100	35.2

* Same as Table 1; the ratio of PCL to 75% deacetylated PVA is 4 to 1.

5. Insulin Release from Passive Matrix

Around pH 6-7, insulin is essentially insoluble in water, and indeed very little protein was detected after 30 days in the *in vitro* run from the 1/4 piece of the pellet disc made of palmitic acid containing 20% insulin. However, at pH 2.4 insulin is readily soluble, and another 1/8-size piece assayed in the 0.1 M orthophosphate solution showed that close to 60% (i.e., *c.* 3 mg) of the protein content was released in about 14 days (Table 6). As guided by these release studies observed *in vitro*, it

Table 6. Insulin released at pH 2.4 from a compressed palmitic acid admixture.

Time (days)	Insulin* Released (% of total)
1	7.9
2	19.1
3	19.3
4	20.3
7	30.1
9	36.4
11	47.2
14	56.1
16	57.4

* From a 25 mg piece cut from the 200 mg pellet disc containing 20% insulin.

was inferred that insulin overdose should not occur if a piece of the pellet disc was implanted. Bioassays in several diabetic Wistar rats were then used to determine the adequacy of insulin release from the lipid disc. The 1/8-size piece selected contained about 5 mg bovine insulin (24 U/mg) or a total of 120 U. At a demand of about 2 U/day for normalization of hyperglycemia the insulin supply would be sufficient for about 60 days, if the release efficiency was 100%. Sustained release of insulin did occur for over 40 days as indicated in the near normoglycemic condition of the otherwise diabetic animal (Table 7).

DISCUSSION

Drugs with molecular weights less than 850 daltons can be dispensed by many means. For polypeptide hormones, especially somatotropin (Mol. Wt. = 22,000) and insulin (Mol. Wt. = 6,000), subcutaneous injection remains the most common mode of administration. Recently, delivery by external[5] or implantable[6] pumps has clearly demonstrated their advantages over daily injection. But the size of the hardware, frequency of refill, presence of an indwelling catheter or the complex implantation surgery required necessitates the continued search for a suitable implant. In addition to the compact size and simple insertion, the solid admixture can retain ample amounts of a drug sufficient for a long period of sustained release. Although still on a trial basis after over a decade, the non-degradable silicone capsule which releases steroid hormone for long-term contraception has clearly demonstrated the advantages and feasibility of drug delivery by diffusional implants.[7]

Recent improvements using biodegradable polyesters of glycolic or lactic acid have shown that zero-order release of steroids can be achieved,[8] but matrix erosion does not readily occur in step with release kinetics. However, as diffusion by bioactive polypeptide is slow through

Table 7. Typical Reduction of Hyperglycemia in a Diabetic Wistar Rat by 20% Insulin in a Compressed Palmitic Acid Admixture*

Time (days)	Blood Glucose (mM/mL)
0	>22
1	2.4
3	7.0
5	3.0
10	2.2
15	5.0
20	4.1
25	7.2
30	3.6
35	4.7
40	5.2
45	>22

* Implanted as 1/8 size piece cut from a 200 mg pellet disc.

a solid medium, catalysts have been incorporated therein to enhance hydrolysis of several specially synthesized polyesters.[9] Alternatively, an elaborate casting procedure must be used to create porous channels for insulin diffusion through the non-erodible ethylene:vinyl acetate copolymer medium, but over 90% of the polypeptide hormone may be irreversibly trapped.[10] A magnetic or inductive mechanism has been explored to enhance the release.[11,12]

Ideally, a diffusional implant should be erodible without any adverse effect, and be able to release large or small drug molecules steadily for several months. These two criteria are very difficult to achieve together. However, very few attempts have been made to combine the Type A and B polymers for drug delivery. It is believed that a combined matrix should attenuate somewhat the tissue response to the erosion products from either polymer types, because a lowered amount of one of the compounds in an implant will be required when a second is added.

The initial study was designed to determine the optimal composition of the combined matrix components, using PVA and PCL as the model Type A and Type B polymers. It was observed that with 75%-acetate hydrolyzed PVA in combination with PCL at a ratio of 1 to 4 in a 200-mg pellet disc, release of the incorporated MB could be sustained at 20°C. The data also shows that at a set temperature, the release rate can be changed by the weight and the hydrophobic substituent groups on the Type A polymer, i.e. the acetyl group in PVA used in the present study. In contrast, increase in the loading of the model drug caused its quick initial release, but did not prolong the duration of release referred to as the service life.

However, the data revealed several interesting characteristics of a combined matrix system. Firstly, it was found that an additive such as maleic anhydride could facilitate the release of MB from the otherwise seemingly impermeable PCL matrix without erosion by ester hydrolysis. Secondly, as indicated by MB release and analyses of the composition, at 20% by weight or less, a polymeric component of low solubility, such as partially hydrolyzed PVA, could be released from a PCL pellet disc which did not erode and acted as a passive structural component. Finally, the passive component could essentially be selected from any compound, polymeric or otherwise, as well as being permanently or even temporarily insoluble. Therefore, it was inferred that a bioactive polypeptide like insulin or somatotropin could also be safely delivered on a sustained basis from an implant made of a passive structural component as aforementioned.

Insulin is a rather unique drug, and its therapeutic dosages vary with several parameters. Particularly in clinical practice, a single subcutaneous injection of as much as 100 U of some long acting preparations can normalize hyperglycemia for 20-30 hours. Therefore, it was decided that the release of this bioactive polypeptide from a diffusional implant should be evaluated by bioassay.[13] Although the data in the model study suggest that the delivery is feasible, a composition for the pellet disc Containing insulin must still be selected for the initial testing. Because insulin is practically insoluble in water, it is taken as equivalent to the 75%-acetate hydrolyzed PVA at 21°C. Since lipids are water insoluble, but biocompatible, palmitic acid was chosen as a reasonable substitute for PCL. The weight ratio of the two components was set at 40 mg insulin/160 mg palmitic acid which was similar to the ratio evaluated for PVA/PCL. Only an 1/8-size piece of the whole pellet disc was implanted, because the *in vitro* study at pH 2.4 showed that a maximum of 8 U insulin/day would be released which should not be fatal to the test animal. As the results showed, the selection made from limited information and the precautions taken were, perhaps, still within the physiological capability of the diabetic animal to compensate for any inadequacy in the release by the small implant. Because no artificial material was used, no explantation would be required. The fatty acid component, after depletion of insulin, will be absorbed by the tissue thereafter.

In conclusion, the model study using a combined PVA/PCL polymer system has shown that the sustained delivery of a bioactive polypeptide does not require a synthetic polymer as a structural component. Therefore, many natural materials can be used to form a compressed admixture with the bioactive polypeptide for sustained delivery.

ACKNOWLEDGMENT

I thank the Medical Research Council of Canada for support and Health and Welfare Canada for a contract; D. Horton and C. Streutker for technical assistance.

REFERENCES

1. P. Y. Wang. "*Proc. 11th Internat. Symp. Controlled Release Bioact. Materials*", Controlled Release Soc., Lincolnshire, IL, 1984, p. 121.
2. P. Y. Wang, & C. Chambers in: "*Polymeric Materials and Artificial Organs*", C. G. Gebelein, Ed., ACS Symp. Ser. 256, Washington, DC, 1984, p. 31.
3. H. W., Coover, Jr. & J. M. McIntire in: "*Tissue Adhesives in Surgery*", T. Matsumoto, Ed., Med. Exam. Publishing, Flushing, NY, 1972, p. 154.
4. A. Schiffrin, M. Desrosiers & M. Belmonte, Diabetes Care. 6, 166 (1983).
5. E. B. Marliss, D. Caron, A. M. Albisser & B. Zinman, Diabetes Care, 4, 325 (1981).
6. H. Buchwald. J. Barbosa & R. L. Varco, Lancet, 2, 1233 (1981).
7. H. B. Croxatto, S. Diaz, P. Miranda, K. Elamsson & E. D. B. Johansson. Contraception, 23, 197 (1981).
8. C. G. Pitt, T. A. Mark & A. Schindler in: "*Controlled Release of Bioactive Materials*", R. Baker, Ed., Academic Press, 1980, p. 19.
9. J. Heller in: "*Recent Advances in Drug Delivery Systems*", J. M. Anderson & S. W. Kim. Eds., Plenum Press, NY, 1984, p. 101.
10. H. M. Creque, R. Langer & J. Folkman, Diabetes, 29, 37 (1980).
11. E. R. Edelman, J. Kost, H. Bobeck & R. Langer. J. Biomed. Mater. Res., 19, 67 (1985).
12. J. Kost, K. Leong & J. Langer. "*Proc. 12th Internat. Symp. Controlled Release Bioact. Materials*", 1985, p. 73.
13. P. Y. Wang, Diabetes, 36, 1068 (1987).

METAL-PROMOTED HYDROLYSIS OF POLYMERIC CHELATING AGENTS: CHELATORS ON DEMAND

C. G. Pitt*, Z-W Gu, J-H. Zhu, and Y. T. Bao

Research Triangle Institute
Research Triangle Park, NC 27709

The feasibility of designing polymer-chelator conjugates from which release of the chelator is triggered reversibly by the appearance of the target (toxic) metal in the circulatory system was tested by synthesis and measurement of the rates of metal-catalysis hydrolysis of the ester of poly(vinyl alcohol) and quinaldic acid at pH 7.5. Hydrolysis in 50% aqueous ethanol solution in the presence of the four metals, Cu(II), Ni(II), Co(II) and Zn(II) at pH 7.5 was first order, with half lives of 67, 71, 172 and 476 min., respectively. The rate of hydrolysis in the absence of metals was not measurable. A double reciprocal plot of k_{obs} vs. [M] for Ni(II) exhibited the expected linearity. For films of the ester, the deviation from first order kinetics was consistent with a contributing diffusion process.

INTRODUCTION

Problems of chronic and acute metal overload are long-standing and varied in nature. They include exposure to heavy metals in the industrial work place and the environment, metabolic disorders (e.g. Wilson's disease) and their treatment (e.g. Cooley's Anemia), and accidental ingestion by children.[1,2] The fact that success in identifying chelating agents for the treatment of metal excess has been mixed is a reflection of two problems. First, many of the more potent chelators exhibit toxic signs which limit their dose or prohibit their use.[3] Second, the metabolism and excretion of the chelator can proceed independently of the metal chelation process; because metal binding may be kinetically limited by slow metal redistribution from tissue depots, a high proportion of the chelator can be lost prior to metal binding. Desferrioxamine B, which is the only prescription drug now available for treatment of iron overload, exemplifies this problem. Its plasma half-life is very short,[4] and negative iron balance can only be achieved in man if the relative rates of iron binding versus drug metabolism and excretion are changed by slow administration of the drug using a constant infusion pump.[5]

---

* Present address: Amgen, Inc.
                   Thousand Oaks, CA 91320

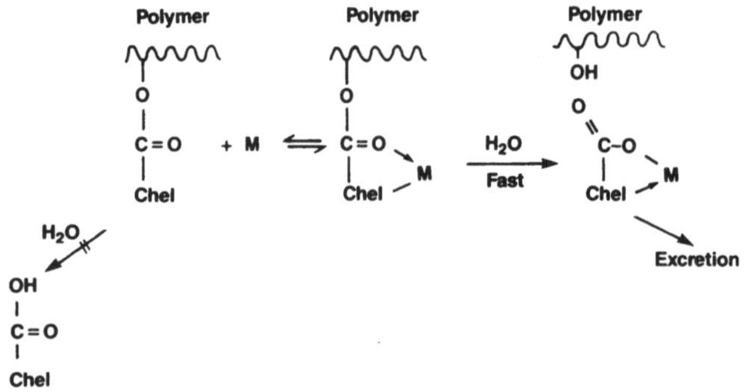

Figure 1. Self-regulated delivery of metal chelating agents.

We have been interested in the feasibility of designing polymer-chelator conjugates from which release of the chelator is reversibly triggered by the appearance of the target (toxic) metal in the circulatory system, occurs at a rate which is directly proportional to the metal concentration, and is sustained over a long period of time.[6] The potential advantages of such a system include both reduced toxicity and increased efficiency. The basis of the method, summarized in Figure 1, is the long known observation that when carboxylate and phosphate esters and amides are incorporated into, or are proximate to a chelating site, their hydrolysis can be accelerated by metals by factors of 10^6 or greater.[7] A decrease in the half-life of hydrolysis from months to minutes may be achieved in the presence of metals at physiological pH. The application of this approach to chelation therapy depends on the ability to achieve the same magnitude of rate enhancement in a polymeric environment, where diffusion or steric hindrance of the chelating site can become rate limiting. To establish feasibility, we have studied the synthesis and rates of metal-catalyzed hydrolysis of the ester of poly(vinyl alcohol) and quinaldic acid (PVA-QA), which is structurally related to 8-hydroxy-quinoline (Figure 2).

EXPERIMENTAL

Coupling of quinaldic acid and poly(vinyl alcohol)

8-Acetoxyquinoline-2-carboxylic acid[8] (1.2 g, 5.2 mmol), benzotriazole (0.62 g, 5.2 mmol), and DCC (1.07 g, 5.2 mmol) in dry THF (8 mL) were stirred at 0°C (2h), then 25°C (1h). After filtration and concentration, the residual solid (1.79 g), PVA (MW = 25000; 88% hydrolyzed; 1.02 g, 20.8 mmol) and triethylamine (0.61 g) in DMSO (17 mL) were heated at 60°C for 48 hr. under nitrogen. The product was precipitated by pouring onto ice water, filtered, and washed with acetonitrile. Yield 1.35 g. Unchanged QA and other low molecular weight species were removed by precipitation from DMF with acetonitrile, then dialysis in 50% aq. ethanol using an Amicon YM10 membrane (10,000 cutoff). The QA incorporation was determined to be 5 mole-% by comparison of the UV absorbance at 258 nm with a calibration curve derived from standard solutions of QA in 50% aq. ethanol; this result was verified qualitatively by ^{1}H-NMR spectroscopy. A satisfactory elemental analysis was not obtained. Analysis calculated for 5 mole-% QA in PVA: C, 61.4; H, 6.39; N, 3.58. Found: C, 55.27; H, 6.87; N, 1.63. Films of the polymer were solution cast from DMF.

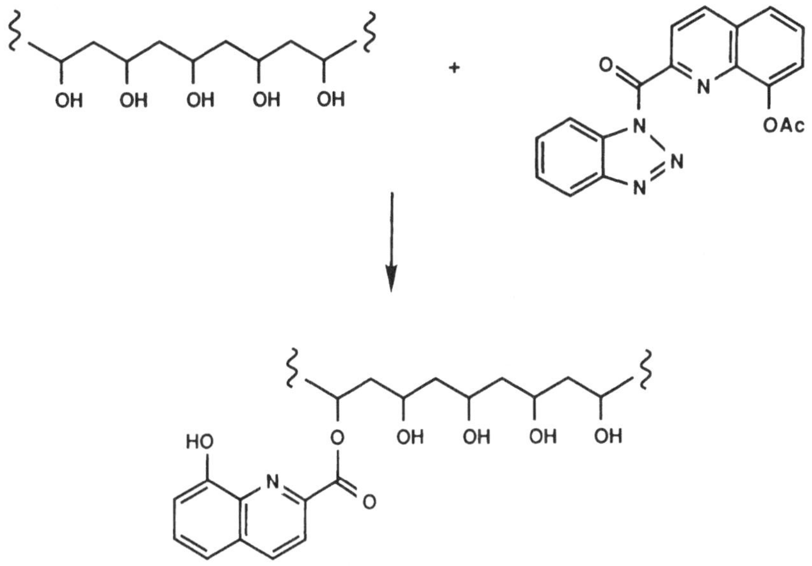

Figure 2. Synthesis of the ester of poly(vinyl alcohol) and quinaldic acid.

Rates of hydrolysis were determined spectrophotometrically at 37.5°C using a Beckman DU-2 instrument. An aliquot of a standard solution of the metal salt was added to 3 mL of a 0.5 x 10⁻⁴ molar solution of PVA-QA in 50% aq. ethanol buffered with 0.05M HEPES at pH 7.5 in a standard cuvette, and the change in absorbance as a function of the time was measured for at least 3 half-lives at the following wavelengths: Ni(II) acetate 287 nm. Co(II) acetate 277 nm, Cu(II) nitrate 286 nm, Zn(II) sulfate 280 nm. The rates of hydrolysis of PVA-QA films were measured at 37.5°C in water buffered with 0.05M HEPES at pH 7.5. The rate constants were derived from the kinetic data by the method of Swain et al.[9] or by a non-linear least square curve fitting program capable of deconvoluting consecutive and simultaneous first order processes.[10]

RESULTS AND DISCUSSION

PVA-QA was insoluble in water and ethanol but soluble in mixtures of the two solvents. Therefore, the solution kinetics were determined in 50% aq. ethanol buffered at pH 7.5 with HEPES. It has been demonstrated that this buffer does not bind to the metals studied, or modify the kinetics of metal-promoted hydrolysis.[11]

By analogy with the behavior of low molecular weight amino acid esters, the metal-promoted hydrolytic cleavage of PVA-QA may be described as a two-step process (Equation 1). The equilibrium formation of the intermediate polymeric metal complex, PVA-QA-M is followed by hydroxide ion cleavage of the ester bond and liberation of the free metal chelate. At constant pH and [M]>>[Ester], and provided steady-state conditions apply to the intermediate, the kinetics of formation of the product are first-order and the observed rate constant is given by Equation 5.[12] If the intermediate PVA-QA-M is not fully formed under the reaction conditions, both Equations 5 and 6 require that a plot of $1/k_{obs}$ versus $1/[M]$ be linear with an intercept of $1/k_3$.

$$PVA \cdot QA + M \underset{k_2}{\overset{k_1}{\rightleftharpoons}} PVA \cdot QA \cdot M \xrightarrow{k_3} PVA + QA \cdot M \qquad \text{(Equation 1)}$$

$$k_1/k_2 = [PVA \cdot QA \cdot M]/[M][PVA \cdot QA] \qquad \text{(Equation 2)}$$

$$-d[PVA \cdot QA \cdot M]/dt = k_3[PVA \cdot QA \cdot M][OH] \qquad \text{(Equation 3)}$$

$$-d[PVA \cdot QA \cdot M]/dt = k_3 k_1/k_2 [M][PVA \cdot QA][OH] \qquad \text{(Equation 4)}$$

Then integrating,[12]

$$k_{obs} = k_1 \cdot k_3 \cdot [M]/(k_1 \cdot [M] + k_2 + k_3) \qquad \text{(Equation 5)}$$

If $k_2 \gg k_3$:

$$k_{obs} = k_1 \cdot k_3 [M[/(k_1[M] + k_2) \qquad \text{(Equation 6)}$$

The hydrolysis of PVA-QA was measured in the presence of four metals, Co(II), Zn(II), Cu(II), and Ni(II). The first order rate constants (k_{obs}) observed in the presence of a 5:1 or greater excess of each metal are listed in Table I. The rate of hydrolysis at pH 7.5 in the absence of metals was not measurable. The kinetics of hydrolysis in the presence of a 4:1 ratio of Cu(II) was biphasic, consisting of two simultaneous first order processes. The contribution of the faster component diminished as the Cu(II):PVA-QA ratio was decreased to 1:1. A single first order process was observed in the presence of Ni(II), Co(II), and Zn(II). A double reciprocal plot of k^{-1}_{obs} vs. $[M]^{-1}$ for Ni(II) exhibited the expected linearity. Utilizing Equation 6, the value of k_3 derived from the intercept of this plot was 0.013 min^{-1}. Similar but less reproducible results were obtained for Co(II)-promoted hydrolysis. Precipitation of Zn(OH)$_2$ prevented the use of this metal above a concentration of 1.7×10^{-4} M, and a maximum zinc(II):chelator ratio of 7:1.

Comparison of k_{obs} for PVA-QA with the rate constants reported for metal promoted hydrolysis of methyl quinaldate (Table 1) shows the latter is more rapid and the difference between metals is greater.[11] The difference in the solvent (water vs. 50% aq. ethanol) and the ester alkyl groups does not allow any conclusions about the contribution of the polymeric environment to the kinetics.

Table 1. Equilibrium and first order reaction constants of metal complexes of methyl quinaldate and PVA-QA.

Metal	Methyl Quinaldate		PVA-QA	
	log K_{eq}	k_3 (min^{-1})	k_{obs} (min^{-1})	$t_{1/2}$ (min)
Cu(II)	>8.3	12.0	0.015	67
Ni(II)	5.7	0.19	0.014	71
Co(II)	5.5	0.21	0.0058	172
Zn(II)	6.6	0.049	0.0021	476

Film Hydrolysis

The complete kinetic expression for the metal-promoted hydrolysis of PVA-QA in the solid state requires the inclusion of terms for the rates of diffusion of the metal ion into the film and diffusion of the cleaved metal chelate out of the film into external buffer. The limited case of metal influx coupled to hydrolysis may be solved by assuming the diffusion is Fickian and the reaction rate is proportional to the average concentration of the metal in the film.[13] Then, combining the kinetic expression for sorption from a fixed volume by a film with that of metal promoted hydrolysis, and integrating, leads to Equation 7, which is only valid if the rate of egress of the metal-chelate is rapid relative to its formation.[14]

$$[M \cdot QA]_t / [M \cdot QA]_\infty = 1 - \exp\{-k(t + \sum_{n=0}^{n=\infty} 8(2n+1)^{-4}(C\pi^2)^{-1}\{\exp(-(2n+1)^2 Ct)-1\})\}$$

(Equation 7)

Where:

k = pseudo 1st order rate constant, $k_3[M]_\infty[OH]$

$C = \pi^2 D/l$, where D is the diffusion coefficient and l is the half film thickness.

Evidence of the minor role of diffusion was provided by the rate of hydrolysis of PVA-QA films after addition of 20×10^{-4} M nickel(II) acetate. The rate of appearance of the hydrolyzed metal chelate in the aqueous buffer conformed to the kinetics predicted by Equation 7 but was not greatly different when the diffusion terms were neglected (Figure 3).

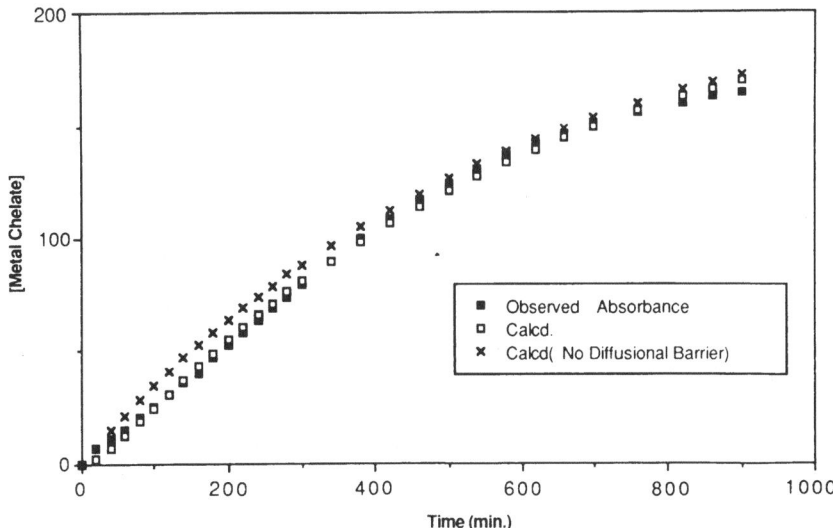

Figure 3. Comparison of the observed rate of formation of the nickel(II) chelate of quinaldic acid from a film of PVA-QA with the rate calculated from Equation 7 with and without a diffusional barrier.

It was evident from these preliminary results that the rate of hydrolysis was sufficiently great in the solid state for practical applications of these and other polymer-bound chelators.

ACKNOWLEDGMENT

Scholarships to Z-W. Gu and J-H. Zhu by the World Health Organization are gratefully acknowledged.

REFERENCES

1. A. Catsch & A. E. Marmuth-Hoene, "*The Chelation of Heavy Metals*", W. G. Levine, Ed., Pergamon Press, Oxford, 1979, p 107-224.
2. A. E. Martell, Ed., "*Inorganic Chemistry in Biology and Medicine*", ACS Symposium Series, No. 140, American Chemical Society, Washington, DC, 1980.
3. C. G. Pitt & A. E. Martell in: "*Inorganic Chemistry in Biology and Medicine*", A. E. Martell, Ed., ACS Symposium Series, No 140, Washington, DC, 1980, p. 279-312.
4. G. Peters, H. Keberle, K. Schmid & H. Brunner, Biochem. Pharm., **15**, 93 (1966).
5. R. D. Propper & N. G. Nathan in: "*Chronic Iron Overload*", E. C. Zaino & R. H. Roberts, Eds., Stratton Int. Medical Book Corporation, New York, 1977, p 17-36.
6. C. G. Pitt, Z-W. Gu, R. W. Hendren, J. Thompson & M. C. Wani, J. Controlled Release, **2**, 363 (1985).
7. D. A. Buckingham in: "*Biological Aspects of Inorganic Chemistry*", A. W. Addison, W. R. Cullen, D. Dolphin & B. R. James, Eds., Wiley-Interscience, New York, 1976, p. 141-196.
8. R. W. Hay and C. R. Clark, J. Chem. Soc., **1977**, 1993.
9. C. G. Swain, M. S. Swain & L. F. Berg, J. Chem. Inf. Comput Sci., **20**, 47 (1980).
10. D. W. Marquard, J. Soc. Ind. Appl. Math., **11**, 431 (1963): IBM Share Program No. 3094.
11. R. W. Hay & C. R. Clark, J. Chem. Soc., **1977**, 1866.
12. S. Strickland, G. Palmer & V. Massey, J. Biol. Chem., **250**, 4048 (1975).
13. C. E. Reese & H. Eyring. Textile Res. J., **20**, 743 (1950).
14. C. Crank, "*The Mathematics of Diffusion*", Oxford University Press, Oxford, 1956, p 42-61.

FORMATION OF POLYMERIC ANTIMICROBIAL SURFACES FROM ORGANOFUNCTIONAL SILANES

R. L. Gettings & W. C. White

Dow Corning Corp.
2200 West Salzburg Road
Midland, MI 48686-0994

Organofunctional reactive silanes offer unique monomers for the formation of bioactive polymers. This paper discusses the ability of 3-(trimethoxysilyl)-propyloctadecyldimethyl ammonium chloride to polymerize on a wide variety of surfaces and for these surfaces to be active against a broad spectrum of microorganisms. These silane modified surfaces have led to a broad array of use applications ranging from the control of microorganisms that cause odor, discoloration and deterioration, to aiding in the control of microorganisms associated with nosocomial infections and allergies. This unique technology has presented a new dimension in antimicrobial compounds and the test methodologies used for their evaluation.

INTRODUCTION

During the late 1960s, Dow Corning began a screening project to identify silicone and silane chemicals which exhibited antimicrobial activity against a broad spectrum of microorganisms. As particular chemistries were being evaluated in the culture vessels, unexplainable problems were encountered in that some of the vessels, subsequently continued to kill microbial cells. Investigation of these phenomena revealed a unique polymerization of a silane-quaternary compound on the solid surface which continued to exhibit antimicrobial activity.

CHEMISTRY

Researchers discovered that antimicrobial organofunctional silanes could be chemically bound to receptive substrates by what were believed to be Si-O linkages. The method was described as orienting the organofunctional silane in such a way that hydrolyzable groups on the silicon atom were hydrolyzed to the silanols and formed chemical bonds with each other and to the substrate. The resultant surface modification, when an antimicrobial moiety such as a quaternary nitrogen was included, provided for the antimicrobial group to be oriented away from the surface.[1]

The attachment of this monomer to the surface appears to involve two processes. First, and most important, is a very rapid process which coats

91

the substrate with the cationic species one molecule deep (physico-adsorption). This is an ion exchange process by which the cation of the silane quaternary ammonium compound replaces protons from the water on the surface. It has long been known that most surfaces in contact with water generate negative electrical charges at the interface between water and the surface. It is also well known that all surfaces have some form of water on their surfaces, the so-called Stern Layer. This mechanism is further supported by data generated with a radioactive silane quaternary ammonium compound. During this treatment, depletion of the radioactivity from solution was almost immediate by the amount corresponding to that sufficient to cover the surface one layer deep, even on surfaces which contain no reactive functionality.[2] Similar results are published for many organic quaternary ammonium compounds.[3] The second process is unique to materials, such as silane quaternary ammonium compounds which have methoxyfunctional silane functionality, enabling them to homopolymerize, after they have coated the surface, to become almost unremovable, even from surfaces on which they cannot react. On those surfaces where the methoxyfunctional silane functionality can react, covalent bonding to that surface will also occur (chemi-adsorption) and it is also possible to have intermolecular polymerization.[2]

This complex polymer, silane monomers polymerized onto a surface and homopolymerized, provides a most unique polymeric coating. The number and types of monomers that have utility in this process vary from hydroxyl-functional, acid-functional and ester-functional to organic and inorganic materials.[4] Although most of the historical work on this class of unique materials has been done with simple organo-functional silane monomers, recent work on emulsions has expanded our view of these polymerizable materials. Work by Blehm, Malek and White has shown that a large variety of organofunctional silanes are capable of acting as emulsifiers to make water in oil and oil in water emulsions. These emulsions, when exposed to surfaces, react as if they are "monomers". In effect, they treat surfaces, show the same durability profiles and manifest the same antimicrobial properties as the monomer treatment. The nature of these reactions and associations have not yet been fully characterized, but the probability of oligomer formation at the emulsion interface can be predicted.[5]

APPLICATIONS

The value of these silane polymers is only just beginning to be realized. Our work has focused on the antimicrobial properties of certain of these materials and includes a variety of delivery techniques to substrates where bioactive polymers satisfy industrial, commercial and consumer needs.

Degradation, defacement, odors, and health related problems can all be caused by microbes. Bacteria, fungi and algae all have the ability to impact humans, their dwellings, their food sources, their clothing and, in general, their well being negatively. Antimicrobial polymers based on 3-(trimethoxysilyl)-propyldimethyloctadecyl ammonium chloride have been effective at dealing with many of these problems.

In 1976, Dow Corning received EPA registration for the use of the immobilized antimicrobial on socks. This opened the door to the broad base of uses on both woven[6] and nonwoven[7] textiles, as well as carpeting.[8,9] More recently, this technology has been used as an *in situ* additive for urethane foam. In this use the antimicrobial serves to protect a wide variety of stabilized foams from the negative effects of microorganisms.[10] All of these applications take advantage of the safety and durability of the polymerized form of the 3-(trimethoxysilyl)-propylocta-decyldimethyl ammonium chloride.

In another recent development, an EPA registration has been received for the SYLGARD[R] Antimicrobial Treatment [3-(trimethoxysilyl)-propylocta-decyldimethyl ammonium chloride] to be used by commercial applicators as an aftercare treatment to carpeting and basement walls.[11-13] Expansion of this use to other surfaces will allow us to address some major building environmental concerns such as the microbial influences associated with the "sick building syndrome".

Uses of the SYLGARD[R] Treatment and other types of antimicrobial poly-mers are limited only by our imaginations. The opportunity to devise unique delivery techniques for durable or nondurable, safe and effective bioactive agents is just beginning to unfold.

Silane surface active antimicrobial polymers offer unique advantages not available with the slow release types of polymer systems. The SYL-GARD[R] Treatment is antimicrobial without degradation of the surface treating polymer. Slow release antimicrobials are based on trapping the active agent in a polymer matrix so that the rates of release are appro-priate for the end use. This bursting release of a "filled" matrix con-stantly erodes the characteristics of the polymer. As fillers are lost from the polymers, properties, such as tensile strength, elongation, rebound, gloss, etc., are altered. The reservoir concept for long term use of antimicrobials must be approached very carefully. In a similar manner, slow release mechanisms based on pH, hydrolysis, UV, or other energy caused bond cleavages, can do considerable damage to the base polymer and to the properties of the polymer treated surface. These approaches still have considerable utility when their effects on the treated surfaces are of little or no consequence.

EVALUATION OF ANTIMICROBIAL SURFACES

In order to demonstrate antimicrobial activity it is absolutely necessary to initiate contact between the microbial cell and the anti-microbial compound. For decades traditionally known antimicrobial com-pounds, and substrates treated with them, have been subjected to classi-cal microbiological test techniques such as the determination of the minimum inhibitory concentration (MIC) or the zone of inhibition. MIC tests determine, in solution, the minimum concentration of a chemical that will inhibit the growth of a particular microorganism. In solution, the silane-quat is a very dynamic polymer which is constantly bonding with and detaching from itself and any reactive surface available. Con-sequently, data generated in solution tests are variable and virtually impossible to extrapolate to the real world. The most popular test for determining the antimicrobial activity associated with a treated sub-strate is the zone of inhibition. A measureable zone indicates that the antimicrobial is not durable on the substrate. A substrate treated with the silane-quat will not show a zone of inhibition due to the durable polymeric surface that has been created. This immobilized polymeric anti-microbial surface has led to the development of new and novel tests to demonstrate the interruption of microbial growth or life functions.

Surfaces treated with such a polymer-bound antimicrobial have to be mobile or there has to be a dynamic presentation of the microorganisms to the test surface. Uniform distribution of the microbial cells is also necessary to allow intimate contact with the treated surface for inacti-vation of the cells. These criteria have been built into the dynamic shake flask test used as a quality assurance test to determine if a surface treated with the silane-quat is bioactive. A standard weight of the treated substrate is shaken for a specified time interval in a prescribed volume of phosphate buffer which has been inoculated with bacteria. Comparison of the bacterial counts before and after shaking yields the percent reduction achieved by the surface treatment. Because the shake flask test only provides data in a state of dynamic solution movement, it may or may not provide insights into the antimicrobial activity of various end-use situations.

This can be exemplified very well for a carpet fiber. Carpeting as a substrate provides a habitat for a large variety of microorganisms, some of which may produce putrid or mildew odors and may contribute to unsightly defacement and deterioration of the carpet components. Carpet fiber treated with the silane-quat, when tested in the shake flask test, will exhibit 95-100% reduction of microorganisms as compared to the untreated control. In order to gain further knowledge/data representing the real world, treated and untreated carpet were subjected to a second level of tests. By spraying the carpet with fungal spores and incubating under high humidity conditions, the treated carpet can be evaluated for its resistance to fungal attack which may cause odor, defacement and deterioration. Parallel to this test, treated and untreated carpet can be carefully inoculated with bacterial populations according to AATCC Method 100 and evaluated for its inhibition of bacterial growth or the production of foul odors generated during the metabolism of nutrients.[14] Each of these tests provides a small piece of the overall informational picture needed for a complete evaluation of the benefits of treating the substrate with the antimicrobial agent.

REGULATORY CONCERNS

No paper including antimicrobials would be complete without some discussion of the regulatory realities of antimicrobials. Whether a sanitizer, a paint film preservative, a wood preservative, or a fabric protectant, all antimicrobials are pesticides and, therefore, regulated by the Environmental Protection Agency (EPA) under the provisions of the Federal Insecticide, Fungicide, Rodenticide Act (FIFRA), as amended, and the Federal Environmental Pollution Control Act (FEPCA). Under these two laws the EPA has promulgated a large number of provisions and regulations which must be met before a pesticide can be sold in commerce. Although the use of polymerics as delivery mechanisms for pesticides seems attractive, this tactic is a new approach to the EPA and considerable scutiny can be expected.

CONCLUSION

The ability to create essentially irreversible polymeric coatings of cationic silanes on surfaces and the ability of these modified surfaces to kill and/or control microorganisms has been demonstrated in laboratory and real world situations. A large number of microbological techniques have been found useful in determining the antimicrobial activity of a wide variety of surfaces with polymeric antimicrobials. This has provided considerable insight into the mode of antimicrobial action of these compounds.

ACKNOWLEDGEMENT

The authors wish to acknowledge and thank Jane Oberhellman for the preparation of this document.

REFERENCES

1. P. A. Walters, E. A. Abbott & A. J. Isquith, Applied Microbiology, 25, 253 (1973).
2. J. R. Malek & J. L. Speier, J. Coated Fabrics, 12, 38 (1982).
3. G. Domagk, Dent. Med. Wochn., 161, 829 (1935).
4. C. Roth, Can. Patent No. 2,010,782 (May 24, 1977).
5. L. M. Blehm, J. R. Malek & W. C. White, U. S. Patent No. 4,631,273 (December 24, 1986).
6. R. L. Gettings & B. L. Triplett, AATCC Book of Papers, AATCC National Technical Conference, 259, 1978.
7. S. F. Hayes & W. C. White, Amer. Dyestuff Reporter, 36, June, 1984.
8. J. B. McGee, J. R. Malek & W. C. White, Amer. Dyestuff Reporter, 24, June, 1983.
9. W. C. White & J. B. McGee, "*SYLGARD Antimicrobial Treatment for Carpets: Effectiveness and Durability in Field and Laboratory Testing*", Dow Corning Corp., Midland, MI, Form No. 24-181-85.
10. D. R. Battice & M. G. Hales, Proc. 30th Annual Technical/Marketing Conf. for the Society of the Plastics Industry, 332, October, 1986.
11. M. G. Hales, M. E. Sorkin & W. C. White, Cleaning & Restoration, 14, March, 1986.
12. M. G. Hales, M. E. Sorkin & W. C. White, Cleaning & Restoration, 13, April, 1986.
13. M. G. Hales, M. E. Sorkin & W. C. White, Cleaning & Restoration, 18, May, 1986.
14. "*Technical Manual*", American Association of Textile Chemists and Colorists, P. O. Box 12215, Research Triangle Park, NC.

DEVELOPMENT OF POLYMERS WITH ANTI-INFECTIOUS PROPERTIES

B. Jansen, G. Peters, S. Schareina, H. Steinhauser*,
F. Schumacher-Perdreau, and G. Pulverer

Hygiene-Institute
University of Cologne
Goldenfelsstr. 19 - 21
D-5000 Cologne 41, FRG

*Institute of Physical Chemistry
University of Cologne
Luxemburger Str. 116
D-5000 Cologne 41, FRG

The significance of foreign-body infections caused by bacteria is discussed. The aspects of bacterial adhesion to polymeric materials, which is regarded as a first important step in the development of foreign-body infections, are discussed. With this background, possible strategies for the prevention of bacterial adhesion to polymers are presented. Hydrophilic surface modification of polymers, performed by radiation-grafting or glow discharge treatment, reduces the number of bacterial cells *in vitro*. The possibility of surface modification for the selective adsorption of blood proteins and its effect on bacterial adhesion is considered. As another approach, attachment or incorporation of antibiotic drugs onto or into polymers, with the aim to prevent adhesion or to kill adhered bacteria, is presented. Preliminary experiments with antibiotic-loaded polymers show that the released drugs still possess their activity. A reduction of bacterial adhesion is observed for polymers into which the antibiotic was incorporated.

INTRODUCTION

Polymeric materials are frequently used in the diagnostic and therapeutic procedures of modern medicine. Their use as prostheses and different kinds of catheters has rapidly increased. This has led to medical progress for the benefit of many patients. On the other hand, special complications associated with the foreign-body materials have occurred. One of the most frequent complications, which is now considered as a major problem in prosthetic medicine, is the infection of the materials.[1] These foreign-body-associated infections are clinical routine phenomena, although the consequences for the individual patient may be very severe, e. g. development of septicemia and the necessity for the removal of the

97

prosthetic material. Various kinds of bacteria, but also fungi, can be found as etiological agents for foreign-body infections. In the majority of the cases staphylococci are the most frequently isolated bacteria. Other bacteria isolated from infected materials are *Pseudomonas*, non-fermenting gram-negative rods, *Enterobacteriaceae* and fungi of the Candida group.

One can find differences in the incidence of microorganisms due to the various types of prostheses and catheters . In infections of liquor shunt systems,[2-4] intravascular catheters,[5-8] catheters for continuous ambulant peritoneal dialysis,[9,10] and heart valves,[11-13] coagulase-negative staphylococci are by far the most frequently isolated bacteria. They are also predominantly responsible for "late-onset" infections of trans-venous endocardial pacemaker electrodes[14,15] and joint prostheses.[16] *S. aureus* is the most important causative agent in hemodialysis shunt and vascular prostheses infections,[17] but is also found in "early-onset" infections of joint prostheses[16] and pacemaker electrodes.[14] *Enterobacteriaceae* (*E. coli*) are nearly exclusively found in "early-onset" infections associated with urinary catheters, whereas in "late-onset" infections *Pseudomonas aeruginosa* dominates.[18] From the clinical point of view foreign-body infections can be characterized according to their onset and to their clinical course. "Early-onset" infections occur within days or weeks after surgery or catheterization. In those cases the inoculation of the pathogen takes place during surgery or insertion of the catheter with the skin of the patient or the surgeon as common source.[19] "Late-onset" infections start after a much longer interval of several weeks or months.[14] The inoculation of the pathogen may also happen at the time of surgery or during a septicemia of other origin or during a clinically inapparent bacteremia.

While foreign-body infections caused by e.g. *S. aureus* or *Enterobacteriaceae* show a more or less dramatical clinical course, infections with coagulase-negative staphylococci appear less dramatical, and sometimes marked clinical symptoms are missing. The long-lasting nature of the infection is a further characteristic, especially if the infected device is not removed. In most cases antimicrobial therapy alone cannot cure the infection and the removal of the infected device becomes necessary. Depending on the kind of infected device, this can be a very threatening situation for the patient, e.g. the case of removal of an infected prosthetic heart valve. It is a special clinical phenomenon of these "chronic" foreign-body infections that the host is not able to overcome this type of opportunistic infection despite a normal immune system and the low virulence of bacteria involved.[20,21] The same is true for the failure of chemotherapy, despite the use of substances with proven high *in vitro* activity.

There is evidence from many investigations that bacterial adhesion to biomaterials (mainly synthetic polymers) is the first step in the pathogenesis of foreign-body infections. Subsequent colonization and production of extracellular substances ("slime") lead to the formation of a compact matrix on the polymer surface capable of protecting the embedded bacteria against antibiotics and host defense mechanisms (Figure 1). Therefore, bacterial adhesion to polymers has been the subject of numerous investigations. Most of the studies have been performed on the adhesion of coagulase-negative staphylococci as the predominantly causative organisms.

Recently, an extensive review on bacterial adhesion to biomedical polymers has been given by Dankert,et al., summarizing most of the important work done in this field.[22] It was concluded by these authors that,

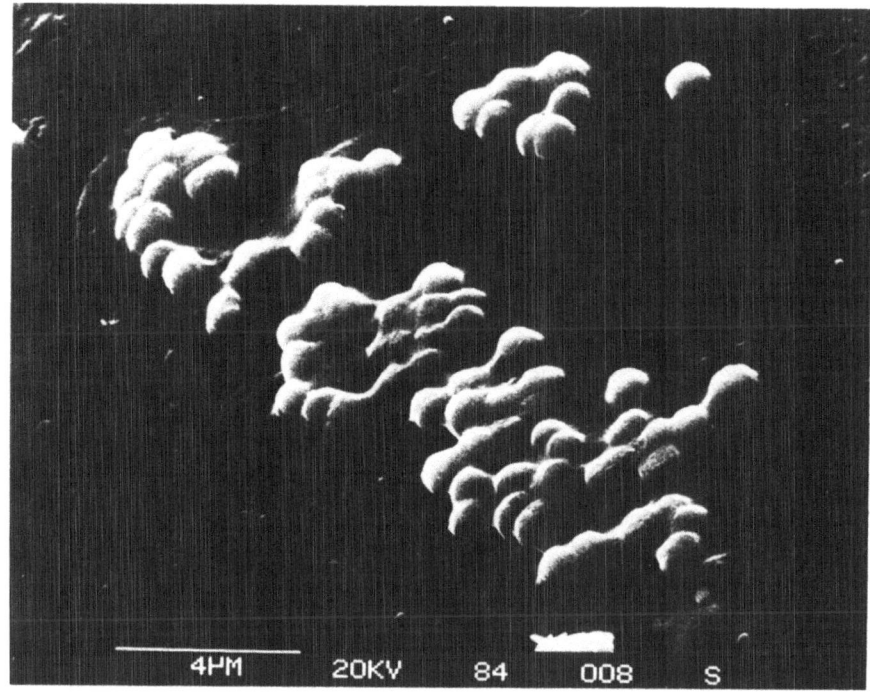

Figure 1. Adhering microcolonies of *S. epidermidis* on a
polyethylene catheter after 6 - 12 hr. incubation
in bacterial solution in PBS. A thin slime layer
covers the adhered cells.

despite numerous studies, the mechanisms of bacterial adhesion to polymers are not understood.

While the *in vitro* adhesion can partly be described by theoretical
models, the *in vivo* situation may be completely different. Both, polymers
and bacteria, undergo changes in the dynamic environment of the living
organism, e.g. by protein adsorption to their surfaces, and this may
affect the adhesion process. It is very likely that under *in vivo* conditions specific interactions between bacterial structures and the polymer
may overrule the non-specific forces which regulate the adhesion *in
vitro*.

Figure 2 shows a summary of the factors which influence the bacterial
adhesion process. In the following we will discuss the principles of
bacterial adhesion to polymers focusing on coagulase-negative staphylococci and biomedical polymers. The knowledge of the basic adhesion
mechanisms is necessary for the development of possible strategies for
the prevention of foreign-body infections other than the classical way of
using antibiotic therapy.

MECHANISMS OF BACTERIAL ADHESION TO POLYMERS

Physico-chemically the bacterial adhesion to a polymer can be regarded as the adhesion of a colloid particle to a solid surface in a liquid
environment. Besides the hydrodynamic conditions of the liquid medium
which regulate the transport of the particle to the surface, the adhesion
is governed by attractive or repulsive forces including electrostatic,
van der Waals, dipole-dipole and hydrophobic interactions.[23] Provided

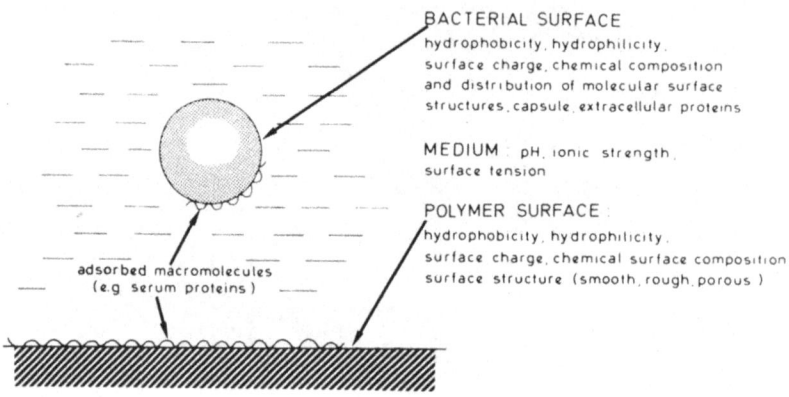

BACTERIAL SURFACE
hydrophobicity, hydrophilicity,
surface charge, chemical composition
and distribution of molecular surface
structures, capsule, extracellular proteins

MEDIUM : pH, ionic strength,
surface tension

POLYMER SURFACE :
hydrophobicity, hydrophilicity,
surface charge, chemical surface composition,
surface structure (smooth, rough, porous)

adsorbed macromolecules
(e.g serum proteins)

Figure 2. Factors influencing the adhesion of bacteria to polymers.

only van der Waals and electrostatic interactions are present, the DLVO-theory of lyophobic colloid stabilization can be applied to the adhesion process.[24,25] If a negatively charged bacterial cell approaches an also negatively charged surface (e.g. a mammalian cell), the adhesion is a balance between van der Waals attraction and electrostatic repulsion. Depending on the electrolyte concentration of the liquid medium, a secondary and a primary minimum in total energy is observed, at which interactions between bacteria and surface can take place (Figure 3). The DLVO-theory is useful for a qualitative description of bacterial adhesion to polymers *in vitro*. Quantitative calculations are difficult due to the problems in obtaining the necessary parameters in practice.[23,26] For the description of the *in vivo* adhesion the DLVO model is not suitable because other interactions may occur in addition to those considered in the DLVO theory.

Another model for the adhesion of cells to solid surfaces was developed by Neumann and Absolom, et al. and is based upon thermodynamical

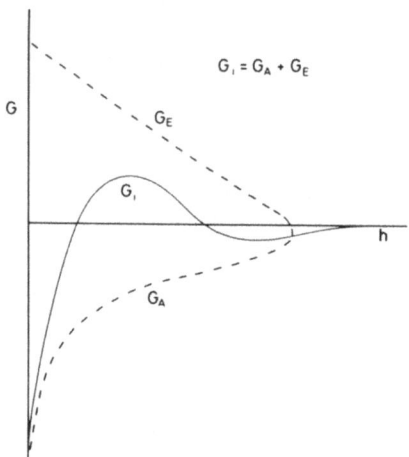

Figure 3. Interaction free energy, G, plotted against distance, h, from the surface in the case of a negatively charged particle approaching a negatively charged surface at medium electrolyte concentration (developed from the DLVO theory).

considerations.[27,28] If electrostatic interactions are neglected, adhesion is controlled by a change in the free energy of adhesion, ΔF_{adh}, and depends on the interfacial tension between solid and bacteria, γ_{SB}, solid and liquid medium, γ_{SL}, and bacteria and liquid medium, γ_{BL}.

$$\Delta F_{adh} = \gamma_{SB} - \gamma_{SL} - \gamma_{BL} \qquad \text{(Equation 1)}$$

The adhesion is thermodynamically favored if ΔF_{adh} becomes negative. Absolom, et al.,[28] distinguished three cases which depend on the magnitudes of bacterial and liquid surface tension:

(1) $\gamma_{LV} > \gamma_{BV}$ ΔF_{adh} increases with increasing γ_{SV}; adhesion decreases with increasing γ_{SV} of the solid substrate.

(2) $\gamma_{LV} < \gamma_{BV}$ adhesion decreases with decreasing γ_{SV} of the substrate.

(3) $\gamma_{LV} = \gamma_{BV}$ adhesion should be independent of the surface tension of the substrate.

The thermodynamic model is, like the DLVO theory, only applicable for the adhesion *in vitro*. Both models are based upon non-specific interactions occurring between particles (cells) and solid surfaces. *In vivo*, or under *in vivo* like conditions, specific interactions also have to be taken into account. Such specific interactions have been shown to mediate adhesion between bacteria and natural substrata, such as adhesion of streptococci to dental enamel,[29] γ adhesion of *E. coli* to uroepithelial cells.[30] Although not clearly demonstrated for the bacterial adhesion to synthetic polymers, it is highly possible that specific interactions, e.g. between bacterial surface proteins and protein layers adsorbed on the polymer surface, play an important role as well.

In most of the *in vitro* studies which were performed in saline or other nutrient- or protein-free media, it was demonstrated that the adhesion is mainly governed by electrostatic and hydrophobic interactions.[31-34] In a previous work we investigated the adhesion of several *S. epidermidis* strains with varying surface properties onto several basic polymers used for medical implants and devices.[35,36] We found that in general the more hydrophobic strains adhered better to the polymers. If the surface free energy (surface tension) γ_{SV} of the polymers was plotted against the number of adhered bacteria, a decrease in adhesion was observed for hydrophobic strains with increasing γ_{SV} of the polymers (Figure 4). This is in accordance with the thermodynamical model of Absolom, et al.[28] for the case in which $\gamma_{LV} > \gamma_{BV}$ (see above). If the polar contribution γ_{PS} to the surface free energy of the polymer was plotted against the bacterial number, a clear correlation was found such that adhesion was reduced with increasing γ_{PS}. The increase in surface hydrophilicity of the polymers obviously leads to a weakening of hydrophobic interactions between bacteria and polymer.

In a more recent study on adhesion of two different *S. epidermidis* strains (KH 6 and KH 11) onto polyetherurethanes, the importance of hydrophobic interactions was confirmed: the more hydrophobic strain KH 6 adheres stronger to the polyetherurethanes BIOMER[R] and TUFTANE[R] which have quite similar surface free energies.[37] Similar results, stressing the role of hydrophobic bonding in *in vitro* adhesion, were found by other

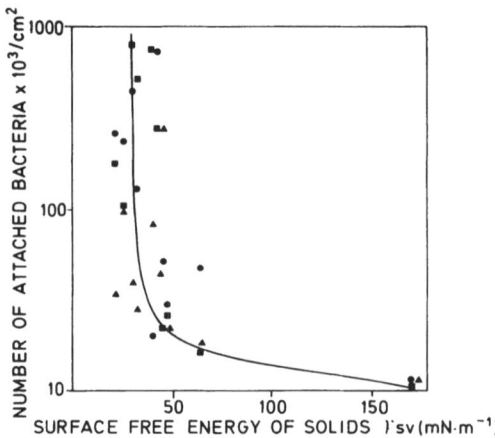

Figure 4. Influence of the polymer surface free energy γ_{SV} on the adhesion of hydrophobic *S. epidermidis* strains to various polymers.

investigators, especially by Hogt, et al. in earlier studies on adhesion of *S. epidermidis* onto fluorinated polyethylene (FEP) and cellulose acetate.[31]

The influence of polymer surface charge onto bacterial adhesion was also studied by Hogt, et al.[38] They investigated the adhesion of coagulase-negative staphylococci to methacrylate/2-hydroxyethylmethacrylate copolymers and methyl methacrylate copolymers with positive or negative charges.

Adhesion was highest on positively charged copolymers, intermediate on negatively charged copolymers and lowest on copolymers with a high surface hydrophilicity. We could show that the *in vitro* adhesion of *S. epidermidis* to a negatively charged surface (polyvinylfluoride grafted with acrylic acid) was strongly reduced, which is likely due to a repulsion effect between the two negatively charged surfaces.[35]

If polymers come into contact with body fluids (blood, tissue fluid), they are rapidly coated with proteins or other substances.[39] Bacteria also become coated by substances from body fluids and undergo changes in their surface properties. In both cases the surface properties can be markedly altered in comparison with the original state. A number of studies has been done on the influence of adsorbed macromolecules on the adhesion, mainly using plasma, serum or proteins.[40-44] In almost all studies, it was found that the presence of serum or plasma leads to a strong decrease in bacterial adhesion. Fletcher, et al. found a relationship between the increase in surface hydrophilicity of polystyrene surfaces due to protein adsorption and the decrease in adhesion of *Pseudomonas spp.*.[42] It was assumed by these authors that the decreased adhesion is caused by a change in surface properties from hydrophobic to hydrophilic as measured by the water contact angle. In our studies on the adhesion of *S. epidermidis* onto polyetherurethanes, we also found a decrease in adhesion in the presence of 10% serum or plasma.[45] Contact angle measurements and xylene tests with serum treated polyurethanes and bacteria revealed that the surface properties of both, polymer and bacteria, had become more hydrophilic. Thus it can be speculated that the decrease in adhesion is due to a decrease of hydrophobic interactions. However, if the precoating of the polymers is done with single serum proteins (albumin, fibrinogen or IgG), in the case of one particular strain (KH 11), we found a decrease only after precoating with albumin, whereas on fibrinogen-coated polyurethane an increase in adhesion was noticed.[45] This enhancement of adhesion suggests specific interactions between *S. epidermidis* KH 11 and the polymer-adsorbed fibrinogen molecule.

From the literature, little is known about specific interactions in bacterial adhesion to polymers. In the adhesion of *S. sanguis* to saliva-coated hydroxyl apatite (HA), the existence of two specific receptor sites on HA could be demonstrated to which sialic acid lectins can bind.[46] Vaudaux, et al., found in adhesion experiments of *S. aureus* to fibronectin-coated PMMA coverslips, that presumably a specific site in the amino-terminal region of fibronectin is involved in the adhesion process, and that collagen may play a role as an adhesion cofactor.[47]

It is obvious that the ability of several bacterial species, especially of *S. epidermidis*, to adhere to almost all kinds of polymers used in modern medicine is a major pathogenic factor in the development of a foreign-body infection. Furthermore, the capability of *S. epidermidis* to produce extracellular substances which protect polymer-adhered bacteria against host defense and antibiotics is another feature which has to be considered in developing new strategies of prevention and treatment of foreign-body infections. One possible solution to this problem would be the prevention of the adhesion of microorganisms to the polymer itself. This could be achieved by developing polymers with anti-adhesive properties either through synthesizing novel polymers or through modifying the original polymer surface. However, reduction or inhibition of adhesion to modified surfaces *in vitro* does not necessarily lead to a reduction or inhibition under *in vivo* conditions, where protein coating and cofactors from blood or tissue may play an important role in adhesion. Surfaces which preferentially adsorb albumin are regarded as relatively anti-thrombogenic, because they adsorb almost none or only small amounts of blood platelets. It has also been shown for bacteria that the adhesion to albumin-coated surfaces is reduced. Therefore another approach to developing anti-adhesive surfaces might be modification of the polymer surface to achieve selective adsorption of a particular blood or serum component, e.g. albumin.

Regarding specific interactions between bacteria and polymers which are likely to occur between bacterial surface proteins and protein layers on the polymer surface, the knowledge of the participating components (lectins, sugars, proteins) and the mechanisms of specific adhesion could be used for the inhibition of adhesion by blocking the specific structures involved. This has been recently demonstrated in the adhesion of bacteria to organ cells, e. g. inhibition of the adhesion of *S. pneumoniae* to lung and meningeal cells by blocking bacterial lectins with specific sugars.[48]

Another possibility to preventing foreign-body infections is the development of devices or implants with antimicrobial properties. This could be performed either by synthesizing polymers with functional groups exhibiting antimicrobial activity or by attaching or coupling antimicrobial substances (e. g. antibiotic drugs) to the polymers. The effect of such materials could be the prevention of adhesion or the killing of already adhered microorganisms. The systemic antibiotic therapy of catheter or prostheses infections is usually insufficient, so that materials releasing antibiotics and thus leading to a high local antibiotic concentration might be more successful. There have been several studies in the past dealing with the bonding of antibiotics to catheters or vascular prostheses, but with the exception of the PMMA-Gentamicin beads for the treatment of osteomyelitis none of these materials are routinely used.

Especially in the field of *S. epidermidis* foreign-body infections the mechanisms, how antibiotic-loaded polymers could work, are not yet investigated. Table 1 summarizes the possible strategies of prevention of foreign-body infections based on the modification of polymeric materials. Other possibilities, e. g. the modulation of the bacterial cell (surface) or the development of novel antibiotics, perhaps with slime-penetrating ability, are not considered.

We have begun the development of infection-resistant polymers based upon the above discussed considerations. Forced by previous results on the blood compatibility of modified polyetherurethanes,[49-52] we have investigated the bacterial adhesion on radiation-grafted hydrophilic polyurethanes. We also use glow discharge treatment for the modification of polyurethane surfaces in order to obtain functional groups with antiadhesive properties. In another approach we try to fix antibiotics to polymers to obtain polymeric devices which continuously release the antibiotic to inhibit adhesion or to kill already attached bacteria.

EXPERIMENTAL

1. Modification of polymer surfaces

Polyetherurethanes "WH8" (Biosearch Inc., Raritan, NJ) and "WALOPUR" (Wolff, Walsrode, FRG) were extracted in an EtOH/H$_2$O mixture prior to use. Liquid monomers 2-hydroxyethylmethacrylate (HEMA), 2-epoxypropyl-methacrylate (GMA), 2-dihydroxypropylmethacrylate (GOMA) and acrylic acid (AAc) were distilled under reduced pressure. Acrylamide (AAm) was recrystallized from methanolic solution. Gases for glow discharge treatment

Table 1. Strategies in the prevention of foreign body infections.

Development of materials with antiadhesive properties.	Modification of the polymer surface with chemical, radiation or glow discharge methods in order to create functional groups which –
	exhibit antiadhesive properties.
	selectively adsorb particular blood or tissue components.
Development of materials with antimicrobial properties.	Synthesis of polymers with antimicrobial functional groups.
	Surface modification of polymers to introduce functional groups –
	with antimicrobial activity.
	to which antimicrobial substances can be attached or coupled.

were used without further purification. Acrylic acid was degassed in repeated freeze-thaw cycles. Radiation-grafting of polyetherurethane WH8 was performed as described previously.[30] Briefly, the polymer films were swollen in pure monomer or monomer solution for certain lengths of time, blotted between two filter sheets and irradiated in a ^{60}Co γ source in an argon atmosphere. The dose rate was usually 1.8×10^5 rad/hr. After irradiation the films were extracted in appropriate solvents (EtOH, H_2O or EtOH/H_2O 1:1) to remove monomer and homopolymer. After drying, the grafting yield was determined gravimetrically. Glow discharge treatment of WALOPUR films was performed in a parallel plate reactor. Discharge was driven with a audiofrequency generator. Discharge pressure was usually 0.4 mbar, the discharge time 1 min. at an electrode temperature of 30°C. No extraction was done following the glow discharge treatment. Both sides of the polymer films were modified.

2. Contact angle measurements

The water contact angles of the modified polymers were measured using a Lorentzen & Wettre goniometer and triply distilled water as the contact angle liquid. At least 5 measurements were performed for each sample and the mean value was taken as the final result.

3. Bacterial adhesion to modified polymers

Bacterial adhesion to the surface-modified polyetherurethanes was measured using the bioluminescence assay described by Ludwicka, et al.[33] Polymer discs (d = 6 mm) were incubated in bacterial solution in PBS, usually containing 10^8 colony forming units (cfu), at room temperature. After a given adhesion period, the polymer discs were washed three times in PBS and then treated in 100 µL 2% trichloroacetic acid to extract bacterial ATP. Next, 50 µL of the ATP extract were diluted with 450 µL TRIS-EDTA buffer (pH 7.75), and to an aliquot of 50 µL 200 µL ATP monitoring reagent (LKB Wallac, Finland) and 400 µL TRIS-EDTA buffer were added. The ATP monitoring reagent converts ATP to AMP and light which was measured in a bioluminometer (LKB Wallac, Finland). The light emission is proportional to the ATP-concentration and by establishing a standard curve bacterial concentration vs. ATP-content, the number of adhered bacterial cells per cm^2 polymer could be calculated. The mean value of 5 measurements per sample was taken as the final result.

4. Coating of polymer surfaces with proteins

Bovine serum albumin, fibrinogen and IgG (Serva, Heidelberg, FRG) were dissolved in PBS (pH = 7.2) at room temperature or, in the case of fibrinogen, at 37°C. Polymer discs were incubated in 1% solutions of the proteins for 1 or 24 hr. and washed afterwards with PBS. Contact angles of protein-coated surfaces were measured as described above.

5. Coating of polymers with antibiotics

Unmodified and glow discharge-treated polyetherurethane WALOPUR pieces were incubated 24 hr. in aqueous solutions containing 1 to 5 mg antibiotics per mL. Clindamycin (Upjohn, USA), vancomycin (Lilly, USA), ciprofloxacin (Bayer, FRG) and oxacillin (Bayer, FRG) were used as antibiotics. After incubation, the antibiotic-loaded discs were washed once with PBS. In the case of the unmodified polyetherurethane, antibiotics dissolved in EtOH/H₂O (1:1) were also used to achieve a better swelling of the polymer in the solution.

6. Incorporation of antibiotics into polyetherurethanes

WALOPUR was dissolved in dimethylformamide and various amounts of clindamycin (Upjohn, USA) and flucloxacillin (Beecham, UK) added to the solution. After careful evaporation of the solvent at ~50°C in air, the antibiotic-containing films were evaporated under reduced pressure to remove dimethylformamide completely.

7. Measurement of the bioactivity and the drug release kinetics of antibiotic-loaded films

As a screening test, antibiotic-loaded films were placed on a solid agar plate inoculated with a bacterial test strain (in most cases *S. epidermidis* KH 11). After overnight incubation at 37°C, the occurrence of an inhibition zone around the polymer disc indicated that the released antibiotic was still active. To obtain the drug release-kinetics, especially of the antibiotic-incorporated polymer films, polymer discs (d = 6 mm) were investigated in a standard bioassay using Isosensitive agar (Oxoid, UK). *S. epidermidis* KH 11 and *S. aureus* SG 511 were used as bacterial test strains. The polymer discs were eluted in 0.9% NaCl solution and aliquots of the elutions were introduced into punched wells of the agar which was previously inoculated with the test strain. The amount of the released antibiotics was calculated by comparing the resulting inhibition zone diameters with those of standard antibiotic solutions of known concentration.

RESULTS AND DISCUSSION

We and others have shown in previous investigations that the *in vitro* adhesion of coagulase-negative staphylococci is mainly governed by hydrophobic bonding. E. g., adhesion of two *S. epidermidis* strains differing in their hydrophobicity onto polyetherurethane reveals that the more hydrophobic strain (in this case *S. epidermidis* KH 6) adheres stronger to polyetherurethanes with similar surface properties (Figure 5). Radiation-grafting of a polyetherurethane with the hydrophilic monomer HEMA leads to a reduction of adhesion in comparison with the unmodified polymer (Table 2). Obviously the increase in surface hydrophilicity (as indicated by the decreasing water contact angles) due to the grafting with HEMA leads to a weakening of hydrophobic interactions and thus to a reduction in adhesion. The same is observed for polymer films grafted with other monomers (Figure 6). In the case of the hydrophilic monomers acrylamide (AAm) and 2,3-dihydroxypropylmethacrylate (GOMA), hydrophilic surfaces are created and bacterial adhesion decreases, whereas in the case of the hydrophobic monomer 2,3-epoxypropylmethacrylate (GMA) no increase in surface hydrophilicity and no decrease in bacterial adhesion is observed.

Somewhat different results are obtained with glow discharge treated polyurethanes (Figure 7). The glow discharge modification with the gases O₂, N₂, NH₃ and Freon leads, under standard discharge conditions (P ~0.4 mbar, discharge time 1 min.), to hydrophilic surfaces, as measured with the water contact angle. Surprisingly, this also occurred in the case where Freon was used. However, bacterial adhesion to these surfaces is increased compared to the untreated polyetherurethane.

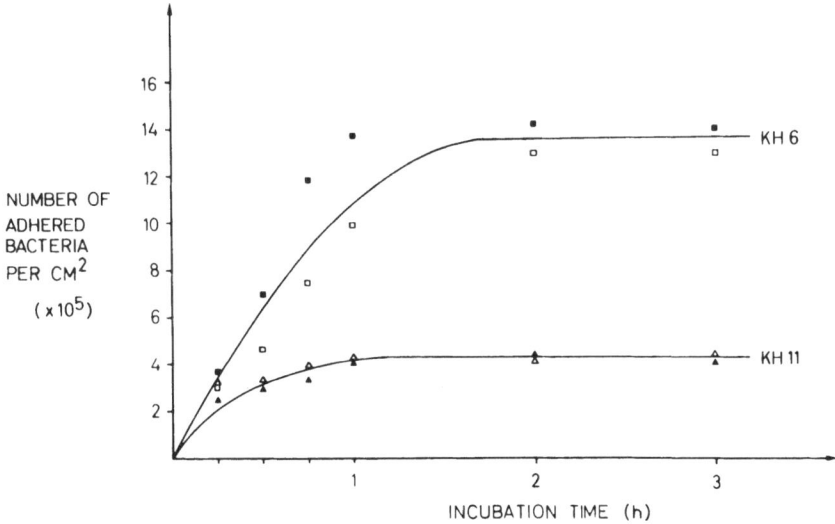

Figure 5. Adhesion of *S. epidermidis* KH 6 and KH 11 onto the
polyetherurethanes BIOMER (△ , □) and TUFTANE
(▲, ●).

If monomeric acrylic acid, in the vapor phase, is used for glow discharge modification, both, an increase in surface hydrophilicity and a
decrease in bacterial adhesion is seen. It is likely that the treatment
with the gases leads to an etching effect of the polymer surface. The
increase in surface roughness might be the reason for the enhancement of
bacterial adhesion, although from thermodynamical considerations adhesion
to the more hydrophilic surface should be reduced. Treatment with acrylic
acid leads to a smoother surface modification, and bacterial adhesion is

Table 2. *In vitro* bacterial adhesion onto HEMA-grafted
polyetherurethane films.

	water contact angle ($^\circ$)	Bacterial adhesion (cells/cm^2 x 10^{-5})	
		Strain 1*	Strain 2**
PUR unmodified	107	1.46	0.6
PUR grafted with HEMA, graft yield = 20%	88	0.26	0.07
PUR grafted with HEMA, graft yield = 130%	72	0.27	0.07
* *S. epidermidis* Gloor 1/1 ** *S. epidermidis* Gloor 99			

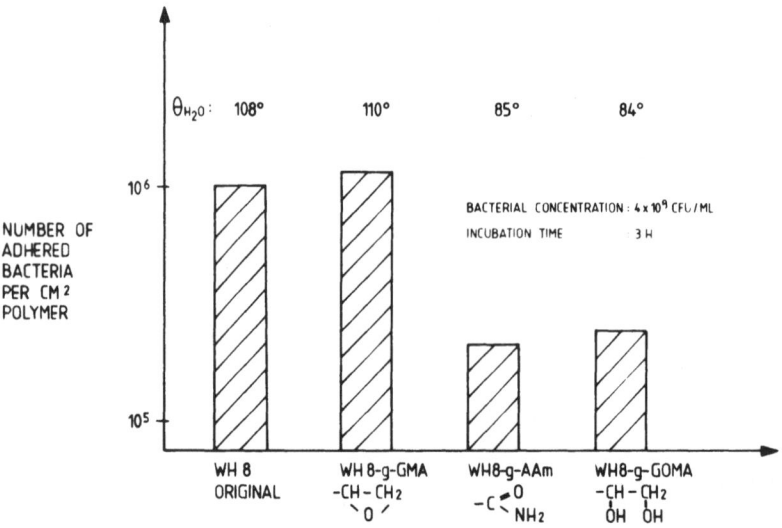

Figure 6. Adhesion of *S. epidermidis* KH 11 onto polyetherurethane grafted with different monomers, GMA =
2,3-epoxypropylmethacrylate, AAm = Acrylamide, GOMA
= 2,3-dihydroxypropylmethacrylate, where Θ_{water} =
water contact angle.

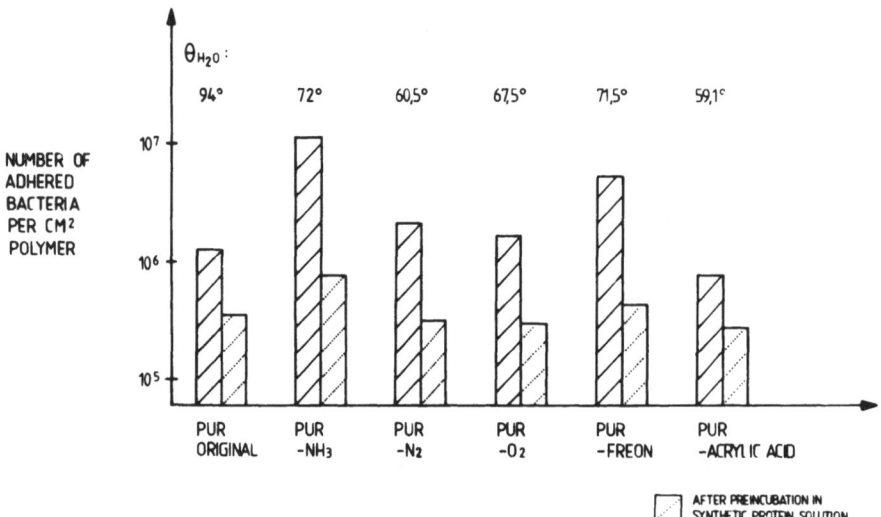

Figure 7. Adhesion of *S. epidermidis* KH 11 onto polyetherurethane modified in a glow discharge treatment
with different gases and acrylic acid (smaller
columns: adhesion after precoating of the polymer
surfaces with a synthetic protein solution) where
Θ_{water} = water contact angle of the modified polyetherurethanes.

reduced as the surface hydrophilicity is increased. Figure 6 also shows the bacterial adhesion to the modified surfaces coated with a synthetic protein solution (4.5% albumin, 1.2% IgG and 0.3% fibrinogen in PBS).

Adhesion is reduced in all cases, even onto the unmodified, protein-coated polyurethane. This decrease in adhesion could be due to an increase in surface hydrophilicity caused by a hydrophilic protein layer. Indeed, the surface hydrophilicity increases after protein-coating, demonstrated by contact angle measurements. In case of the glow discharge-modified samples the protein layer obviously "smoothens" the formerly roughened surfaces, leading also to a reduced adhesion.

In other studies on the bacterial adhesion to protein-coated surfaces, a relationship between bacterial adhesion and the nature of the adsorbed protein was detected.[45] If polyetherurethane samples were pre-coated with albumin or serum, a decrease in bacterial adhesion was always obtained for all strains tested compared to the uncoated polymer. However, precoating with fibrinogen led to an increase in adhesion for at least for one bacterial strain. Also, incubation of the polymer in 10% blood plasma for 1 hr. increased bacterial adhesion, while a 24 hr. plasma incubation did not have this effect. It is known that polyetherurethanes preferentially adsorb albumin from serum or plasma.[50] In the case of blood plasma, we found that after 1 hr. incubation fibrinogen is the major protein adsorbed. However, this is replaced by albumin after a 24 hr. incubation period. We believe that the increase in adhesion is likely due to specific interactions between the fibrinogen layer and the particular bacterial strain.

In the future we plan to clarify the role of adsorbed proteins and their influence on bacterial adhesion, involving studies with fibronectin which seems to play a key role in cellular adhesion processes. As the composition of the original polymer surface determines the nature of the adsorbed protein layer, it might be possible to modify the polymer surface in a way that proteins with antiadhesive properties are selectively adsorbed. Such an effect is known for albumin on platelet adhesion; in a former study we could show that albumin is preferentially adsorbed onto radiation-modified hydrophilic surfaces.[49] Bacterial adhesion to such surfaces is considerably reduced.

Besides the approaches to prevent bacterial adhesion to polymers by modifying the polymer surface, we also investigated the possibility to inhibit bacterial adhesion by attaching or incorporating antibiotics to or into the polymers. First experiments with the polyetherurethane WALOPUR dipped into antibiotic solutions (in water or ethanol/water) showed that the antibiotics are attached to the polymer surface. Antibacterial activity could be demonstrated for almost all samples in an agar disc diffusion test. However, the major amount of attached antibiotic is released within the first ten minutes as was shown in an elution assay, indicating that the antibiotics were very weakly attached to the surface. To obtain stronger interactions and thus prolonged antibiotic release, we used glow discharge treated polyetherurethanes in the attachment assay. Table 3 shows some of the results obtained with the antibiotics clindamycin, vancomycin and ciprofloxacin. It can be seen that the amount of drug attached to the surfaces is considerably increased after modifying the polymer surface with acrylic acid in a glow discharge. Using oxacillin, no difference was seen between the modified and unmodified polyurethanes. It is likely that the antibiotics clindamycin, vancomycin and ciprofloxacin, which were supplied as hydrochloride salts, bind ionically to the negatively charged acrylic acid groups on the polymer surface. In contrast, oxacillin was not used in the salt form.

Table 3. Drug release from polyurethane discs incubated 24
hrs. in antibiotic solutions (5 mg/mL) at room
temperature. The amount of released drug was
determined in a bioassay.

Polymer	Release of antibiotic from polymer after 30 min. elution (µg/cm² polymer)		
	Clindamycin	Vancomycin	Ciprofloxacin
Walopur, unmodified	1.70	0.0	7.64
Walopur, glow discharge modified with acrylic acid	7.62	8.41	18.46

Much higher amounts of the drug fixed to the polymer and a more prolonged release are obtained with our method of incorporating antibiotics
by the solvent casting method. Figures 8 and 9 show the drug release of
polyurethane discs loaded with the antibiotics clindamycin and flucloxacillin at different loading concentrations. The sample with clindamycin
initially shows a high release rate, which drops after 3 to 4 days to
almost zero. In the case of the polyurethanes loaded with flucloxacillin,
a more constant release is seen, lasting for at least five days. We have
now succeeded in changing the release pattern of the clindamycin device
by crosslinking the polymer surface so that also a more constant release
of clindamycin, over a longer period than 4 days, is obtained.

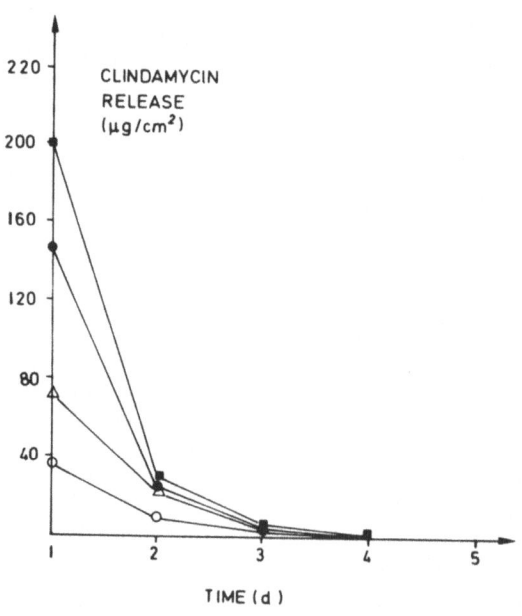

Figure 8. Release of clindamycin from polyetherurethane at
different loading concentrations.   ■ 4.4%; ● 2.8%;
△ 1.5%; ○ 0.75%).

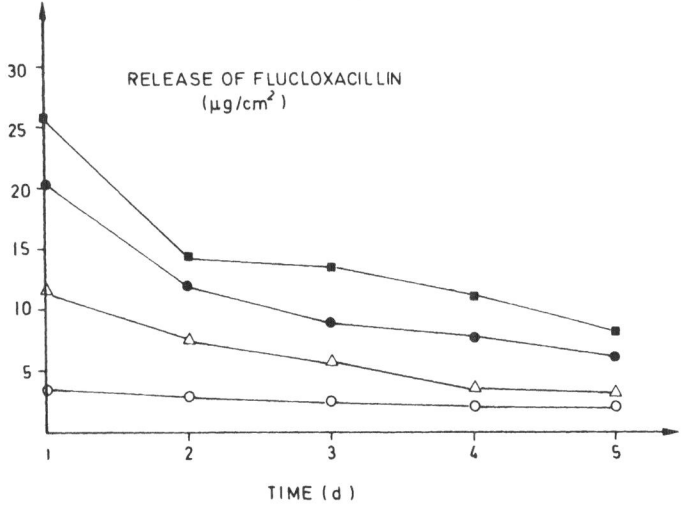

Figure 9. Release of flucloxacillin from polyetherurethane at different loading concentrations. (■ 4.4%; ● 2.8%; △ 1.5%; ○ 0.75%).

The effectiveness of such antibiotic-loaded polymers on bacterial adhesion is now being tested under *in vitro* conditions. In preliminary experiments we have found that flucloxacillin loaded polyurethane leads to a considerable reduction of adhesion in PBS or nutrient-medium in the first 24 hr. Studies with the clindamycin devices revealed that adhesion is not reduced compared to the control polymer, but that a killing effect on adhered bacteria can be seen after 72 hr. We are now studying the incorporation of other antibiotics, with various modes of action, and their effect on bacterial adhesion.

REFERENCES

1. B. Sugarman & E. J. Young, "*Infections associated with prosthetic devices*", CRC Press, Boca Raton, 1984.
2. R. P. Callahan, S. J. Cohen & J. T. Stewart, Brit. Med. J., 14, 860 (1961).
3. R. T. Schimke, P, H. Black, V. H. Mark & M. H. Schwartz, N. Engl. J. Med., 264, 264 (1961).
4. S. C. Schoenbaum, P. Gardner & J. Shillito, J. Infect. Disease, 131, 543 (1975).
5. R. J. Duma, J. F. Warner & H. P. Dalton, New Engl. J. Med., 284, 257 (1977).
6. J. W. Bender & W. T. Hughes, John Hopkins Med. J., 146, 13 (1980).
7. R. J. Sherertz, R. J. Falk, K. A. Huffman, C. A. Thomann, & W. D. Mattem, Arch. Intern. Med., 143, 52 (1983).
8. G. Peters, G. Pulverer & R. Locci, Dtsch. Med. Wochenschr., 106, 822 (1981).
9. R. Gokal, J. Antimicrob. Chemother., 9, 417 (1982).
10. J. Rubin, W. A. Rogers, H. M. Taylor, E. D. Everett, B. F. Prowant, L.V. Fruto & K. D. Nolf, Ann. Int. Med., 92, 7 (1980).

11. R. A. Amoury, F. O. Bouman & R. J. Mahn, J. Thorac Cardiovasc. Surg., **51**, 36 (1966).
12. H. Masur & W. D. Johnson, J. Thorac. Cardiovasc. Surg., **80**, 31 (1980).
13. J. E. Okies, J. Viroslaw & T. W. Williams, Chest, **59**, 198 (1971).
14. M. H. Choo, D. R. Holmes, B. J. Gersh, J. D. Maloney, J. Meridith, J. R. Pluth & J. Trusty, Am. J. Cardiol., **48**, 559 (1981).
15. G. G. Lemire, J. E. Morin & A. R. C. Dobell, Can. J. Surg., **18**, 181 (1975).
16. F. P. Patterson & C. S. Brown, J. Bone Joint Surg., **54A**, 257 (1972).
17. W. G. Liekweg & L. J. Greenfield, Surgery, **81**, 335 (1971).
18. J. W. Warren in: "*Infections Associated with Prosthetic Devices*", B. Sugarman & E. J. Young, Eds., CRC Press, Boca Raton, 1984.
19. R. M. Kluge, F. M. Calia, J. S. McLaughlin & R. B. Hornick, JAMA, **230**, 1415 (1974).
20. G. Peters, F. Schumacher-Perdreau & G. Pulverer, Med. Microbiology, **5**, 209 (1986).
21. G. Peters in: "*The Staphylococci*", J. Jeljaszewicz, Ed., Zbl. Bakt. Hyg., Suppl. 14, Gustav Fischer Verlag, 1985.
22. J. Dankert, A. H. Hogt & J. Feijen in: "*CRC Critical Reviews in Biocompatibility*", D. F. Williams Ed., Vol. 2, Issue 3, CRC Press, Boca Raton, 1986.
23. P. R. Rutter & B. Vincent in: "*Microbial Adhesion to Surfaces*", R. C. W. Berkeley Ed., Ellis Horwood Ltd., 1980.
24. B. V. Derjaguin & L. D. Landau, Acta Phys. Chim. U. S. S. R., **14**, 633 (1941).
25. E. J. W. Verwey & J. Th. G. Overbeek, "*Theory of Stability of Lyophobic Colloids*", Elsevier, 1948.
26. Th. F. Tadros in: "*Microbial Adhesion to Surfaces*", R. C. W. Berkeley, Ed., Ellis Horwood Ltd., 1980.
27. A. W. Neumann, D. R. Absolom, C. J. van Oss & W. Zingg, Cell. Biophysics, **1**, 79 (1979).
28. D. R. Absolom, D. W. Francis, W. Zingg, C. J. van Oss. & A. W. Neumann, J. Coll. Interf. Sci., **85**, 168 (1982).
29. R. J. Gibbons, J. van Houte in: "*Bacterial Adherence, Receptors and Recognition*", E. H. Beachey Ed., Series B, Vol. 6" Chapman and Hall, 1980.
30. C. Svanborg-Eden, B. Ericksson & L. A. Hanson, Infect. Immun., **18**, 767 (1977).
31. A. H. Hogt, J. Dankert, J. A. deVries & J. Feijen, J. Gen. Microbiol., **129**, 4959 (1983).
32. R. J. Gibbons & I. Etherden, Infect. Immun., **41**, 1190 (1983).
33. G. Westergren & J. Olsson, Infect. Immun., **40**, 432 (1983).
34. W. E. Nesbitt, R. J. Doyle & K. G. Taylor, Infect. Immun., **38**, 637 (1982).
35. A. Ludwicka, B. Jansen, G. Uhlenbruck, J. Jeljaszewicz & G. Pulverer in: "*Biomaterials and Biomechanics 1983*", P. Ducheyne, Ed., Elsevier, 1984.
36. A. Ludwicka, B. Jansen, T. Wadstrom, L. M. Switalski, G. Peters & G. Pulverer in: "*Polymers as Biomaterials*", S. W. Shalaby, Ed., Plenum Publ. Corp., 1984.
37. B. Jansen, F. Schumacher-Perdreau, G. Peters & G. Pulverer, Adv. Biomaterials, **7**, 693 (1987).
38. A. H. Hogt, J. Dankert & J. Feijen, J. Biomed. Mater. Res., **20**, 553 (1986).
39. A. Bantjes, Brit. Polym. J., **10**, 267 (1978).
40. G. Kronvall, A. Simmons, E. B. Myhre & S. Jonsson, Infect. Immun., **25**, 1 (1979).
41. P. Kuusela, Nature, **276**, 718 (1978).
42. M. Fletcher, J. Gen. Microbiol., **94**, 400 (1976).

43. A. H. Hogt, J. Dankert & J. Feijen, J. Gen. Microbiol., **131**, 2485 (1985).
44. A. Fleer, J. Verhoef & A. P. Hernandez, Am. J. Med., **80**, Suppl. 6B, 161 (1986).
45. B. Jansen, F. Schumacher-Perdreau, G. Peters & G. Pulverer, Abstract No. D-62, ASM Annual Meeting, Atlanta, 1987.
46. E. J. Morris, B. C. McBride, Infect. Immun., **43**, 556 (1984).
47. P. E. Vaudaux, F. A. Waldvogel, J. J. Morgenthaler & U. E. Nydegger, Infect. Immun., **41**, 768 (1984).
48. J. Beuth, H. L. Ko, H. Schroten, J. Solter, G. Uhlenbruck & G. Pulverer, Zbl. Bakt. Hyg., **A261**, 160 (1987).
49. B. Jansen & G. Ellinghorst, J. Biomed. Mater. Res., **18**, 655 (1984).
50. B. Jansen & G. Ellinghorst, J. Biomed. Mater. Res., **19**, 1085 (1985).
51. B. Jansen, A. Ludwicka & L. W. Storz, Radiat. Phys. Chem., **25** (4-6), 529 (1985).
52. B. Jansen, H. Steinhauser & W. Prohaska, Adv. Biomaterials, **6**, 207 (1986).
53. A. Ludwicka, L. M. Switalski, A. Lundin, G. Pulverer & T. Wadstrom, J. Microbiol. Meth., **4**, 169 (1985).

SYNTHESIS AND CHARACTERIZATION OF POLYMERS HAVING STEROID SEX HORMONES AS PENDENT MOIETIES

Malay Ghosh

Department of Chemistry & Chemical Engineering
Stevens Institute of Technology
Hoboken, NJ 07030

Steroids are widely known for their versatile biological activities and they are being used by physicians all over the world since the 1930s. These drugs have some major disadvantages. A large number of polymeric compounds have been found to be efficient as chemotherapeutic agents. This paper describes the synthesis and characterization of two new monomers derived from two steroid sex hormones - estrone and androsterone, and their subsequent polymerization.

INTRODUCTION

The discovery of any new class of compounds has always resulted in a high level of research activities in the history of chemistry and medicine. No other class of compounds are more spectacular, diverse in nature, and have influenced the daily lives of people, than the steroids and antibiotics. Steroids are complex tetracyclic systems that are widely available both in the animal and the plant kingdoms.[1,2] They have been known to chemists for a long time, but the finding, that a large number of them act as vitally important effectors in the physiological processes, led to in depth investigations.[3] Sex hormones are an important subclass of the steroid family.[2] Their applications to treat various types of cancer and to correct disorders associated with fertility and menstruation began as early as 1930.[4-6] Preparation of orally active contraceptives from steroid sex hormones has virtually opened a new direction in medicinal chemistry.[6] The steroid hormone therapy, however, is not free from problems. Some of the drugs exhibit high immunogenicities towards human subjects. Besides, most of them are fast removed from the bloodstream after their administration, i.e., the concentration of the drug in the plasma decreases rapidly.[7] This means that the bioavailability of the drugs are not acceptable. Among the several different approaches to solve these problems, two are noteworthy. A number of semi-synthetic steroids have been made which exhibit a better pharmacodynamic profile than the naturally occurring ones.[6] The other approach taken by various groups is the well known "soft drug" approach.[8-10]

Recently, polymeric compounds have been found to be a powerful paradigm for the development of various structures that possess the desired physiological properties with acceptable pharmacokinetic properties.[11-13]

However, very few attempts have been made to synthesize and investigate the bioactive polymeric steroidal compounds.[14,15] We, as a part of our continuing investigations on polymeric drugs, planned to prepare some new macromolecules possessing biologically active steroids in every repeat unit.[16,17] For this purpose, two steroids have been chosen. They are 3-hydroxy-1,3,5(10)-estratrien-17-one and 3-α-hydroxy-5-α-androstan-17-one, commonly known as estrone [1] and androsterone [4], respectively. Estrone is a strong estrogen and is used to treat cancer of the prostate, prevent pregnancy, and treat menstrual cycle irregularities.[18] On the other hand, androsterone finds its applications in the treatment of breast cancer, to gain weight, for stimulation of growth, and, in a few cases, to help red blood cell production.[4,18]

From the point of view of a synthetic polymer chemist, there could be four viable routes available for preparing polymeric drugs. They have been described elsewhere.[17] We planned to make use of one particular strategy which requires the synthesis of the steroid based monomers first and finally to polymerize this monomer under appropriate conditions. In this case, each repeat unit of the polymer will carry the steroid moiety. The retrosynthetic analysis[19] is shown in Scheme 1.

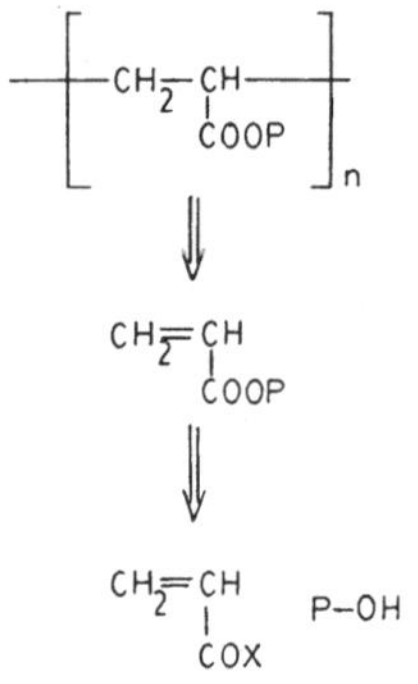

$$
\begin{array}{c}
\left[-CH_2-\underset{\underset{COOP}{|}}{CH}-\right]_n \\
\Downarrow \\
CH_2\!\!=\!\!\underset{\underset{COOP}{|}}{CH} \\
\Downarrow \\
CH_2\!\!=\!\!\underset{\underset{COX}{|}}{CH} \quad P\!-\!OH
\end{array}
$$

Scheme 1. Retrosynthetic Analysis Procedure.

The retrosynthetic study clearly shows that the steroid molecule could be transformed into monomers by easy chemical manipulation and the monomers eventually could be polymerized by standard polymerization methods.

EXPERIMENTAL

Materials

Acrylic acid, triethylamine, dicyclohexylcarbodiimide and N,N-dimethylaminopyridine were obtained from BDH Chemical Company. Androsterone and estrone were purchased from Sigma Chemical Company. AIBN was received from Aldrich Chemical Company. Dioxane, ether, chloroform and tetrahydrofuran were purified and dried by following the standard procedures.[20]

Methods of Characterization

Melting points were taken on a Buchi 510 M.P. apparatus. Infrared (IR) spectra were run on a Perkin-Elmer Model 1310 instrument using either KBr pellets or a nujol mull. Proton NMR spectra were recorded on a Varian EM-390 or a Bruker AF-200 (200 MHz) spectrometer using TMS as an internal standard. ^{13}C-NMR spectra were taken on a Jeol FX-200 or a Bruker AF-200 (50.08 MHz) spectrometer using TMS or CHCl$_3$ as internal standards. INEPT spectra were obtained according to the pulse sequence as reported by Shoolery.[21]

TLC were carried out on SiO$_2$-gel layers (0.25 mm) containing 15% gypsum and activated at 100°C (5 hrs.) and using ethyl acetate-hexane as the solvent system. Flash chromatography was performed following the method described by Clarkstill and coworkers.[22]

Synthesis of Monomers

Both the monomers [2] and [5] were prepared either by reaction of acryloyl chloride with the steroids in the presence of an acid acceptor (Method A) or by the reaction of the steroids with acrylic acid, using N,N-dicyclohexylcarbodiimide and a catalytic amount of N,N-dimethylaminopyridine as condensing agents (Method B).

Preparation of Monomer [2]

Method A

Estrone [1] (2.7 g, 0.01 m) was dissolved in chloroform (250 mL) and triethylamine (3 mL, 0.02 m) was added. The reaction mixture was magnetically stirred at -10°C under a nitrogen atmosphere. To this was added a solution of acryloyl chloride (1.35 g, 0.015 m) in chloroform (50 mL) over a period of 30 min. The reaction mixture was stirred at -10°C for another hour and then allowed to come to room temperature. After 8 hrs. the reaction product showed complete conversion of the starting material to a new compound. Then the reaction was quenched by adding a large excess of ice water. The organic layer was washed with 3N HCl, 5% aqueous NaHCO$_3$, water and brine, successively, and then dried over anhydrous Na$_2$SO$_4$. Evaporation of the solvent afforded a thick black oil. The monomer was then purified by flash chromatography using ethyl acetate:hexane (1:2) as the eluting solvent system. Finally, the monomer was crystallized from a chloroform:hexane solvent system to give the analytically pure sample. The yield of the reaction was 73%. The monomer is soluble in most of the polar organic solvents (Table 1).

Method B

A solution of estrone [1] (2.7 g, 0.01 m), acrylic acid (0.072 g, 0.01 m) and N,N-dimethylaminopyridine (0.12 g, 0.001 m) in tetrahydrofuran (250 mL) was stirred at -20°C under a nitrogen atmosphere. To this was slowly added a solution of N,N-dicyclohexylcarbodiimide (2.00 g, 0.01 m) in tetrahydrofuran (50 mL) over a 30 min. period. After complete addition, the solution was allowed to warm up to 20°C and was stirred overnight. The precipitated urea derivative was filtered out and subsequent removal of the solvent afforded a sticky mass which was dissolved in ethyl acetate. The organic layer was washed with 5% aqueous NaHCO$_3$, water, brine and then dried over anhydrous NaSO$_4$. The solvent was removed under reduced pressure to yield an oil. The monomer was finally purified by flash chromatography. The yield of this reaction was 89%. The mixed melting point was undepressed.

Table 1. Physical Properties of Monomers.

	Compound	
	[2]	[5]
Melting point, °C	151	141
Solvents	ethyl acetate chloroform p-dioxane	ethyl acetate chloroform tetrahydrofuran
Non-solvents	n-pentane n-hexane cyclohexane	n-pentane n-hexane cyclohexane
Elemental Analysis; %		
C (calcd.)	77.77	76.74
C (obs.)	77.63	76.60
H (calcd.)	7.40	9.30
H (obs.)	7.31	9.14

Preparation of Monomer [5]

Method A

Androsterone [4] (2.9 g, 0.01 m) was reacted with acryloyl chloride (1.35 g, 0.015 m) in the presence of triethylamine (3 mL) in chloroform (250 mL) according to the procedure described for the preparation of [2]. The monomer was purified by flash chromatography using ethyl acetate: hexane (1:2) as the eluting solvent system. The yield of the reaction was 69%.

Method B

Acrylic acid (0.72 g, 0.01 m), androsterone [4] (2.9 g, 0.01 m), dicyclohexylcarbodiimide (2.06 g, 0.01 m) and N,N-dimethylaminopyridine were reacted in tetrahydrofuran (250 mL) to afford monomer [5] in 72% yield. The usual work up, followed by purification, produced the analytically pure sample.

Synthesis of Polymers

Homopolymerization of the steroid monomers [2] and [5] was carried out in p-dioxane solvent, using AIBN as the initiator. In a typical experiment, monomer [2] or [5] was dissolved in p-dioxane (15% w/w). To this was added the AIBN initiator (1.00m%). The reaction vessel was first evacuated and then purged with dry nitrogen gas. This process was repeated several times. Then the reaction vessel was placed in an oil bath maintained at 60°C for 48 hrs. Afterwards, the solution was cooled and diethyl ether was added; a white solid separated out from the solution. This solid material was filtered and was purified by repeated reprecipitation from dimethylformamide and ether. The yield of the polymers were 85-92%.

Characterization of Monomers and Polymers

The physical properties and elemental analyses of the synthesized monomers are given in Table 1.

The spectroscopic information are in good agreement with the proposed structure of monomers [2] and [5]. Thus the IR spectra of [2], taken in a nujol mull, exhibits two sharp bands at 1645 and 1725 cm^{-1}. The first band corresponds to an olefinic group whereas the second band arises due to the combined ester and ketone functionalities. Later, we observed that taking the IR spectra in CHCl$_3$ solution would permit resolution of the ester and ketone bands into bands at 1725 and 1720 cm^{-1} for [2]. Similarly, the IR of [5], in a nujol mull, showed bands at 1650 and 1720 cm^{-1}.

The ^{1}H-NMR of [2] has a sharp singlet at 1.0δ due to the methyl protons in the steroid system, and complex multiplets in the region 1.1 to 3.0δ, which are associated with the protons due to the steroid framework. The three vinylic protons show signals as complex multiplets in the region 6.05, 6.45 and 6.7δ, respectively. The ^{13}C-NMR and INEPT spectra are shown in Figure 1. The bottom spectra corresponds to the ^{13}C (PND), which shows a peak at 220δ for the keto carbonyl and another peak at 166δ for the ester carbonyl group. The saturated carbons of the steroid moiety (methyl, methylene, methine) exhibit signals from 13 to 50δ. The top spectra in Figure 1 is the INEPT spectra of monomer [2]. One interesting point we observed was that the olefinic CH$_2$ peak occurs downfield (132.40δ) from their normal spectral position.

The ^{1}H-NMR spectra of [5] is similar to that of [2]. It showed three multiplets for the vinylic protons at 5.2, 6.1 and 6.30δ values. The C-3 proton appears at 4.7δ as a complex multiplet. The other protons show signals from 0.95 to 2.65δ. The ^{13}C-NMR (PND and INEPT) spectra of [5] are shown in Figure 2. The carbonyl carbon appears at 221.11δ and the ester carbon shows a signal at 166.06δ. From INEPT spectra it is clear that the olefinic carbons possess peaks at 130.55 and 129.24δ values. The other carbons appear in their usual positions.

The IR spectra of polymers [3] and [6], taken in a nujol mull, exhibit a band at about 1730 cm^{-1}. The absence of the band due to the olefinic double bond is indicative of the formation of the target polymers.

The ^{1}H-NMR spectrum of [3] shows the disappearance of the olefinic protons and the appearance of a new multiplet at 4.45δ, which is indicative of a methine proton. Aromatic protons appear in their characteristic position at 7.0 to 7.5δ, and a new methylene proton peak merged with the signals of the steroidal protons. Similarly, the ^{1}H-NMR of [6] has a multiplet at 4.6 for CH and at 4.85δ for the C-3 proton, while the remaining steroidal protons came from 0.9 to 2.9δ values, respectively.

DISCUSSION

The polymers bearing steroid sex hormones as pendent moities are rare in the literature. These kinds of compounds, however, do possess high promise in hormone therapy. We have prepared two such polymers - one having estrone and the other androsterone as the pendent group connected with the main polymeric network via an ester bond. The monomers required for the preparation of these polymers were synthesized by following either Method A or Method B.

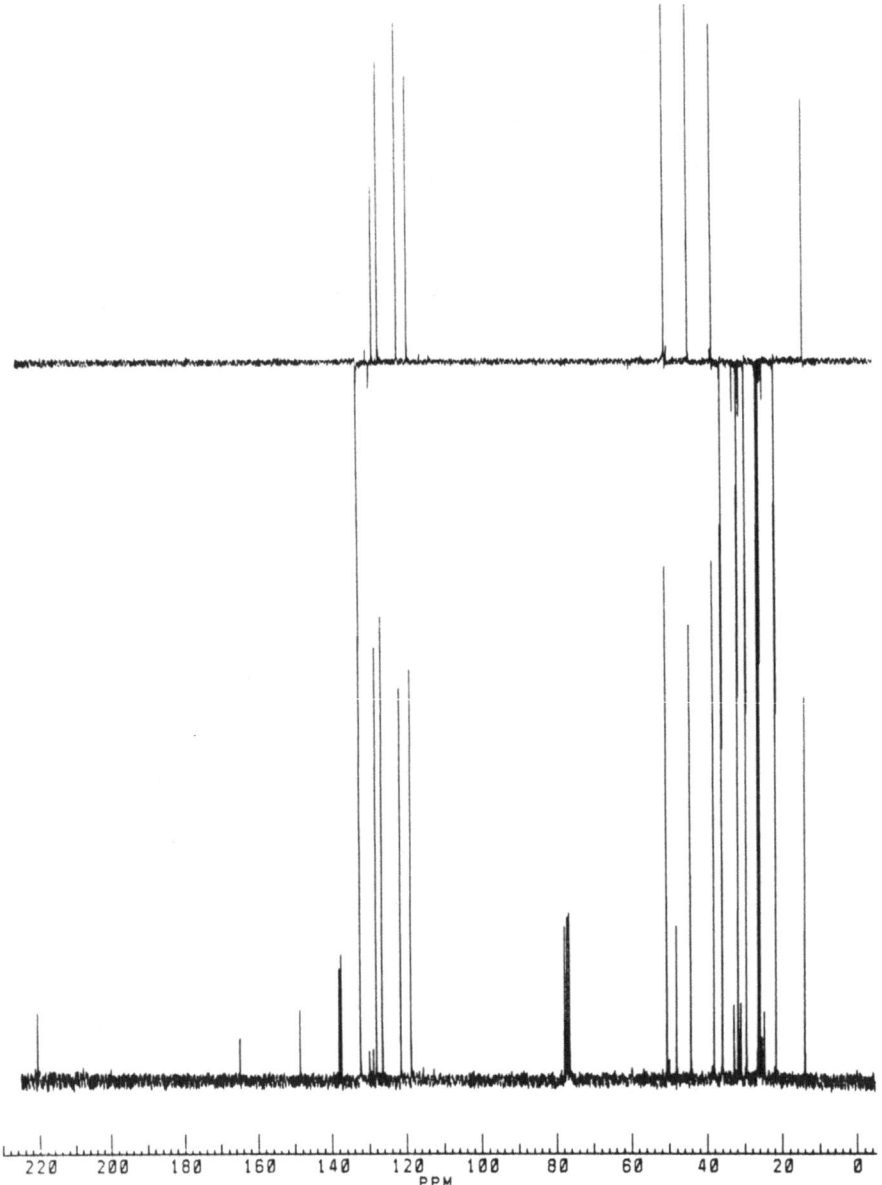

Figure 1. ^{13}C-NMR (PND, INEPT) of Monomer [2].

In Method A, the steroids are reacted with acrlyoyl chloride in the presence of triethylamine at low temperatures to provide the desired monomers. In Method B, acrylic acid is condensed with the steroids in the presence of dicyclohexylcarbodiimide and N,N-dimethylaminopyridine to give the same monomers. In both cases the crude monomers need to be purified first by flash chromatography and, finally, by recrystallization. Method B has been found to be more efficient and the crude products obtained are cleaner than those obtained from Method A. The monomers are

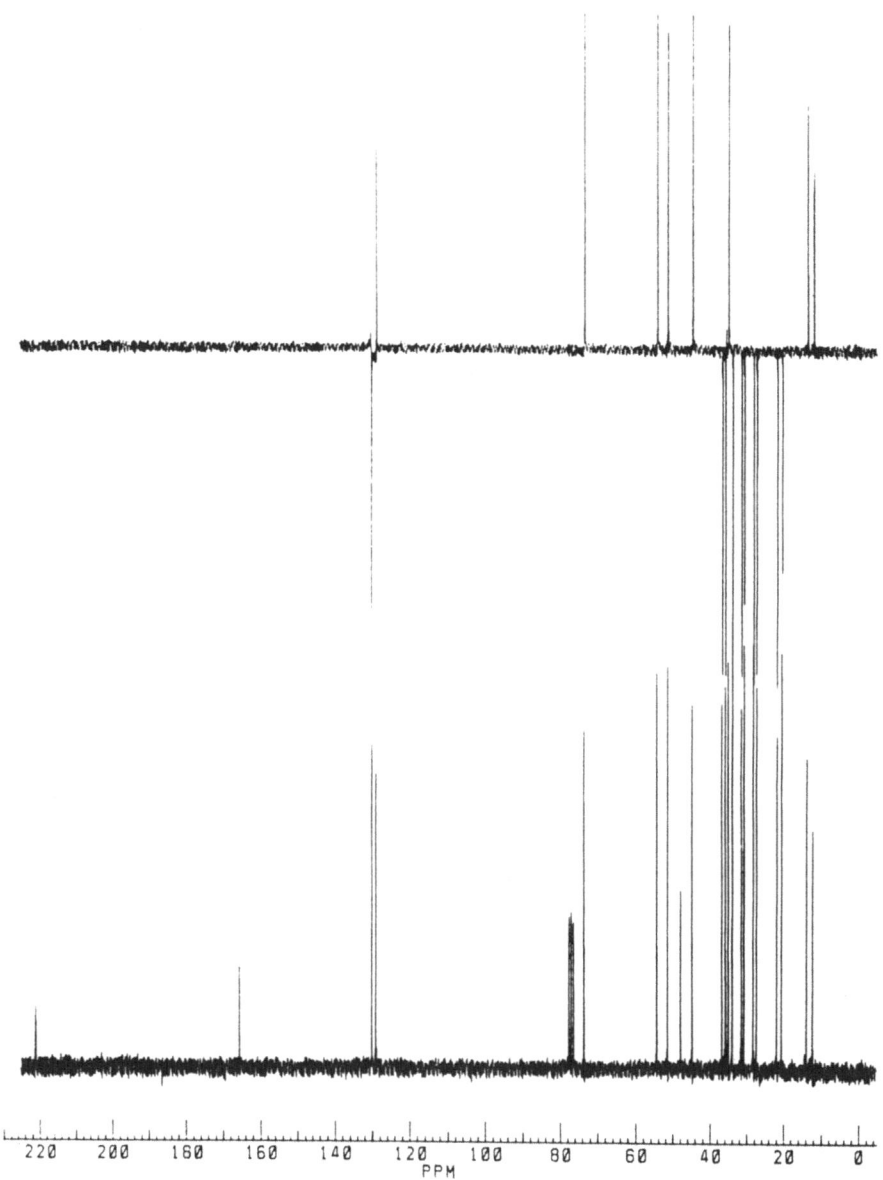

Figure 2. ^{13}C-NMR (PND, INEPT) of Monomer [5].

then polymerized under free radical conditions in p-dioxane using AIBN as the initiator. The overall synthetic scheme for the preparation of the monomers and the polymers in shown in Scheme 2. (The yields of the monomers and the polymers varied in the range of 70-90%.)

Any kind of biological response due to the compound, either *in vivo* or *in vitro* systems, is associated with the interaction of the appropiate receptor and the compound. This is one of the most important steps.[23] In the case of the steroidal hormones, formation of the receptor - hormone complex is essential. So the polymeric derivative needs to be hydrolyzed

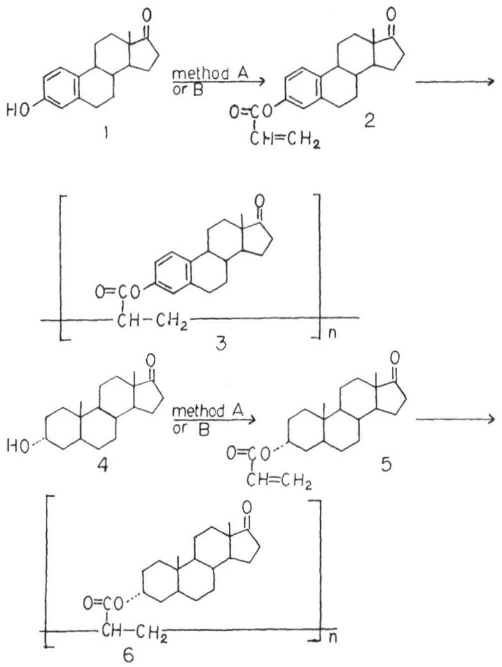

Scheme 2. The Synthesis and Polymerization of the Steroid
Monomers by Methods A or B.

in vivo to provide steroids which eventually could exhibit the biological
properties via the receptor-drug complex. Various types of enzymes, for
example hydrolases, esterases, etc., that are present in the human system
have been proven to be highly efficient in cleaving the ester bonds,[24-26]
and the polymeric steroid derivatives synthesized here should elicit
biological properties after their administration.

The solubility of these polymeric steroid derivatives could be
changed by copolymerizing steroid monomers with other monomers. For
instance, copolymerization with acrylic acid, acrylamide, and/or N-vinylpyrrolidone could result in water soluble copolymers.

CONCLUSION

This paper describes the synthesis of new steroid based monomers and
polymers. The chemistry adopted for that purpose provides a framework by
which different other steroid based monomers and polymers could be synthesized in a relativley concise fashion. The physiological activities of
the synthesized polymers are currently underway and will be reported in a
future article.

ACKNOWLEDGEMENT

The author wished to express his thanks to Mrs. Prarthana Bose for
her invaluable help. The valuable help rendered by Dr. Animesh Bose is
gratefully acknowledged. Dr. C. G. Gebelein and Dr. A. K. Bose are
thanked for their suggestions. The Council of Scientific and Industrial
Research, Government of India is thanked for the partial support of this
work.

REFERENCES

1. T. Kemeetani & H. Nemoto, Tetrahedron, **37**, 3 (1981).
2. L. F. Fieser & M. Fieser, "*Steroids*", Reinhold, New York, 1959.
3. A journal has been established named "*Steroids*", which publishes papers on the chemical and biological aspects of steroids only.
4. N. Applezweiz, "*Steroid Drugs*", Vol. I & II, Holden-Day, Inc., San Francisco, 1964.
5. "*Annual Reports in Medicinal Chemistry*"; a multivolume treatise, Academic Press, Orlando.
6. A. Burger in: "*Medicinal Chemistry*", A. Burger, Ed., Interscience Publishers, New York, 1960.
7. G. J. H. Melrose, Rev. Pure Appl. Chem., **21**, 83 (1971).
8. N. Bordor in: "*Drug Metabolism and Drug Design: Quo Vadis?*", M. Briot, W. Cantreels & R. Roncucci, Eds., Center de Recherches Clin-Midy, Montpellier, France, 1981, p. 217.
9. N. Bodor in: "*Strategy in Drug Research*", J. A. Keverling Buisman, Ed., Elsevier, Amsterdam, 1982, p. 137.
10. N. Bodor in: "*Advances in Drug Research*", Vol. 13, Academic Press, London, 1984, p. 255.
11. C. G. Gebelein & F. F. Koblitz, "*Biological and Dental Applications of Polymers*", Plenum Publ., New York, 1981.
12. C. E. Carraher, Jr. & C. G. Gebelein, "*Biological Activities of Polymers*", American Chemical Society Symposium Series No. 186, 1982.
13. D. A. Tirrell, L. G. Donaruma & A. B. Turek, "*Macromolecules as Drugs and as Carriers for Biologically Active Materials*", Ann. New Academy of Science, Vol. **446**, New York, 1985.
14. R. V. Peterson, J. M. Anderson, S. M. Fang, J. Regin, D. E. Gregonis & S. W. Kim, Polymer Prepr., **26 (2)**, 20 (1979).
15. K. V. Nguyen, L. Jung, G. Coupin & P. Poindron, J. Poly. Sci., Polymer Chem., **24**, 359 (1986).
16. M. Ghosh, Proc. Polymer Mater. Sci. & Eng., **55**, 755 (1986).
17. M. Ghosh, Polymer News, **13**, 71-77 (1988).
18. C. R. Baker, "*Physician Desk References*", Medical Economics Co., Oradell, NJ, 1982.
19. E. J. Corey, Quart. Revs., **25**, 455 (1971).
20. D. D. Perrin, W. F. F. Armareo & D. R. Perrin, "*Purification of Laboratory Chemicals*", Pergamon Press, London, 1966.
21. J. N. Shoolery, J. Nat. Prod., **47**, 226 (1984).
22. W. Clarkstill, M. Kahn & A. Mitra, J. Org. Chem., **43**, 2923 (1978).
23. R. R. Ruffolo, J. Auton. Pharm., 2, 277 (1982).
24. G. M. Whiteside & C. Wong, Angew. Chem. Internat. Ed., **24**, 617 (1985).
25. M. Dixon, E. C. Webb, C. J. R. Thorne & K. F. Tripton, "*Enzymes*", 3rd Ed., Longman, London (1979)
26. G. M. Whiteside & C. Wong, Aldrichimica Acta, **16**, 27 (1983).

NOVEL APPROACHES AND APPLICATIONS OF STEROID HORMONE DELIVERY VIA POLY(DIMETHYLSILOXANE)

D.J. Kesler

Physiology Research Laboratory
Reproductive Engineering & Biotechnology
Department of Animal Sciences
University of Illinois
Urbana, Illinois 61801

Poly(dimethylsiloxane) has been used to deliver steroid hormones to animals since the 1960's and commercial poly-(dimethylsiloxane) based delivery systems for estradiol and progestins are currently available. Studies were conducted with androgens to develop poly(dimethylsiloxane) delivery systems that would maintain relatively constant blood testosterone concentrations in ruminant females for six months. All androgens tested passed through the poly(dimethylsiloxane) *in vivo* at rates proportional to surface area and increased blood testosterone concentrations relatively proportionally to the secretion rate. Implants with testosterone propionate incorporated in poly(dimethylsiloxane): (1) maintained relatively constant blood testosterone concentrations *in vivo* for six months and maintained more constant blood testosterone concentrations than commercially available implants (non-poly(dimethylsiloxane) containing testosterone propionate, (2) evoked an anabolic effect in heifers, (3) maintained male sexual behavior in female ruminants and (4) prenatally androgenized female ruminants. The poly(dimethylsiloxane) implants not only facilitated therapy but also enhanced efficacy and in some cases eliminated side effects.

INTRODUCTION

The development of chronic drug delivery systems began when Folkman and Long noted, while performing *in vitro* studies on artificial heart valves, that silicone elastomers absorbed lipid-soluble dyes from solution and subsequently gave off these dyes.[1-3] Dziuk and Cook demonstrated in 1966 that several classes of steroid hormones penetrated silicone membranes and suggested that silicone implants might be quite useful in chronic administration of steroids because the silicone elastomer also was known to be non-antigenic and non-irritating.[4]

Previously, sustained delivery of steroids was accomplished by one of two primary methods. In one case the steroids were mixed with carriers, such as oils, and injected intramuscularly.[5] Such carriers, however, did not yield satisfactory results since the rate of release was so rapid that frequent injections were still necessary. The second method of prolonging the delivery of steroids consisted of subcutaneously implanting the desired steroid in the form of compressed pellets. Absorption of these steroid pellets varied greatly. Regardless of these limitations, however, numerous commercial products have been developed utilizing these methods and many are available on the market today.[5]

Early research conducted with steroid/silicone implants suggested that steroids were approximately 10 times more effective via subcutaneous implantation than by subcutaneous injection. It was further demonstrated that only minimal local tissue reaction occurred, no significant migration of the implants occurred and steroids could be released over a period of years.

Silicone elastomers are based upon the poly(dimethylsiloxane) structure shown below:

$$CH_3 - Si - O - \left[Si - O \right]_n - Si - CH_3$$

The release of steroids from silicone implants follows Ficks' law of diffusion with the flux of diffusion being affected by a diffusion coefficient, membrane surface area, thickness of the membrane and the concentration gradient across the diffusion path in the membrane.

The silicone elastomers have been fabricated into various forms of controlled release drug/hormone systems. In their patent application, Long and Folkman injected a silicone elastomer suspension of drug and polymerizing catalyst and permitted polymerization to occur *in situ*.[3] This prototype was a matrix-type silicone implant. Currently, it is more common to mix the desired steroid thoroughly with a commercially available elastomer followed by mixing this mixture with a polymerizing catalyst and extruding the mixture into an appropriate mold. In the matrix-type silicone implant, the desired steroid is homogeneously dispersed as crystals or as a powder in a matrix formed by the crosslinking of linear polymer chains. The encapsulated steroid particles are first dissolved and then diffuse through the polymer structure with the crystals on the surface layer of the matrix being the first eluted followed by the next layer but only after the first layer becomes exhausted. A elution profile, therefore, decreases over time due to an increase in the thickness of the membrane.[6]

Silicone implants can also be fabricated as capsule-type implants. These implants are generally manufactured from commercially available medical grade silicone tubing. The desired diameter of tubing may be cut into various lengths, one end sealed with silicone medical adhesive and allowed to cure. Crystalline steroid may then be added to the tube and the open end can then be sealed with silicone medical adhesive. The crystalline drug/hormone is enclosed in a capsule/reservoir and those in contact with the inner surface dissolve into the polymer structure and diffuse through it to the exterior. A constant drug/hormone release profile should be obtained since the membrane thickness, which remains the same, is the limitation on diffusion. Long term implantation of a compound with a high diffusion flux, however, may decrease over time like the matrix type implant due to reduced crystalline compound in the reservoir resulting in reduced membrane contact.

A third type of silicone implant fabrication is a hybrid of the capsule and matrix-type implants such as microsealed drug delivery system.[7] This system consists of a matrix-type silicone implant with microsealed compartments containing drug/steroid dissolved or suspended in a hydrophilic solvent. Addition of solvents in the silicone implants changes the physical structure of the silicone network and affects the solubility and diffusivity of drugs/hormones so that release fluxes of drugs/hormones increase.[7]

The most common type of silicone implant used by the biologist is the capsule-type implant whereas the matrix-type of implant is the most frequently employed for commercial products. One reason for this difference is that when a crystalline compound is placed in a capsule it is quite evident after it has been used whether it can be used for further experimentation. However, upon implantation caution must be taken to avoid puncture of the capsule membrane which causes a larger than desired release of the drug/hormone. Less damage is done to matrix-type implants due to punctures.

Upon diffusion through the membrane the drug/hormone must then diffuse into the subcutaneous intercellular fluids. Upon entry into the biological system the drug/hormone encounters additional barriers such as cellular and vascular membranes, cellular and tissue metabolism, inactivation via binding to globulins in the vascular system which are encountered before the compound can initiate its biological effect at its specific target tissue. After subcutaneous implantation additional barriers encountered are the inflammatory and wound healing responses initiated by the implantation process. In addition, a fibrous capsule commonly develops around silicone implants and this fibrous capsule is a new biological barrier with different permeation properties that restricts the diffusion of drugs/hormones into the normal adjacent fluids and tissues.[6,8]

Poly(dimethylsiloxane) has been used extensively in animals and humans as a delivery system for a variety of compounds but most notably for steroid hormones. Steroid hormones are a diverse group of lipophilic compounds synthesized as illustrated in Figure 1 from cholesterol predominantly by adrenal, testicular, ovarian and placental tissues.[9] Upon synthesis by the endocrine tissue, steroids are released into the vascular system whereupon the majority (approximately 95%) bind to blood binding globulins that increases their solubility but renders them inactive. Upon release from binding globulins they become active and are capable of binding to intracellular receptors and initiating biological responses.

There are numerous applications for exogenous steroid therapy for both humans and animals. Poly(dimethylsiloxane) based implants to deliver estradiol and progestins are currently available. To my knowledge, however, no poly(dimethylsiloxane) based implants to deliver androgens are available. The purpose of this paper is to report data collected in my laboratory that demonstrate the efficacy and usefulness of poly(dimethylsiloxane) based implants that deliver androgens to animal.

There are several naturally occurring androgens and probably thousands of synthetic androgens. Some of the more commonly used synthetic androgens are esters. Esterification of steroids bearing a hydroxyl group at the 17-position has been demonstrated to improve duration of biolo-

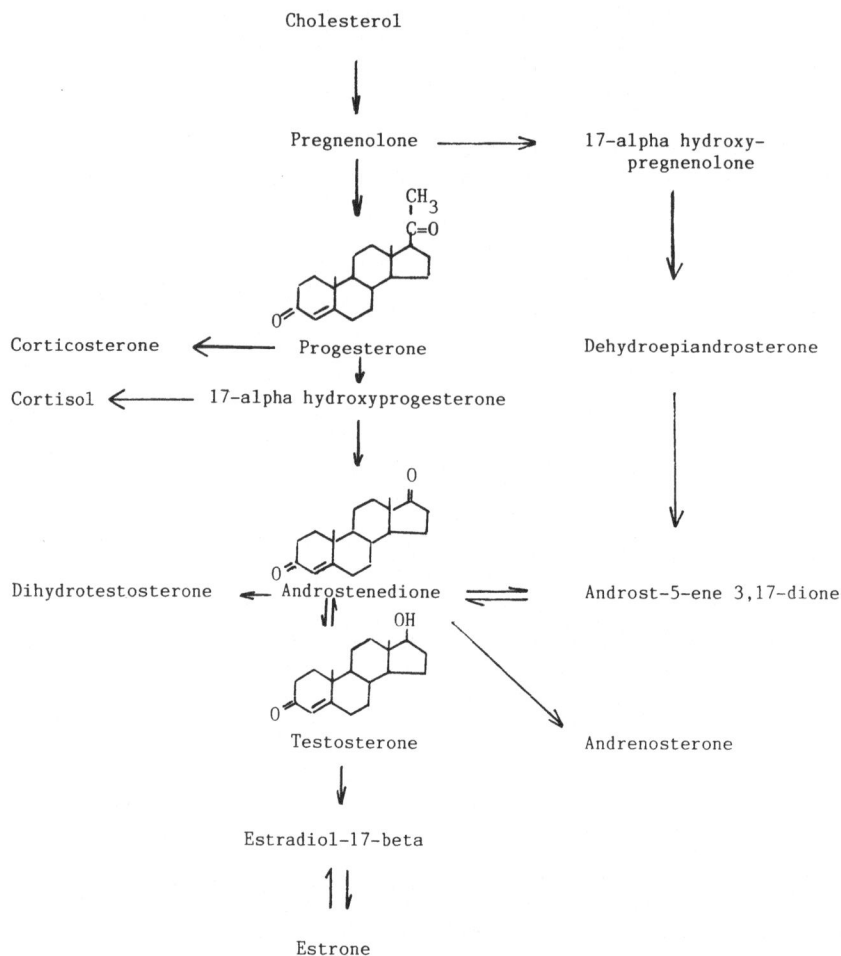

Figure 1. Abbreviated steriod biosynthetic pathway.

gical activity when systematically administered in oil carriers.[10] In general, the duration of effect between a variety of derivatives (such as esters) reside in the alteration of certain physico-chemical properties (solubility and its influence on lipophilic-hydrophilic character) and pharmacokinetic properties. Upon administration it has been shown that the free 17-hydroxyl group is critical for bioactivity. For example, when testosterone propionate was administered to castrated rats pretreated with an esterase inhibitor (an inhibitor of ester/steroid cleavage) their prostate and seminal vesicles showed no weight gain.[10] Administration of testosterone, however, elicited the usual androgenic response. Testosterone enanthate and testosterone cypionate are two testosterone esters that are reputed to be long-acting androgenic compounds. Testosterone propionate, another testosterone ester, is traditionally classified as a short-acting compound but is used in several anabolic implants that are delivered in the form of compressed pellets. All three of these testosterone esters have been shown to be more lipophilic than testosterone (see Figure 2). These three compounds were used in the following studies to develop silicone implants that would maintain relatively constant blood testosterone concentrations in ruminant females for approximately six months.

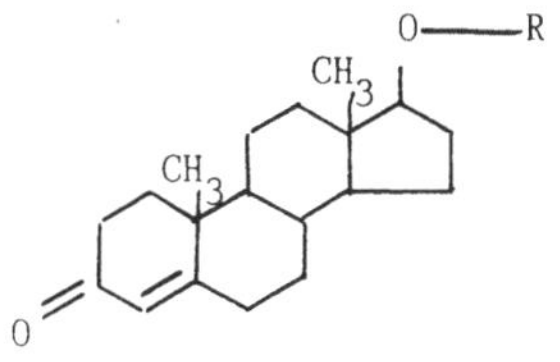

R	Steroid	Solubility[a]
H	Testosterone	40.3
$OCCH_2CH_3$	Testosterone Propionate	3.7
$OC(CH_2)_5CH_3$	Testosterone Enanthate[b]	3.1
$OC(CH_2)_2C_5H_9$	Testosterone Cypionate[c]	10.2

[a]Solubility = ug/ml in water (17)

[b]Also testosterone heptanoate

[c]Also testosterone cyclopentanepropionate

Figure 2. Steroid structure and solubility of testosterone esters used.

EXPERIMENTAL

Experiment 1

Beef females were subcutaneously implanted with 0 to 60 cm of silicone implants containing either testosterone propionate, testosterone cypionate or testosterone enanthate. The implants were made from silicone tubing (6.4 mm i.d., 9.5 mm o.d.) by sealing one end with silicone rubber medical adhesive, filling the tube with a crystalline testosterone ester and sealing the open end with adhesive. Testosterone propionate (melting point = 118-122°C) and testosterone cypionate (melting point = 101-102°C) remain in their crystalline form *in situ*. Testosterone enanthate (melting point = 36-37.5°C), however, melts at body temperature and in a liquid form only fills approximately 75% of what the crystalline form filled. Therefore, testosterone enanthate implants were filled in a hood at approximately 45°C in order that the testosterone enanthate implants would be full *in situ*. Implants were numbered and weighed both before implantation and after implant removal. Implants were subcutaneously implanted behind the shoulder or over the rib cage and were left *in situ* for 12 to 35 days. Blood plasma was collected before and after implantation and assayed for plasma testosterone concentrations by a validated testosterone enzyme immunoassay (described later).

Experiment 2

Fifteen ewes were subcutaneously implanted with 0 to 10 cm of silicone implants containing testosterone propionate. The implants were made as described in Experiment 1. Implants were subcutaneously implanted in the axilla. Blood plasma was collected before and 13 days after implantation and assayed for plasma testosterone concentrations by a validated testosterone enzyme immunoassay (described later).

Experiment 3

Five beef females were implanted with silicone implants containing testosterone propionate. Implants were made from silicone tubing (9.5 mm i.d., 12.7 mm o.d.). A polystyrene rod (4.8 mm in diameter) was fixed in the center of the implant in order to reduce the amount of testosterone propionate required to fill the implants. Two heifers were subcutaneously implanted with 22.5 cm of implants and three heifers were implanted with 45.0 cm of implants. Two blood samples were subsequently collected from each heifer and assayed for plasma testosterone concentrations via a validated enzyme immunoassay (described later). Implants were numbered and weighed both before implantation and after implant removal and secretion rate of testosterone propionate from the implants determined.

Experiment 4

Twenty-four beef heifers were assigned to one of two groups. Twelve heifers were subcutaneously implanted with a commercially manufactured testosterone propionate ear implant on day 0 and re-implanted with another implant on day 84. The other twelve heifers were implanted with two 15 cm silicone implants filled with testosterone propionate. These implants were implanted subcutaneously behind the shoulder or over the rib cage and were left *in situ* for 156 days. Blood samples were collected via jugular venipuncture immediately before implantation (day 0) and 28, 56, 84, 112, 140 and 156 days into the experiment. All samples were assayed for plasma testosterone concentrations via a validated enzyme immunoassayed (described later). The commercially manufactured implants were compressed pellets of testosterone propionate. Each implant consisted of eight compressed pellets and contained a total of 200 mg testosterone propionate (83%) hormone. The silicone implants were capsule type implants and were made as described in Experiment 1.

Testosterone Enzyme Immunoassay

The testosterone enzyme immunoassay was a solid phase double antibody competitive inhibition assay with horseradish peroxidase linked to testosterone-3-CMO. The testosterone antiserum was generated in rabbits against 4-androsten-11-α-17-β-diol-3-one-11-hemisuccinate:bovine serum albumin. Cross reaction of the antiserum was as follows: 17-β-hydroxyl-4,6-androstandien-3-one (60%), 5-α-androstan-17-β-ol-3-one (52%), 19-nortestosterone (19%), 11-α-17-β-dihydroxyl-4-androsten-3-one (8.1%), 5-α-androstane-3-β-17-β-diol (5.0%), 4-androstene-3-17-β-diol (4.0%), 4-androsten-3,17-dione (0.9%), 5-androsten-3-17-β-diol (0.3%), 5-α-androstan-3-17-dione (0.03%), 5-androsten-3-β-ol-17-one (0.02%), progesterone (0.01%), estradiol-17-β (0.01%), estrone (0.01%), deoxycorticosterone (0.01%), cortisol (0.01%), corticosterone (0.01%), cholesterol (0.01%), testosterone propionate (0.01%), testosterone enanthate (0.01%) and testosterone cypionate (0.01%). Anti-rabbit IgG was generated against rabbit IgG. Anti-rabbit IgG was purified by a 50 % ammonium sulfate saturation procedure[11] and treated with the low pH procedure reported by Ishikawa et al.[12] The enzyme labeled testosterone was prepared by coupling horseradish peroxidase to testosterone-3-O-carboxymethyloxime, using a modification of the mixed anhydride method described by Dawson et al.,[13] and later by Munro and Stabenfeldt.[14] Testosterone was extracted from plasma by adding 300 µl of the sample to a 16 x 150 mm glass culture tube. Following the addition of 3.0 mL of anesthesia grade ether, the sample was vigorously shaken on a mechanical shaker for 30 seconds. The mixture was stored at -10 to -20°C and the organic phase was decanted into 12 x 75 mm glass culture tubes. The samples were then placed into a

48 to 52 C water bath. Once dry the testosterone was reconstituted with 300 µl of a phosphate buffer solution and shaken vigorously on a mechanical shaker for 3 seconds. Samples were sealed and stored for one hour or overnight at 2-8°C. All samples were shaken for 3 seconds on a mechanical shaker immediately prior to use.

Standards were prepared from a stock solution of testosterone in ethanol (1 mg/mL). Using this stock solution and a phosphate buffer solution containing gelatin, testosterone standards were created to reflect concentrations of 0, 0.5, 1.0, 2.0, 4.0, and 10.0 ng/mL.

Polystyrene tubes (12 x 75 mm) were coated with 300 µl of the secondary antibody at 37°C for one hour. Following incubation, tubes were poured off, washed with 1 mL of distilled water three times and inverted for 3 minutes. For each assay, a standard curve was established. Each point on the curve was assayed in triplicate with 100 µl of each respective concentration added to specific tubes. For the specific sample extract, 100 µl of each sample was added and assayed in duplicate. Following the standard or sample, 100 µl of the conjugate (1:100,000) was added to each tube. The last addition was 100 µl of the primary antibody (1:10,000) per tube. It should be noted that this is the order in which the components were combined: standard or sample, conjugate and primary antibody.

With a total assay volume of 300 µl, the tubes were placed on a mechanical rotator for 3 hours at 180 rpm. Following the 3 hour period, the tubes were again poured off, washed with 1.0 mL of distilled water three time and inverted for 3 minutes. Four hundred µl of o-phenylene-diamine dihydrochloride (16.8 mM) in a citric acid-phosphate buffer was then added, and incubated in darkness for 30 minutes at room temperature. Following this incubation, 400 µl of 1.0 N sulfuric acid was added. All tubes were then shaken on a mechanical shaker for 3 seconds and read on a spectrophotometer at a wavelength of 492 nm (see Figure 3 for an outline).

Selected plasma samples were analyzed by enzyme immunoassay and by a validated radioimmunoassay.[15] An excellent correlation (r = 0.97: P < 0.01) was observed between the values obtained by both types of assays. The sensitivity of the assay as determined by the smallest amount of unlabeled hormone that was significantly different from zero was 10.0 pg per assay tube. In order to determine if nonspecific materials in the sample interfere with an accurate determination, 50, 100 and 200 µl of plasma samples from two males were assayed in triplicate. The parallelism exhibited by the groups had a correlation coefficient of 0.99 (P < 0.01). Mean concentrations of plasma testosterone were 4.4, 4.1 and 4.4 ng/mL for 50, 100, and 200 µl of plasma, respectively. Aliquots of a pool sample from a bull were assayed in the same assay (intraassay) and different assays (interassay). The intraassay and interassay coefficients of variation for 9 assays were 5.8% and 9.7%, respectively. The accuracy of the assay was tested by adding known amounts of testosterone to a constant volume (100 µl) of a low pool sample before extraction. The percentage recovery was 110%. Pool samples assayed both at the front and end of the assays averaged 3.3 and 3.5 ng/mL, respectively.

RESULTS

Experiment 1

Figure 4 illustrates plasma testosterone concentrations of beef females implanted with silicone implants containing testosterone enan-

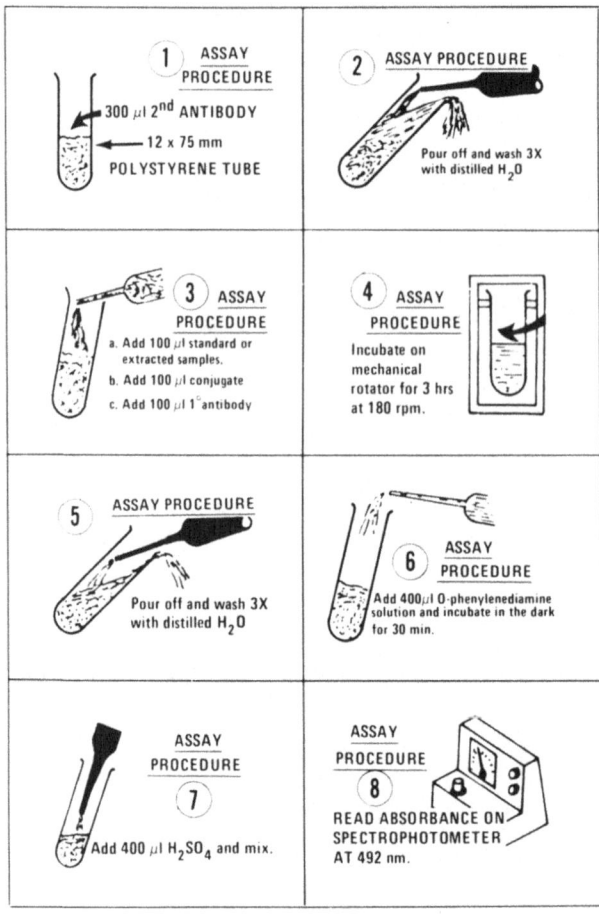

Figure 3. Testosterone enzyme immunoassay procedure.

thate, testosterone propionate and testosterone cypionate and reports secretion rates of the testosterone esters through the silicone implants. Plasma testosterone concentrations increased linearly with implant length (surface area) for all the testosterone esters. Because of increased passage rates, less implant surface area was required to elevate plasma testosterone concentrations to 1.0 ng/mL for testosterone propionate and testosterone enanthate than for testosterone cypionate even though the dosage required was similar (Table 1).

Table 1. Implant length and dosage of tesosterone esters required to elevate blood testosterone concentrations to 1.0 ng/ml.

Testosterone ester	Implant length (cm)	Dosage (mg/day)
Enanthate	10.4	9.05
Propionate	18.9	11.91
Cypionate	70.9	11.34

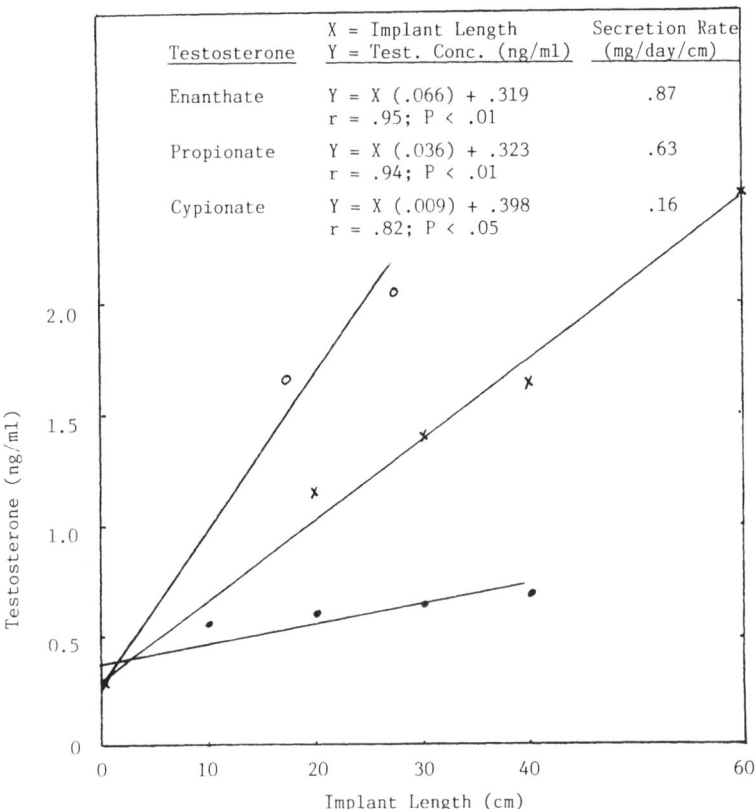

Testosterone	X = Implant Length Y = Test. Conc. (ng/ml)	Secretion Rate (mg/day/cm)
Enanthate	Y = X (.066) + .319 r = .95; P < .01	.87
Propionate	Y = X (.036) + .323 r = .94; P < .01	.63
Cypionate	Y = X (.009) + .398 r = .82; P < .05	.16

Figure 4. Plasma testosterone concentrations of beef females
implanted with testerone enanthate, testosterone
propionate and testosterone cypionate.

Experiment 2

Increasing the length of implants (surface area) increased plasma
testosterone concentrations linearly (r = 0.93; P < 0.01) as in beef
females in Experiment 1 (Table 2).

Table 2. Actual and predicted testosterone concentrations for
various lengths of poly(dimethylsiloxane) implants
containing testosterone propionate implanted in ewes.

Implant length (cm)	Actual testosterone concentrations (ng/ml)	Estimated testosterone concentrations (ng/ml)
0.0	0.15	0.23
2.5	0.83	0.85
5.0	1.65	1.47
10.0	2.63	2.72

Experiment 3

Results in this experiment were similar to Experiment 1 for testosterone propionate in that the secretion rate was directly related to surface area implanted and increased surface area elevated plasma testosterone concentrations (Table 3).

Experiment 4

Mean testosterone concentrations in plasma (1.10 ng/mL) were very similar to predicted concentrations (1.09 ng/mL; based on results in Experiment 1 and corrected for time *in situ*). Concentrations of testosterone in the plasma for the silicone implanted heifers were not only higher than for the heifers implanted with compressed pellets but concentrations were also less variable as illustrated in Figure 5. The coefficient of variation was four times greater for testosterone concentrations in the heifers implanted with compressed pellets than for the silicone implanted heifers.

DISCUSSION

Results in the four experiments clearly demonstrate that testosterone esters pass through poly(dimethylsiloxane). Our *in vivo* results demonstrate that testosterone enanthate passes more rapidly through poly(dimethylsiloxane) than testosterone propionate and both pass more rapidly than testosterone cypionate. We have previously demonstrated that testosterone propionate passed five times more rapidly through poly(dimethylsiloxane) than native testosterone.[16] These *in vivo* results agree with Tojo et al. except in regard to testosterone enanthate.[17] Tojo and coworkers observed that testosterone enanthate passed through poly(dimethylsiloxane) *in vitro* even more slowly than testosterone.[17] The data reported herein, however, more closely agree with our previous

Table 3. Actual testosterone concentrations for various lengths of poly(dimethylsiloxane) implants containing testosterone propionate in beef females.

Implant length (cm)	Testosterone concentrations (ng/ml)		
22.5	1.87		
45.0	2.33		
Testosterone prediction			
Implant size (mm)	Wall thickness (mm)	Secretion rate (mg/cm²)	Equation
6.4 x 9.5	3.15	0.211	$Y = X (0.0119) \pm 0.32$
9.5 x 12.7	3.15	0.199	$Y = X (0.0115) \pm 0.42$
6.4 x 9.5 mm implant data are from Experiment 1.			

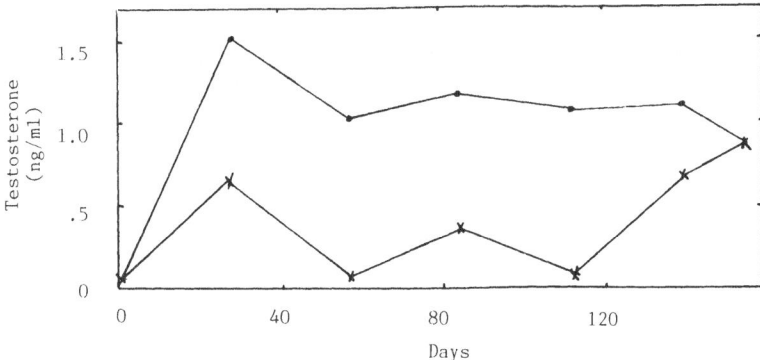

Figure 5. Plasma testosterone concentrations in one heifer implanted with silicone implants containing testosterone propionate (o) and one heifer implanted with pellets of testosterone propionate (x).

reports.[15,16] Therefore, based on *in vivo* data, secretion rate of androgens was inversely related to solubility.[17]

Results in the four experiments also demonstrate that total surface area, regardless of whether by increasing diameter or by increasing implant length, increased secretion rate and elevated testosterone concentrations proportionally.

Since silicone implants containing testosterone propionate were demonstrated to maintain relatively constant blood testosterone concentrations they have been used in several studies to evoke various biological responses. Three such responses are: (1) the induction of and maintenance of male sexual behavior, (2) an anabolic effect and (3) prenatal androgenization.

Accurate estrus detection is essential in order for livestock producers to use artificial insemination and/or embryo transfer. Estrous detector animals as aids in estrus detection have been demonstrated to be helpful in detecting estrus. In the past, the detector animals have been males surgically altered to prevent intromission and/or impregnation of the females in estrus. More recently, testosterone-treated females have been successfully used as estrous detector animals. There are several advantages of testosterone-treated females as estrous detector animals over surgically altered males. First, there would be little, if any, chance of transmitting sexually transmittable diseases. Second, there would be less costs associated with testosterone-treated females than surgically altered males. Furthermore, testosterone-treated females were more gentle to handle than males, they do not become frustrated like some surgically altered males become and they will detect estrous females more quickly than males.

Ten cm silicone implants filled with testosterone propionate induced and maintained male sexual behavior in ewes[16] and 30 cm silicone implants filled with testosterone propionate maintained male sexual behavior in cows.[18] Testosterone-treated ewes, induced and maintained with 10 cm silicone/testosterone propionate implants, began to mount estrus females within two weeks and exhibited males sexual behavior similar to a ram from that time onwards.[16] Under field conditions, testosterone-treated cows, in which the male sexual behavior was maintained with 30 cm silicone/testosterone propionate implants, detected 94% of 342 estrus. These implants were also far more convenient than previously used procedures which consisted of injections every other day for 20 days and every 10 days thereafter. These silicone/testosterone propionate implants, therefore, are a convenient, economical and effective way to develop testosterone-treated females for livestock producers.

Anabolic agents have been desired by livestock producers for some time. Several anabolic implants have been developed that are currently available. Most of these products consist of steroids in the form of compressed pellets. One, however, is a poly(dimethylsiloxane) based implant that delivers estradiol. There are no poly(dimethylsiloxane) based anabolic implants that delivers androgens. We have tested the feasibility of a poly(dimethylsiloxane) based androgen implant for stimulating growth rate and feed efficiency in beef heifers and results reported in Table 4 clearly demonstrate the efficacy of such an implant.

A key to improving the economic competitiveness of mammals as sources of protein in the human and/or animal diet lies in improving the carcass merit (relative ratio of lean meat to fat), growth rate and feed efficiency (i.e., decreasing the amount of feed required per unit of weight gain). Female ruminants grow approximately 6 to 15% slower and are 4 to 12% less efficient in converting feed to weight gain than intact male herd-mates. We have discovered that carcass merit of female mammals can be improved by exposing the female mammal solely during its gestation to androgens.[19] This is conveniently done by administering to the mother during pregnancy an effectively constant amount of androgen sufficient to achieve and maintain a level of circulating androgen in the mother's bloodstream approximately equivalent to that of a normal adult male of the same species. To obtain and maintain a relatively constant level of circulating androgens in the mother's bloodstream, we have used silicone implants filled with testosterone propionate as previously described.

Upon the completion of several trials to date we have reported a 16.4 to 19.5% increase in average daily gain due to prenatal androgenization.[20,21] Furthermore, prenatally androgenized heifers have been 13.6 to 14.6% more efficient in converting feed to gain and have less subcutaneous and internal fat at slaughter. Results to date clearly demon-

Table 4. Daily gain and feed/gain of beef heifers administered Synovex-H and testosteone propionate (TP)/silicone implants.

Treatment	Daily Gain	Feed/Gain
Control	2.47	7.69
Synovex-H	2.61	7.97
TP/silicone implant	2.90	6.87

Synovex-H is a commercially available anabolic implant. (TP is compressed pellets).

There were 30 cm of testosterone propionate/silicone implants implanted in group 3.

TP/silicone implanted heifers had a greater (P < 0.05) daily gain than controls.

TP/silicone implanted heifers were more feed efficient (P < 0.05) than both control and Synovex-H treated heifers.

strate that prenatal androgenization via silicone/testosterone propionate implants improves efficiency of heifers and lambs as red meat producers. It should also be noted that prenatally androgenized offspring have very few phenotypic changes. Early research demonstrated that androgens administrated early in gestation (at a similar time to prenatal androgenization) via injections or poorly controlled implants caused complete masculinization. In fact, ewe lambs treated early in gestation were born with a penis, an empty scrotal sac and not an external vaginal opening.[22] We have never seen any of the responses that were reported earlier in either cattle or sheep.[20,21] We hypothesize that the different exists because our poly(dimethylsiloxane) based implants deliver a much more constant level of androgen to the fetus which avoids completely masculinizing the offspring. This is, to say it mildly, quite advantageous today with increased awareness of animal treatments.

REFERENCES

1. J. Folkman & D. M. Long, J. Surg. Res., **4**, 139 (1964).
2. J. Folkman, D. M. Long, Jr. & R. Rosenbaum, Science, **154**, 148 (1966).
3. D. M. Long, Jr. & J. Folkman, U.S. Patent 3,279,996 (1966).
4. P. J. Dziuk & B. Cook, Endocrinology, **78**, 208 (1966).
5. V. Lee & J. R. Robinson, In: "*Sustained and Controlled Release Drug Delivery Systems*", J. R. Robinson, Ed., Marcel Dekker, Inc., New York, 1985.
6. Y. W. Chien, In: "*Sustained and Controlled Release Drug Delivery Systems*", J. R. Robinson, Ed., Marcel Dekker, Inc., New York, 1978.
7. Y. W. Chien & H. J. Lambert, U.S. Patent 3,946,106 (1976).
8. J. M. Anderson, Proc. Internat. Symp. Controlled Release of Bioactive Materials, Controlled Release Society, Toronto, Canada, 1987, p. 1.
9. R. I. Dorfman & D. C. Sharma, Steroids, **6**, 229 (1965).
10. A. A. Sinkula, In: "*Sustained and Controlled Release Drug Delivery Systems*", J. R. Robinson, Ed., Marcel Dekker, Inc., New York, 1978.
11. K. Heide & H. G. Schwick, In: "*Handbook of Experimental Immunology*", D. M. Weir, Ed., Blackwell, Oxford, England, 1978.
12. E. Ishikawa, Y. Hamaguchi & M. Imagawa, J. Immunoassay, **1**, 385 (1980).
13. E. C. Dawson, A. E. M. C. Dennison & B. K. VanWeemen, Steroids, **31**, 357 (1978).
14. C. Munro & G. Stabenfeldt, J. Endocrinology, **101**, 141 (1984).
15. D. C. Christensen & D. J. Kesler, Anim. Reprod. Sci., **7**, 531 (1984).
16. N. S. Scheffrahn, B. S. Wiseman, R. A. Nowak & D. J. Kesler, Theriogenology, **18**, 1 (1982).
17. K. Tojo, Y. Sun & Y. W. Chien in: "*Proc. Internat. Controlled Release of Bioactive Materials*", Controlled Release Society, Geneva, Switzerland, 1985, p.153.
18. D. J. Kesler, T. R. Troxel, D. L. Vincent, N. S. Scheffrahn & R. C. Noble, Theriogenology, **15**, 327 (1981).
19. L. L. Berger & D. J. Kesler, U.S. Patent (Filed 7/28/1986; U.S. Serial Number 891,151).
20. K. C. DeHaan, L. L. Berger, D. J. Kesler, F. K. McKeith, D. L. Thomas & T. G. Nash, J. Anim. Sci., **65**, 1465 (1987).
21. K. C. DeHaan, L. L. Berger, D. J. Kesler, F. K. McKeith, D. B. Faulkner & G. F. Cmarik, J. Anim. Sci., in press.
22. I. J. Clarke, R. J. Scarmuzzi & R. V. Short, J. Embryol. Exp. Morph., **6**, 87 (1976).

KINETICS OF SYNTHESIS AND DEGRADATION OF THE POLYMER DERIVED FROM

TETRACHLOROPLATINATE AND METHOTREXATE

Charles. E. Carraher, Jr. and Rickey E. Strothers

Florida Atlantic University
Department of Chemistry
Boca Raton, FL 33431

The kinetics of formation and degradation were determined for the coordination polymer formed from tetrachloroplatinate and methotrexate. Synthesis occurs through pseudo-second order kinetics. Degradation occurs rapidly in DMSO, DMSO/H_2O and as a solid in H_2O. Degradation in DMSO occurs through a random scission mechanism.

INTRODUCTION

Malignant neoplasms are the second leading cause of death in the United States. As a result, much research has been devoted to the treatment of these illnesses. The chemotherapeutic treatment of such neoplasms are of interest here.

After thirty years of use, methotrexate, MTX, [1] remains as one of the most important anti-cancer agents.[1] MTX was introduced as an anti-leukemic agent and it was originally designed to inhibit the utilization of folic acid.

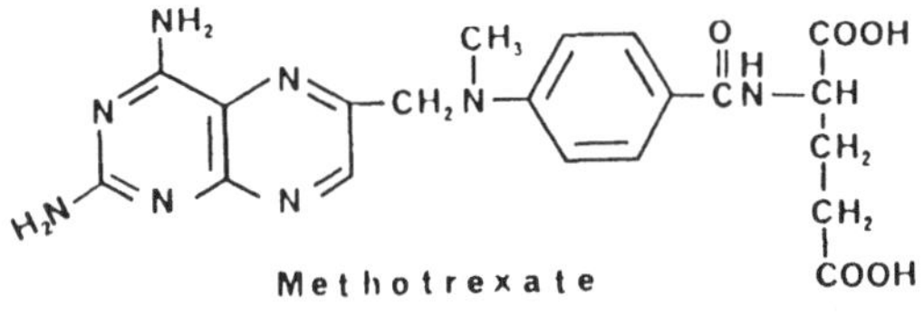

Methotrexate

Structure 1.

In 1964, Rosenberg and coworkers discovered that bacteria failed to divide, but continued to grow into filamentous cells in the presence of platinum electrodes.[2] Later, the cause was traced to certain electrolysis products generated from the platinum electrodes while passing an electric current through the growth medium of the bacteria. Specifically, they were cis-dichlorodiamine Pt (II), (c-DDP), [2] and cis-tetrachlorodiamine Pt (IV), (c-TCP).[3]

$$\begin{array}{ccc} Cl & & Cl \\ & \diagdown\,\diagup & \\ & Pt & \\ & \diagup\,\diagdown & \\ NH_3 & & NH_3 \end{array}$$

Cis — DDP

Structure 2.

C-DDP was licensed in 1980 under the trade name Platinol and is widely used in conjunction with other anticancer agents.[4] The success of c-DDP initiated the synthesis and characterization of a number of structural analogs for potential anticancer activity.[5] In 1974, Carraher and Scott synthesized numerous polymeric derivatives of form [3].[6] Included in the diamines used was 1, 6-hexanediamine.

$$\begin{array}{ccc} Cl & & Cl \\ & \diagdown\,\diagup & \\ & Pt & \\ & \diagup\,\diagdown & \\ & & NH_2-R-NH_2 \end{array}$$

Structure 3. Polymeric derivative studied, [3].

More recently, Carraher and Lopez employed MTX as the diamine.[7] Both products exhibited good antitumor activity and low toxicities. The 1,6-hexanediamine product, Pt-HDA, was found to inhibit L929, WISH, and HeLa cells completely at concentrations greater than 50 µg/mL, with lowered toxicity to the test mice. For example, about twice the LD_{50} dosage, based on c-DDP, has been administered to mice every other day for thirty days without any occurrence of death.

The studies involving the polymeric derivatives of c-DDP, hereafter simply referred to as polyamines, involved only biological and structural characterization. The current study includes the kinetic characterization of the compounds derived from MTX and K_2PtCl_4.

METHOTREXATE

MTX has been used in the treatment of acute leukemia, osteosarcoma, and head, neck and breast cancer with good success.[8] MTX is primarily absorbed from the gastrointestinal tract and delivered mainly to the liver and kidneys. Absorption into the central nervous system is excluded. It is not significantly metabolized, being excreted mostly through the kidneys.[9]

High-dose MTX therapy has been accompanied by serious complications. Although most therapy results in only small side effects, severe prolonged myleosuppression and mucositis have developed in 10% of the patients, and fatalities directly related to MTX drug toxicity have been found in about 6% of the patients.[10]

MTX was designed to inhibit the utilization of the vitamin folic acid. Ten years later, the enzyme dihydrofolate reductase DHFR, was shown to be its primary target.[11] MTX owes its activity to its ability to bind the DHFR almost irreversibly, preventing the formation of tetrahydrafolic acid which is a coenzyme essential for DNA synthesis.

Its close structural appearance to folic acid, along with the fact that it was found to be a competitive inhibitor of DHFR, would lead one to conclude that MTX would bind to the reductase in the same manner as folic acid. However, recently there has been evidence that MTX binds to the reductase in a different manner than that of folic acid. Matthews determined the crystal structure of the binary complex of MTX with DHFR from *Escherichia coli*.[12] The MTX molecule binds in a cavity 15 A deep and a minimum of 13 amine acid residues are involved in the binding. MTX binding to DHFR is about three orders of magnitude greater than that of folic acid. It has been proposed that the substitution of a hydroxyl group with an amine group at C-4 increases the basicity of the pteridine ring by about three pK units. Further, it is thought that the protonation of the ring occurs most readily at N-1, which strongly interacts with the side of aspartic acid-27.

CIS-DICHLORODIAMINE PLATINUM (II)

Cis-dichlorodiamine platinum (II), which is known as Platinol and cis-platin in the literature, has assumed a valuable role in cancer chemotherapy. C-DDP has been used successfully with sensitive tumors such as testicular carcinoma, lymphoma, squamous cell carcinoma of the head, and neck, and ovarian carcinoma. However, the drug has a low therapeutic index and displays a high level of negative side effects. These include gastrointestinal hematopoietic, immunosupression, and auditory and renal dysfunction. The auditory and renal dysfunctions are the most serious side effects. Hearing losses in the 4000-8000 Hz range followed by losses in the spoken range, 1000-4000 Hz, can develop. Total deafness indicates death is imminent. Although nephrotoxicity has been reduced by vigorous hydration, renal damage is cumulative and eventually irreversible.

The exact mode of activity of c-DDP on cells is uncertain, although the bulk of evidence at present favors the theory that DNA damage and synthesis of DNA on a damaged template is directly responsible for its cytotoxic effect. X-ray diffraction studies have shown that a bidentate chelate is formed with the reaction of inosine and c-DDP.[13] The product consists of two hypoxanthine rings bound to the platinum ion at the N-7 position. Other suggestions have been made involving inter-strand and intra-strand crosslinking and DNA-protein crosslinking. Whichever is the case, it is clear that DNA is the primary cellular target of c-DDP.

THE TRANS EFFECT

The trans effect is an empirical rule which is most simply defined as "the effect of a coordinated group upon the rate of substitution reactions of ligands opposite to it in a metal complex".[14]

In 1926, Chugaev introduced the concept of the trans effect in order to correlate many of the reactions of Pt (II) complexes.[15] Since then, numerous explanations have been presented to explain the effect in electronic structural terms. When a good trans directing ligand, in a square planer geometry, is opposite a leaving group, the energy of activation for substitution of that leaving group is lowered. This can be accomplished by either raising the energy of the ground state or by lowering of the energy of the transition state.

Another view to explain the trans effect emphasizes the importance of sigma donor ligands. A good sigma donor ligand will more effectively weaken the trans bond since it will claim a larger share of metal sigma orbits leaving a lesser share for the trans ligand.

MODE OF SUBSTITUTION

Substitution in square planer complexes is thought to proceed through a trigonal bipyramid geometry. In general, Pt^{2+} complexes substitute by an associative mechanism (A-mechanism).[17] For the A-type mechanism the trigonal bipyramid is considered an intermediate rather than a transition state. Hammond's postulate states that the geometry of the transition state (that is not far along the reaction coordinate) will be similar to that of the intermediate. Thus, features that stabilize the transition state will in turn stabilize the trigonal bipyramid intermediate lowering the energy of activation. Sigma donation and pi acceptance offer such stabilization and ligands which possess these characteristics are good trans directors.[18]

Square planer substitution of Pt (II) involves a bimolecular displacement mechanism through the five coordinate intermediates previously described. Arguments for this mechanism can also be given in experimental evidences.

First, a large number of reactions of cis and trans PtA_2LX with E give PtA_2LE products have been studied and, without exception, cis substrates give cis produces and trans substrates give trans products.[19]

The observed high degree of stereospecificity would be unlikely for a dissociative mechanism, since the three coordinated species, which would be involved, would at times be of a nearly regular triangular planer geometry and depending on whether E enters adjacent or opposite to L, it would give the cis and trans isomers, respectively. Therefore, a mixture of both isomers would result. Second, the existence of stable five coordinate Pt(II) species, such as $Pt(SnCl_3)_5^{3-}$ and $Pt(PEt_3)_2H(SnCL_3)_2^-$, argue for the associative mechanism. Finally, kinetic studies of Pt(II) complexes typically give a two term rate law, as shown in Equation 1. This two term rate law indicates a two path reaction mechanism. The rate constant k_1, is associated with the slow displacement of X by the solvent S, which is then rapidly replaced by E. The rate constant k_2 is associated with the direct displacement of X by E.

$$\text{Rate} = k_1 [L_3PtX] + k_2 [PtX][E] \qquad \text{(Equation 1)}$$

EXPERIMENTAL

Chemical

The following chemicals were used without further purification: K_2PtCl_4 (99.9% pure), J & J Materials, Inc. (Neptune City, NJ); Methotrexate, Monsanto Research Corp. (Dayton, OH); 1,6-Hexanediamine, Matheson, Coleman & Bell (Norwood, OH); Dimethylsulfoxide (analytical grade; Mallinckrodt, Inc. (St. Louis, MO); Potassium Iodide, Fisher Scientific Co. (Fairlawn, NJ).

Synthesis

A 250 mL Erlenmeyer flask was employed as the reaction vessel in all syntheses. The Pt-MTX polymer was prepared by heating 1.00 mmole of MTX in 30 mL of distilled water. An equimolar amount of K_2PtCl_4 is added directly to the MTX solution, heating is discontinued, and the solution is magnetically stirred for a specified amount of time. In selected cases, the reaction is "quenched" by addition of K_2PtI_4. The K_2PtI_4 had previously been prepared by heating an aqueous solution of K_2PtCl_4 and KI (in a 1:4 molar ratio) for 20 minutes, and then allowed to cool to room temperature[20].

In the case of Pt-MTX polymers the precipitated products were recovered using vacuum filtration, washed several times with distilled water, and finally transferred to a petri dish at which time they were allowed to air dry.

Physical Characterization

Percentage yields were calculated based on the repeat unit of the polymer [3]. Percentage yields were typically in the range of 80-90%.

Instrumental Methods

Mass spectral analysis was carried out by the Nebraska Mass Spectrometry Service Laboratory. Analysis was carried out using a direct insertion probe connected to a Kratos MS-50 mass spectrometer operating in the E. I. mode, 8 kv acceleration and 10 sec/decade scan rate with a probe temperature of 350 to 450°C.

Infrared spectra were obtained using potassium bromide pellets in a Nicolet 5DX-FTIR. Identification of the peaks was accomplished by using spectra of the monomers and previous assignments from the literature.[21]

Molecular weights were obtained using a Brice-Phoenix model BP-3000 Universal Light Scattering Photometer employing serial dilutions of DMSO-polymer solutions. Refractive index increments, dn/dc, were obtained using a Baush and Lomb Abbe Refractometer model 3-L.

I/Cl ratios were determined by Galbraith Laboratory, Knoxville, TN.

Kinetics

The polymerization kinetics were followed by varying the reaction times and determining the molecular weights by light scattering photometry employing the serial dilution method. Attempts were made to follow the reactions at shorter times by UV/Visible spectrophotometry. The monomers and polymers were scanned from 900-190 nm and in all cases the bands of the monomers and polymers were found to overlap such that the reaction could not be easily monitored by this method.

Degradation

Chemical degradation of the Pt-MTX polymer was carried out in DMSO, DMSO/H_2O (90:10 v/v), and in water. For the solution of DMSO, approximately 0.25 grams of Pt-MTX was dissolved in 250 mL of DMSO. At specific times, 25 mL aliquots of the solution were removed. The aliquot taken was then replaced with an equal amount of DMSO. The weight average molecular weight was then determined using light scattering photometry.

Because the Pt-MTX exhibits such a low solubility in water, the Pt-MTX was placed in water, agitated briefly, and allowed to set for a specified amount of time. Times of 0.5, 1.0, 1.5, 2.0, 2.5, 3.0, 3.5, 4.0, and 5.0 hours were chosen since previous results showed rapid degradation in DMSO and it was expected water would also act in a like fashion.

RESULTS AND DISCUSSION

Structural Characterization

The major purpose of this paper is to present kinetic data, thus physical characterization data will be only briefly presented. Fourier transform infrared spectroscopy, FTIR, was carried out on the reactants and products. Below 600 (all bands are given in cm^{-1}) new bands appear in the polymer at 338, 362, 408, 450, 512, and 521 and most are attributed to the Pt-N stretch which is consistent with complexation occurring at several of the MTX-nitrogens. It is believed that the band at 512 corresponds to the band reported at 508 for the symmetrical Pt-N stretch and the band observed at 521 corresponds to the reported band at 517 for the Pt-N asymmetrical stretch in $Pt(NH_3)Cl_2$.[21] The bands at 324 and 286 are assigned to the Pt-Cl stretch and correspond well to the literature values of 332 and 282 ($Pt(NH_3)_2Cl_2$).[21]

Elemental analysis is consistent with a product as depicted in [3]: %Pt: calcd., 27.1 found 26.6; %Cl: calcd. 9.9, found 11.0; ratio of Cl/Pt = 2.1; %C: calcd. 33.3, found 32.7; %H: calcd. 3.0, found 3.0; and %N: calcd. 15.6, found 14.8.

The mass spectral data is also consistent with [3]. Thus the ion fragments at 367 (all ion fragments given in amu or Daltons) are characteristic of MTX minus two CO_2 groups and 322 characteristic of MTX minus the carboxylic acid containing chain.

KINETICS

Timed Reactions

Reactions of K_2PtCl_4 with MTX were carried out as a function of time. The solid product was removed from solution by vacuum filtration and its weight average molecular weight determined. Sample results appear in Table 1.

The relationship between degree of polymerization, DP, and reaction time varies according to the mechanism of reaction. For chain reaction kinetics, DP is approximately constant as the reaction time increases. Conversely, in stepwise kinetics DP increases steadily throughout the reaction. First order or pseudo-first order reactions give a linear relationship for plots of ln(DP) vs. reaction time; second order re-

Table 1. Weight average molecular weight of Pt-MTX polymers.

Reaction time, hrs.	Product	M_w (g/m)	Average DP_w
6	Pt-MTX	3960	5.5
18		20160	28.0
24		27650	38.4

actions give linear plots of DP vs. reaction time; and third order reactions yield a linear relationship between DP^{-2} and reaction time.[23]

The present system showed a linear plot of DP as a function of reaction time. The relationship of such stepwise order reactions is given by Equation 2, where $[PtCl_4^2] = [MTX] = [A_o]$ and $[A_o]$ is the starting molar concentration, k is the observed rate constant, and t is the reaction time. Regression analysis shows a linear relationship with a correlation coefficient of 0.998 and an observed rate constant of $k = 1.0 \times 10^{-2}$ liter $mole^{-1}$ sec^{-1} (Figure 1). The Y-intercept for the system is not one, as suggested by Equation 3. This indicates additional factors are involved.

$$DP = k[A_o]t + 1 \qquad\qquad \text{(Equation 2)}$$

Previous studies by Carraher and Scott (6) found the relative reaction rates of tetrahaloplatinates with diamines to be $PtI_4^{2-} > PtBr_4^{2-} > PtCl_4^{2-}$ such that yields greater than 80% occur in minutes with PtI_4^{2-} while comparable yields with $PtCl_4^{2-}$ generally took over four hours. It was thought this difference could be used to differentiate between stepwise and chain reaction kinetics. In chain reaction kinetics the monomers are added rapidly and consecutively at the reaction chain end. By filtering off the precipitate and adding K_2PtI_4 to the filtrate, the PtI_4^{2-} would react preferentially over $PtCl_4^{2-}$ and thus, give a high I/Cl ratio for newly precipitated material. In the case of stepwise kinetics,

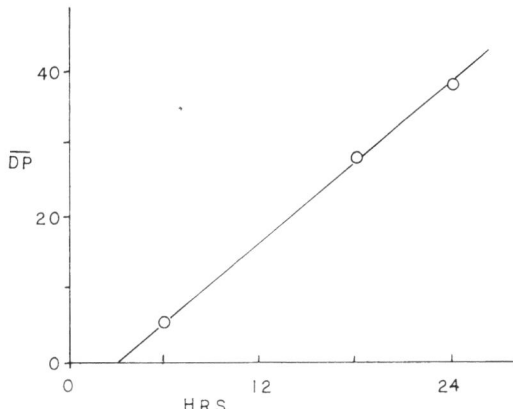

Figure 1. Average degree of polymerization versus reaction time for the Pt-MTX polymer.

most of the monomer disappears early in the reaction forming small chains and the I/Cl ratio should be small for products formed directly after addition of the PtI_4^{2-}; in fact, the ratio should be less than one.

Reactions were run for various times and the %I and %Cl determined. In all cases, the I/Cl ratio is greater than one which is consistent with chain reaction kinetics. However, the I/Cl ratios are dependable for differentiating between stepwise and chain reaction kinetics only if the halides already incorporated in the chains are not capable of exchange with free halides in the solution. In order to determine if exchange was occurring, Pt-HDA polymer (DP = 6) was placed in solution with PtI_4^{2-} and allowed to stir for 10 minutes. The solid product was recovered, washed with distilled water, air dried, and the I/Cl ratio determined. If no exchange occurs, the greatest ratio of I to Cl would be 2:3. An I/Cl ratio of four to every one Cl was found. Thus, the results show the I/Cl ratio method of determining reaction kinetics to be unreliable and any conclusions drawn from this approach are also unreliable.

As discussed in the Introduction, studies of similar systems, except employing monomines (e.g., $PtCl_4^{2-}$ and NH_3), involved two separate pathways, resulting in a two term rate law (Equation 3) where, $k_1 = k'[H_2O]$.

$$\text{Rate} = k_1[PtCl_4^{2-}] + k_2[PtCl_4^{2-}][NH_3] \hspace{2cm} \text{(Equation 3)}$$

The reaction was studied under pseudo first order conditions as described by Equation 4. The rate constants k_1 and k_2 are determined by a plot of k_{obs} versus [Y].

$$k_{obs} = k_1 + k_2[Y] \hspace{4cm} \text{(Equation 4)}$$

Thus, k_1 is the Y-intercept and k_2 the slope of the line. Attempts to determine k_1 and k_2 were unsuccessful. Varying the concentration of the diamine resulted in insoluble, possibly network, polymers and the DP could not be determined; thus no k_{obs} could be determined.

Attempts to follow the reactions at short times employing UV-Vis spectroscopy have failed. However, after precipitation, the kinetic data are consistent with a second order, stepwise polymerization. These results suggest that the replacement of Cl by H_2O has diminished influence on the observed reaction rate at long times, for these particular reactions.

It may be that the precipitated oligomeric product tends to "ward off" water, thereby allowing the direct displacement of Cl with the amine to be the rate determining step. Another possibility is that the formation of the Pt-N bond is now the rate determining step, because at least one of the reactants is already incorporated into the insoluble chain.

Degradation

There are two main aspects of study for the degradation of the platinum polyamines. First, the rate of degradation is important since this should be indicative of the mobility, location, and half life of the polymer in the body. Monomeric platinum compounds typically have more mobility, are less limited to location, and have shorter half lives (less than 24 hours) than their polymeric counterparts. Second, determining the type of degradation is important, since it may allow better structure tailoring to achieve desired release rates of monomeric and/or oligomeric degradation products for biomedical applications.

Random scission can be thought of as the converse of stepwise polymerization. Chain rupture occurs at random points along the chain leaving fragments which are large compared to the monomer units. Chain depolymerization can be considered the reverse of chain polymerization and involves successive release of monomer units from a chain end in a depropagation reaction.

The chemical degradation of the Pt-MTX polymer in DMSO, DMSO/H_2O and H_2O was carried out as described in the experimental section.

The degradation of Pt-MTX in DMSO is rapid (Figure 2). The DP of the polymer decreases from 22.4 to 7.2, a 68% drop, in six hours. By 48 hours, the degradation product has stabilized corresponding to a DP of about 1.2. This indicates that M_w determined in DMSO should be obtained shortly after solution is achieved. This is the case for all results reported, unless otherwise noted.

A second study involved placing known amounts of solid Pt-MTX polymer in water, followed by retrieval of the polymer after a specified amount of time. Over 99% of original solid was retrieved from all studies. The retrieved solid was dried, dissolved in DMSO and the DP determined employing light scattering photometry. Degradation of the solid in water is rapid with the polymer becoming reduced to its stable degradation product within one hour (Figure 3). Degradation of the Pt-MTX polymer in DMSO/H_2O is rapid, reaching its stable degradation product within one hour (Figure 4). The polymer undergoes a DP reduction of 22.4 to about 1. The observation that the polymer degrades when exposed to water, coupled with the previous observations that the DP increases in an aqueous reaction mixture, indicates several possibilities. First, in order for chain length to continue to increase, some MTX or $PtCl_4^{-2}$ may need to be present in the reaction solution. Second, drying the polymer may render it inactive with regards to further reaction. Both of these alternatives have been tested employing HDA as an analogous diamine. The HDA studies, which will be discussed in detail later, showed that increased chain lengths occurred for both "wet" and "dried" products.

Thus, the observations with respect to the Pt-MTX product are currently not fully understood. Also, the Pt-MTX polymer is much less stable in water and DMSO when compared to the Pt-HDA polymer. There may be additional factors related to the Pt-MTX instability, or the presence of additional functional groups may allow alternative pathways for degradation compared to the Pt-HDA polymer, or it may be that degradation occurs more rapidly for the Pt-MTX product compared with chain lengthening steps after some specified time.

In order to determine the route of degradation, relationships have been developed relating DP to time. The Schultz-Flory equation (Equation 5) was developed to describe random chain scission.[24]

$$1/(DP)_t = 1/(DP)_o + 0.5k[K]t. \qquad \text{(Equation 5)}$$

In Equation 5, $(DP)_t$ is the weight average degree of polymerization at time t, $(DP)_o$ is the original weight average degree of polymerization, k is the rate of chain scission and [K] is the catalyst molar concentration. For solution catalyst degradation [K] can be considered to be a

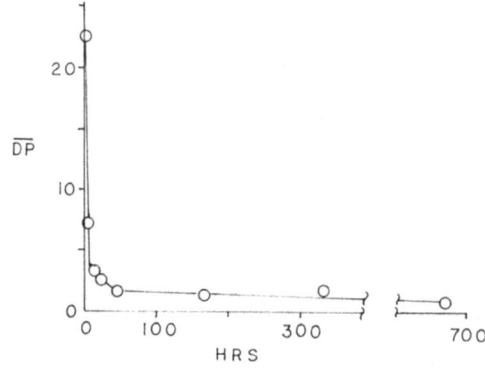

Figure 2. Average degree of polymerization versus time for the
degradation of the Pt-MTX polymer in DMSO.

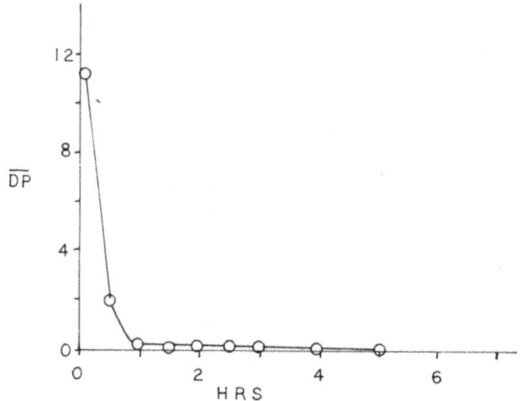

Figure 3. Average degree of polymerization versus time for the
degradation of the Pt-MTX polymer in water.

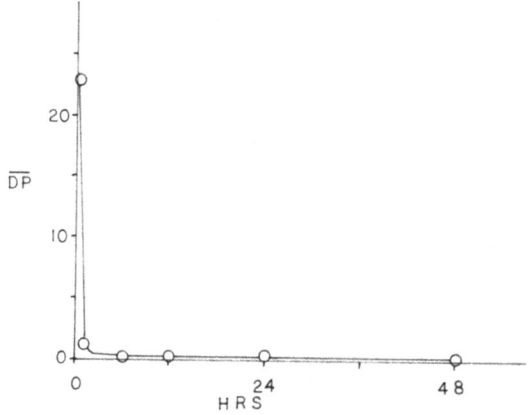

Figure 4. Average degree of polymerization versus time for the
degradation of the Pt-MTX polymer in DMSO/water.

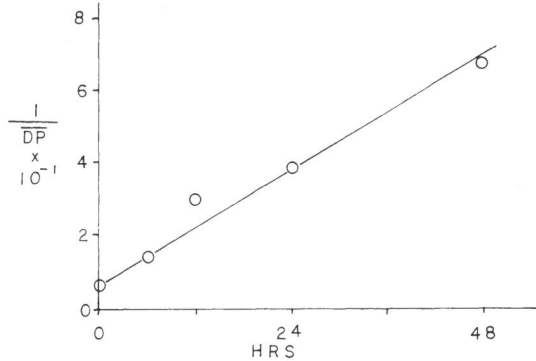

Figure 5. Reciprocal average degree of polymerization versus
time for the degradation of the Pt-MTX polymer in
DMSO.

constant. Thus, a plot of $1/(DP)_t$ vs. time should give a straight line
with a slope of $0.5 k[K]$ and a Y-intercept of $1/(DP)_0$. The plot of
$1/(DP)_t$ vs. t (Figure 5) for the Pt-MTX polymer in DMSO is linear with a
correlation coefficient of $r = 0.980$ from regression analysis, consistent
with random scission degradation.

REFERENCES

1. S. Neidle & M. J. Waring, "*Molecular Aspects of Anti-Cancer Drug
   Action*", Macmillan Press, New York, 1983.
2. B. Rosenbert, L. Van Camp & T. Krigas, Nature, **205**, 698-699 (1965).
3. C. E. Carraher & C. G. Gebelein, "*Bioactive Polymeric Systems: An
   Overview*", Plenum Press, New York, 1985.
4. A. P. Kelman & H. J. Persie, Cancer Chemeother. Rep., **402**, 166-170
   (1975).
5. See for example: A. J. Spear, A. Ridgeway & L. M. Hall, Cancer
   Chemotherapy Reports, **59**, 629-641 (1975); C. E. Carraher, W. J.
   Scott, J. A. Schroeder & D. J. Giron, J. Macromol. Sci. Chem., **A15**,
   625-631 (1981).
6. C. E. Carraher, W. J. Scott, & D. J. Giron in: "*Biologically Active
   Polymers*", Chapter 20, Plenum Press, N.Y. (1984).
7. C. E. Carraher, I. Lopez & D. J. Giron, Polymeric Materials: Science
   and Engineering, **153**, 644-648 (1985).
8. J. Davidson, P. Fisher, R. Fisher, Cancer Chemotherapy. Rep., **59**, 287
   (1975).
9. W. O. Foye, "*Principles of Medicinal Chemistry*", Lea and Febiger,
   Philadelphia, 1981, p. 849.
10. R. G. Stoller & K. R. Hande, New England J. Medicine, **297**, 630-634
    (1977).
11. S. Neidle & M. J. Waring, "*Molecular Aspects of Anti-Cancer Drug
    Action*", Macmillan, New York, 1983.
12. D. A. Matthews, Science, **197**, 452-455 (1977).
13. D. M. L. Goodgame, Biochem. Biophys. Acta, **378**, 153-157 (1975).
14. F. R. Hartley, "*The Chemistry of Platinum and Palladium*", Applied
    Science Publishers Ltd., London, 1973.
15. I. I. Chugaev & S. Krasikov, Ann. Inst. Platine (USSR), **4**, 44 (1926);
    Chem. Abst., **21**, 2620 (1927).
16. A. A. Grinberg, Ann. Inst. Platine (USSR), **5**, 109 (1927).
17. W. W. Porterfield, "*Inorganic Chemistry*", Addison Wesley, Reading,
    MA, 1984.

18. B. Douglas, D. A. McDaniel & J. J. Alexander, "*Concepts and Models of Inorganic Chemistry*", Wiley Press, New York, 1983.

19. See for example: (a) P. O. Mellor, Chem. Revs., **33**, 137 (1943); (b) A. A. Grinberg, "*An Introduction to Complex Compounds*", Addison Wesley, Reading, MA, 1962; (c) F. Basolo and R. Pearson, "*Mechanisms of Inorganic Reactions*", Wiley, New York, 1967.

20. A. J. Hall & D. P. N. Satchell, J. Chem. Soc., Dalton Trans. 1403 (1977): L. Cattalina, R. Ugo & A. Orio, J. Am. Chem. Soc. **90**, XXXX (1968).

21. K. Nakamoto, Inorg. Chem., **4**, 36 (1965); R. Berg & K. Rasmussen, Spectrochimica Acta, **29A**, 319 (1973); A. Grinberg, M. Sermtor & M. Gel'fman, Russian J. Inorg. Chem., **13**, 1695 (1968); G. Barrow, R. Krueger & F. Basolo, Inorg. & Nuclear Chem., **31**, 340 (1956).

22. P. J. Debye, J. Phys. Chem., **51**, 1 (1947).

23. R. Seymour & C. E. Carraher, "*Polymer Chemistry: An Introduction*", Dekker, New York, 1982.

24. H.-G. Elias, Macromolecules, 2, 834-943 (1984).

25. J. W. Moore & R. G. Pearson, "*Kinetics and Mechanisms*", Wiley and Sons, New York, 1981.

THE RELEASE OF 5-FLUOROURACIL FROM POLYCAPROLACTONE MATRICES

Charles G. Gebelein, Mark Chapman and Tahseen Mirza

Department of Chemistry
Youngstown State University
Youngstown, OH 44555

The release of 5-fluorouracil (5-FU) from monolithic dispersions in poly(caprolactone), [FUPC], was studied and compared with the release of 5-FU from the copolymers of 1-(N-2-ethylmethacrylcarbamoyl)-5-fluorouracil, [EMCF], with methyl methacrylate, [MMA]. Whereas the EMCF:MMA copolymers always exhibited zero-order release of the 5-FU (i.e., constant level of drug released with time), the [FUPC] systems did not. Up to about 25% 5-FU, the [FUPC] systems exhibited a profile in which the 5-FU release was dependent on the square root of time. On the other hand, the EMCF:MMA copolymers showed a constant release of the 5-FU regardless of whether the sample was in a powdered or a pellet form. The release rates were also slower for the copolymer systems than for the monolithic FUPC systems, and much higher concentrations of the drug could be incorporated into the copolymer systems. These differences in the release profiles are caused by differences in the basic nature of the two kinds of systems and the mechanisms of the release of the 5-FU from each. These differences and the mechanisms of the release are discussed in detail.

INTRODUCTION

For several years our research group has been studying the synthesis, polymerization and copolymerization of monomers containing 5-fluorouracil (5-FU) and/or 6-methylthiopurine (6-MTP).[1-6] We have observed that the polymeric systems hydrolyzed in an aqueous medium to release the anti-cancer drug in a zero-order kinetic pattern.[4-6] Other studies, by Kaetsu, et al., on the release of 5-fluorouracil have not shown a similar zero-order behavior, but instead have shown a release pattern in which the 5-FU concentration was proportional to the square root of time.[7-10] These studies used highly crosslinked and fairly hydrophilic polymeric materials in which the 5-FU was monolithically dispersed. Our copolymer systems also contain the 5-FU dispersed in a monolithic manner, but, in these cases, the 5-FU is covalently attached to the polymer backbone. In the present study, we have compared the release rates of some monolithic 5-FU dispersions in poly(caprolactone) with the profiles obtained with our 5-FU containing copolymers. These monolithic dispersions in the poly-

(caprolactone) are neither crosslinked nor highly hydrophilic as was the case with the systems studied by Kaetsu, et al.

EXPERIMENTAL METHODS

Materials

Copolymers: The monomeric [EMCF], [1-(N-2-ethylmethacrylcarbamoyl)-5-fluorouracil], was synthesized from 5-fluorouracil and 2-isocyanatoethyl-methacrylate, [IEM], as described previously.[3] This synthetic route is outlined in Figure 1. A 50:50 (molar ratio) copolymer of [EMCF]:[MMA], (methyl methacrylate), was prepared in dioxane solution using an AIBN initiator and the structure of these copolymers is shown in Figure 2.[4,5]

5-Fluorouracil:Poly(caprolactone) Dispersions, [FUPC]: Monolithic dispersions of 5-FU in poly(caprolactone) were prepared by melting the polymer on a hotplate at about 70°C and then mixing the 5-FU into this molten mass. After solidification, the sample was pulverized in a Waring Blendor prior to use.

Hydrolysis Study Samples: Although the copolymers could readily and conveniently be studied in the form of a powder, the [FUPC] monolithic dispersions would tend to have the 5-FU at least partially uncoated by the polymer would not, therefore, be amendable to this approach. Pellets were prepared of the [FUPC] dispersions using an infrared pellet press and die. Pellets were also prepared for the EMCF:MMA copolymer in the same manner so that a direct comparison could be made of both systems, with the same surface area. Carefully weighed 0.2000 g samples of the powdered material were placed in the die and compressed under vacuum at

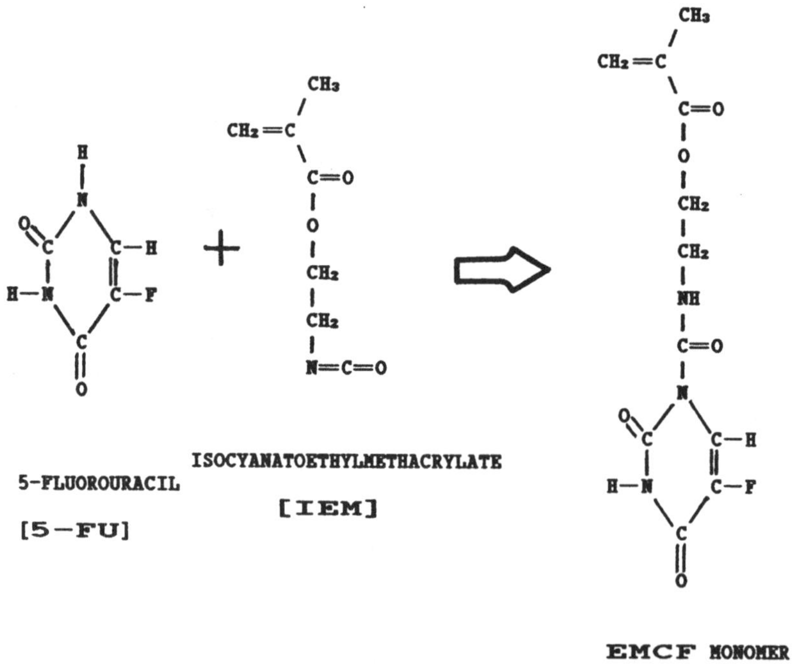

Figure 1. The synthesis of [EMCF] monomer.

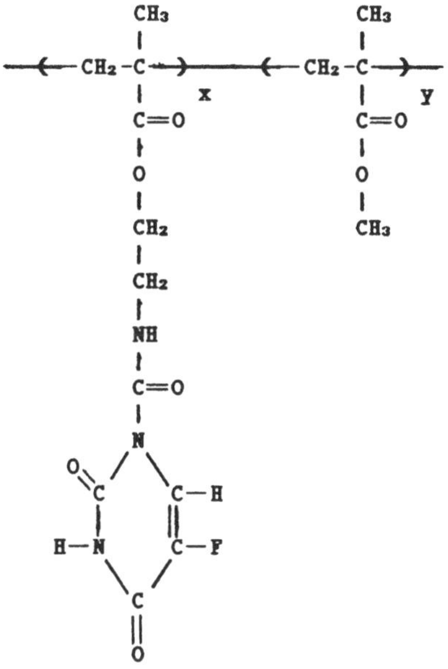

$$CH_3 \qquad\qquad CH_3$$

—(—CH₂—C—)—   —(—CH₂—C—)—
         | x | y
        C=O   C=O
         | |
         O   O
         | |
        CH₂   CH₃
         |
        CH₂
         |
        NH
         |
        C=O
         |
         N
       /   \
      C   C—H
    // ||
   O   C—F
      \   /
    H—N   C
          ||
          O

EMCF:MMA COPOLYMER

Figure 2. The structure of EMCF:MMA copolymers.

room temperature. The resulting pellets appeared homogeneous and could be handled without breakage. Powdered copolymer samples were also studied for comparison with our earlier studies.

Release Studies

The release profiles of the 5-FU from the EMCF:MMA copolymers and the [FUPC] systems were studied using the gas dispersion tube technique previously described.[11,12] These gas dispersion tubes were obtained from Ace Glass and had a 13.0 mm cavity diameter and a 25.0 mm cavity height; the sintered glass thickness was the usual 3.75 mm. The porosity rating was C, which corresponds to a pore size of 25-50 μ. The powdered samples (60-100 mesh) or the pellets of the copolymer or the [FUPC] materials were placed in the gas dispersion tubes in 1000 mL distilled water in a one-liter flask which was fitted with a mechanical stirrer (300 or 600 RPM) and contained in a constant temperature bath at 37.0°C. Aliquots were removed periodically and assayed for the released 5-FU spectrophotometrically at 262 nm using a Beckman DU-7. The release profiles were followed for a minimum of least two weeks. Each sample had its release rate determined at least two different times and these showed good agreement. Typical reproducibility results are shown in Figure 3.

RESULTS AND DISCUSSION

Figure 4, which shows five distinctly curved release profiles, clearly demonstrates that the monolithic [FUPC] systems do not give a zero-order release of the the 5-fluorouracil. The internal 5-FU content varies from 5-25% in these [FUPC] samples. When this same data is replotted according to the Higuchi equation,[13] as shown in Figure 5, some of these [FUPC] samples gave a straight line. The polymeric systems used

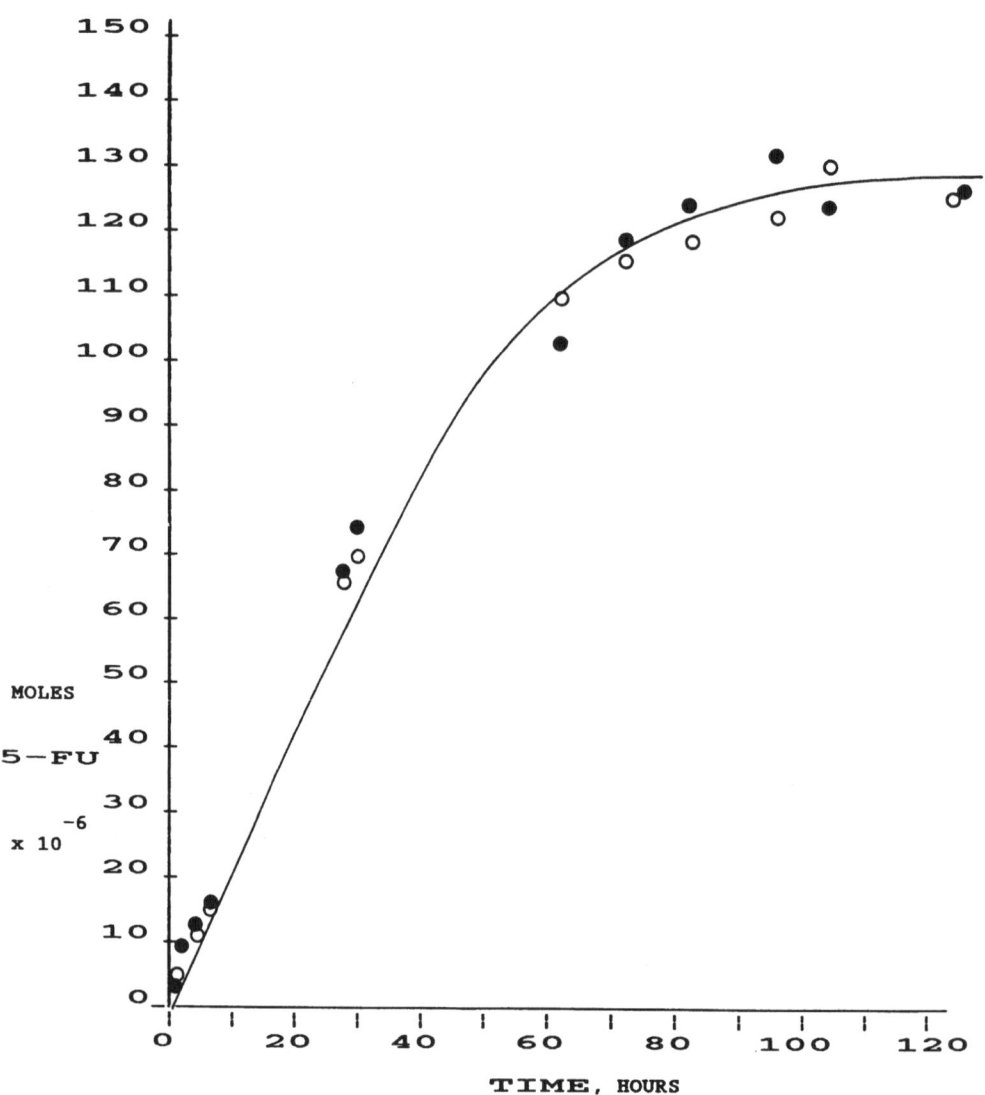

Figure 3. The release of 5-fluorouracil from duplicate runs
of a 0.100 g sample of a EMCF:MMA 50:50 copolymer.

in this study are neither crosslinked nor especially hydrophilic, but
these results are basically in agreement with the conclusions obtained by
Kaetsu with crosslinked, hydrophilic polymeric systems.[7-10] The monolithic systems appear to follow the Higuchi pattern regardless of the
nature of the polymeric system.

There is a maximum amount of internal phase that can be accommodated
before these monolithic [FUPC] systems fail to obey the Higuchi equation.
Figure 5 suggests that this limit is reached at about 25% 5-fluorouracil.
At about this level of internal phase, discontinuities develop within the
sample which lead to pockets of 5-FU rather than a uniform distribution
of this material throughout the poly(caprolactone). Even though the
samples appear homogeneous on visual inspection, the data indicate that
they lack true homogeneity.

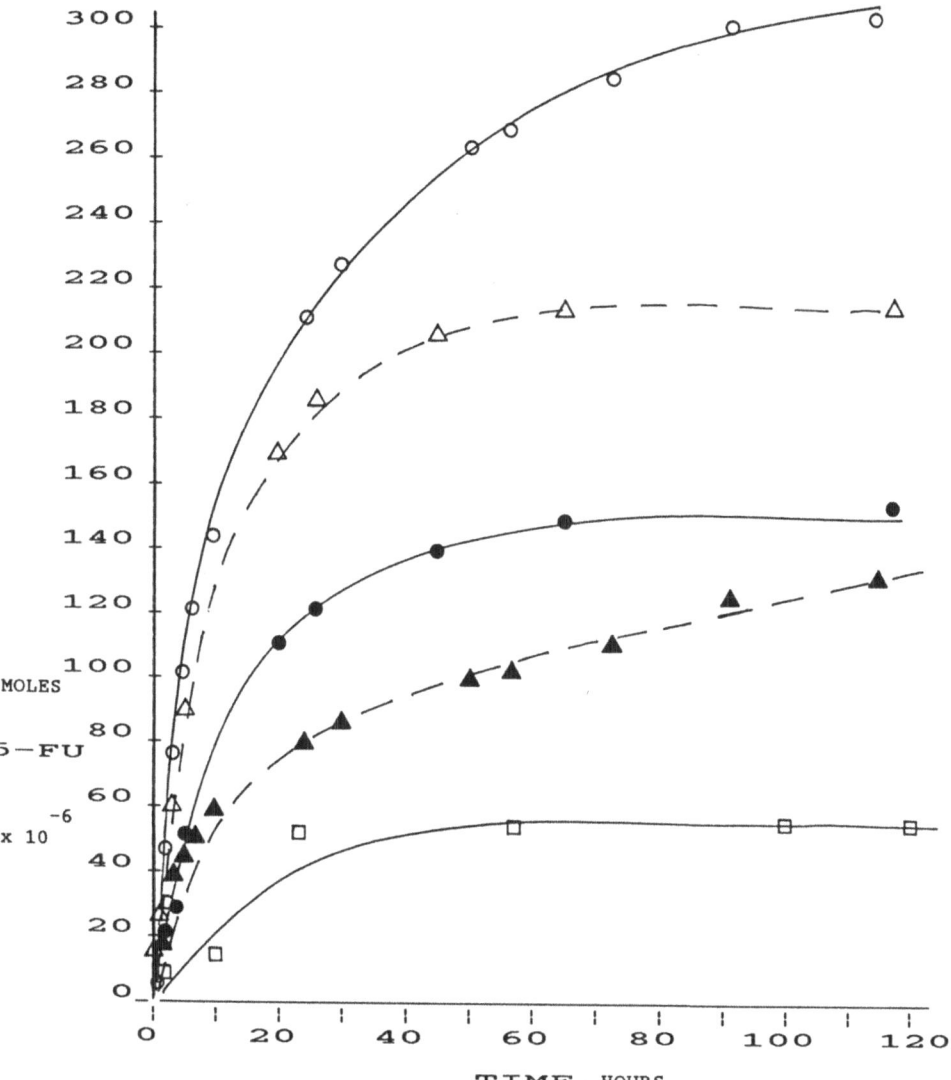

Figure 4. The release of 5-fluorouracil from monolithic dispersions in poly(caprolactone). The individual runs are: (symbol, % 5-FU in matrix); o, 25%; △, 20%; ●, 15%; ▲, 10%; □, 5%.

A direct comparision between the monolithic [FUPC] systems and the EMCF:MMA copolymers is shown in Figures 6 and 7. The copolymers follow zero-order kinetics in both the powdered and the pellet form. The release rate from the pellet form is slower than for the powdered samples, however. This is assumed to be due solely to a smaller surface area for the pellet samples. We must note that the copolymer samples would have the 5-fluorouracil distributed in a completely homogeneous manner within the solid sample. (There would, of course, be some heterogeneity on the molecular scale due to a random distribution of the two monomers along the polymer chain.)

Figures 6 and 7 also show a slower 5-FU release from the copolymeric

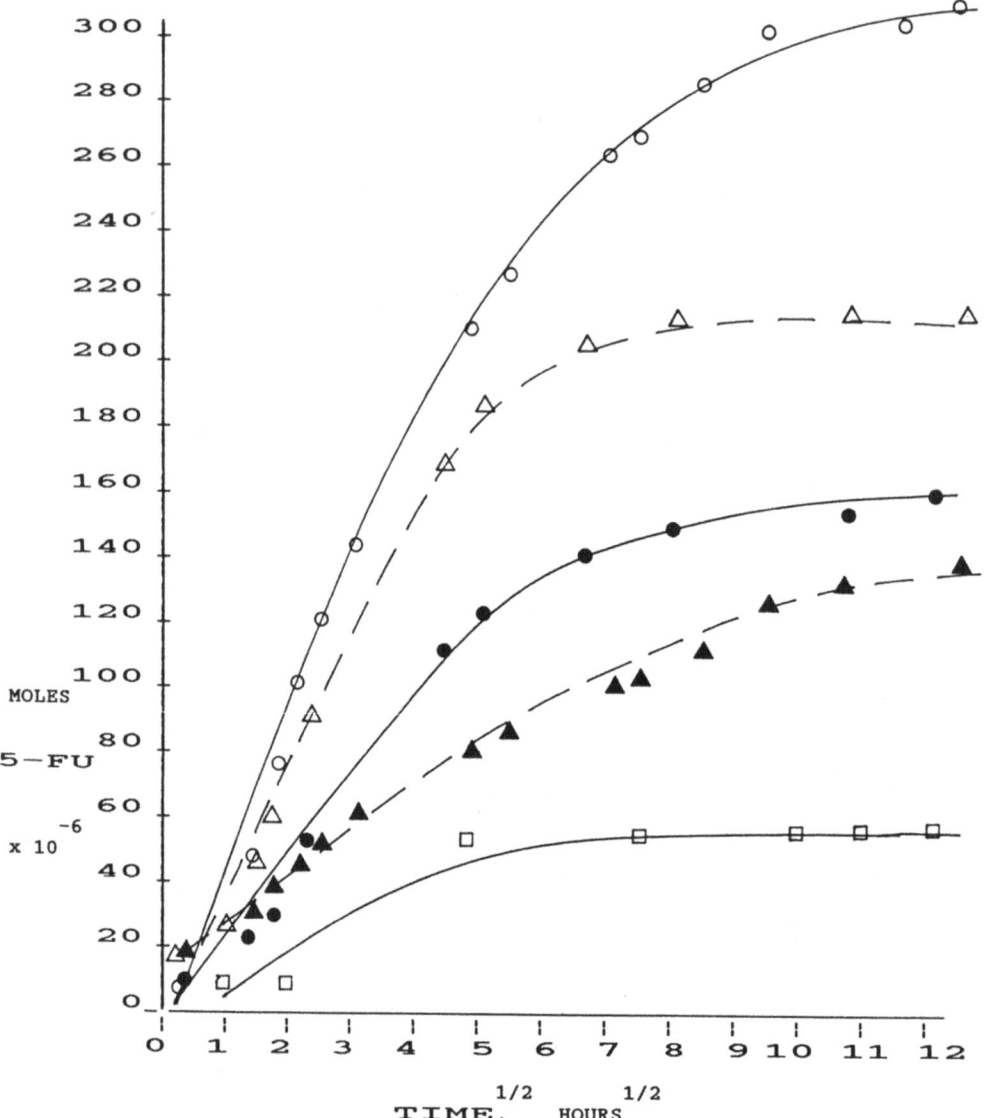

Figure 5. The release of 5-fluorouracil from monolithic dispersions in poly(caprolactone) plotted against the
square root of time (Higuchi kinetics). The individual runs are: (symbol, % 5-FU in matrix); o ,
25%;   △ , 20%;   ● , 15%;   ▲ , 10%;   □, 5%.

system than with a monolithic system of about the same 5-FU level. The
maximum amount of 5-FU in the [EMCF] monomer or homopolymer would be
45.6%. The 50:50 EMCF:MMA copolymer would, therefore, contain 22.8% 5-FU.
It would be difficult, if not impossible to obtain a uniform dispersion
with this amount of internal phase in a typical monolithic system.

    As noted above, the more rapid release of the 5-FU from the powdered
copolymer samples than from the pellet form is believed to be due to the
greater surface area in the powdered form. Significantly, however, both
forms show the same zero-order kinetic profiles. This implies that the

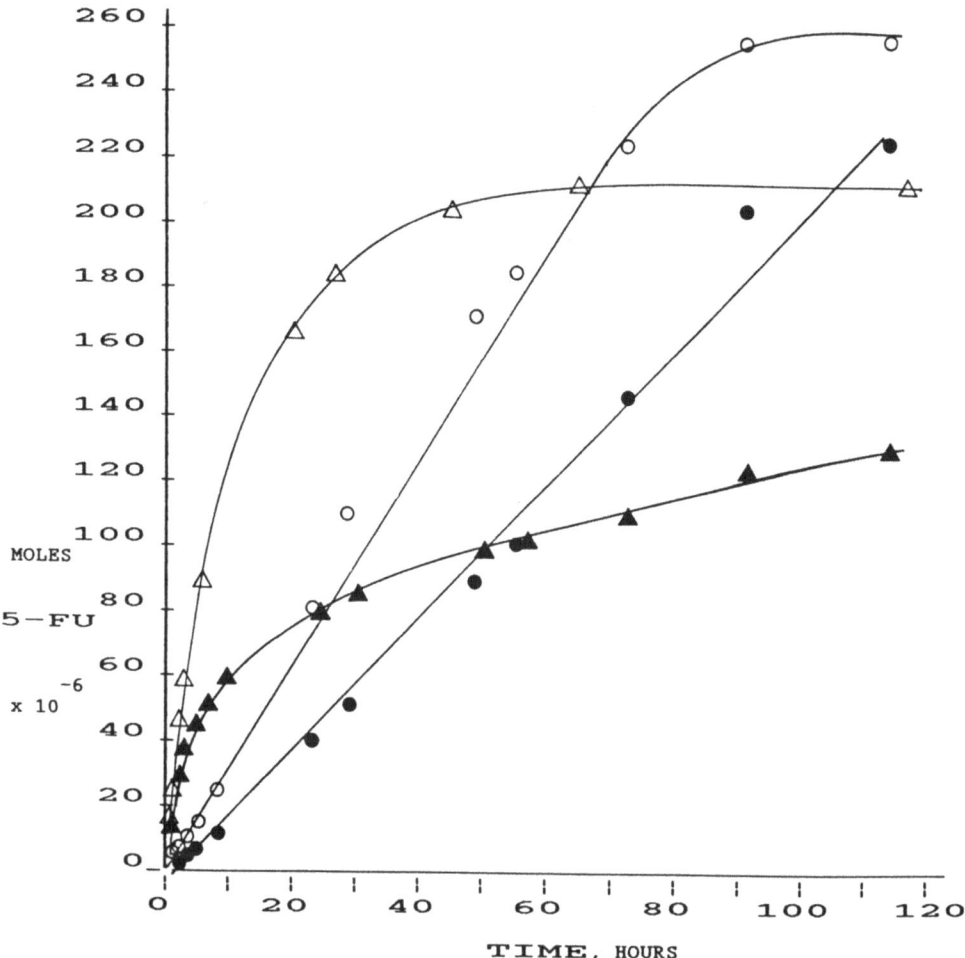

Figure 6. Comparison of the release of 5-fluorouracil from
monolithic dispersions in poly(caprolactone) and
copolymers of EMCF:MMA = 50:50. The individual runs
are: (symbol, sample type); o , EMCF:MMA powdered
material; ●, EMCF:MMA pellet form; △, FU:PC
20:80; ▲, FU:PC 10:90.

mechanism of action is the same for either the powdered or pellet forms
of the copolymers. Likewise, all the [FUPC] samples fail to exhibit a
zero-order kinetic behavior. Most of these [FUPC] systems do follow the
Higuchi kinetic pattern in which the release rate is proportional to the
square root of time.[13] Although only a single shape of pellet was used in
our studies, the results of Kaetsu have shown that their monolithic
systems followed the Higuchi pattern regardless of the shape of the
specimen; only the specific rates depended on the sample shape.[7-10]

The data for the copolymer systems and the 25:75 [FUPC] samples is
plotted according to the Higuchi equation in Figure 8. Although the
[FUPC] sample approximates a straight line, neither the powdered nor the
pellet form of the EMCF:MMA 50:50 copolymer shows such behavior. On the
contrary, both copolymer samples exhibit an S-shaped curve. If a zero-
order system is plotted against the square root of time, the resultant

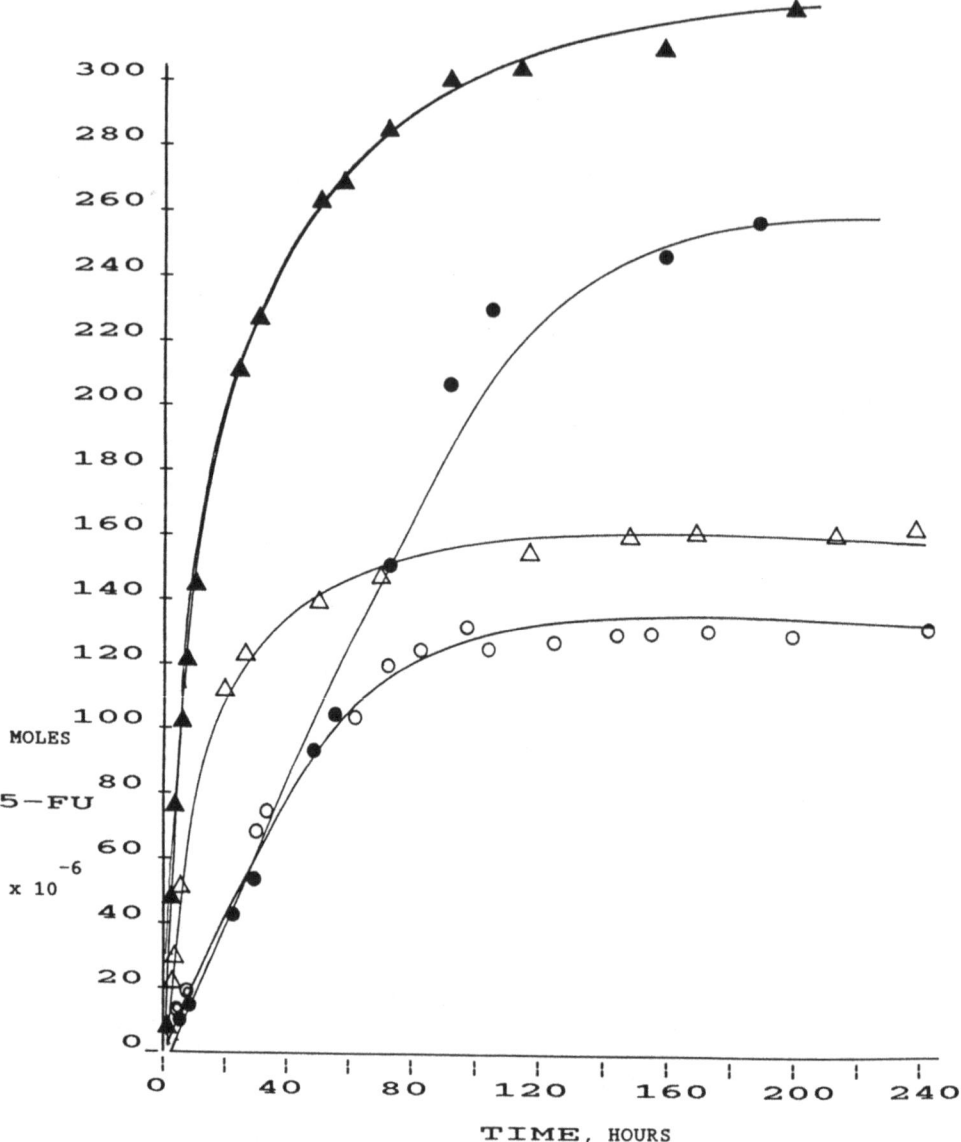

Figure 7. Comparison of the release of 5-fluorouracil from
monolithic dispersions in poly(caprolactone) and
copolymers of EMCF:MMA = 50:50. The individual runs
are: (symbol, sample type); ● , EMCF:MMA powdered
material; o , EMCF:MMA pellet form; ▲ , FU:PC
25:75, pellets; △, FU:PC 15:85, pellets.

curve should be the observed S-shape. This result further shows that the
copolymer and the monolithic [FUPC] systems behave in a different manner
regarding their release kinetics, even though both systems are,
nominally, monolithic in character.

The reason for this difference stems from a difference in the
mechanism of release in each case. The [FUPC] systems obey the conditions
proscribed for a monolithic system and follow this solution of the
Fickian equation. The mode of release in the copolymer system is, how-

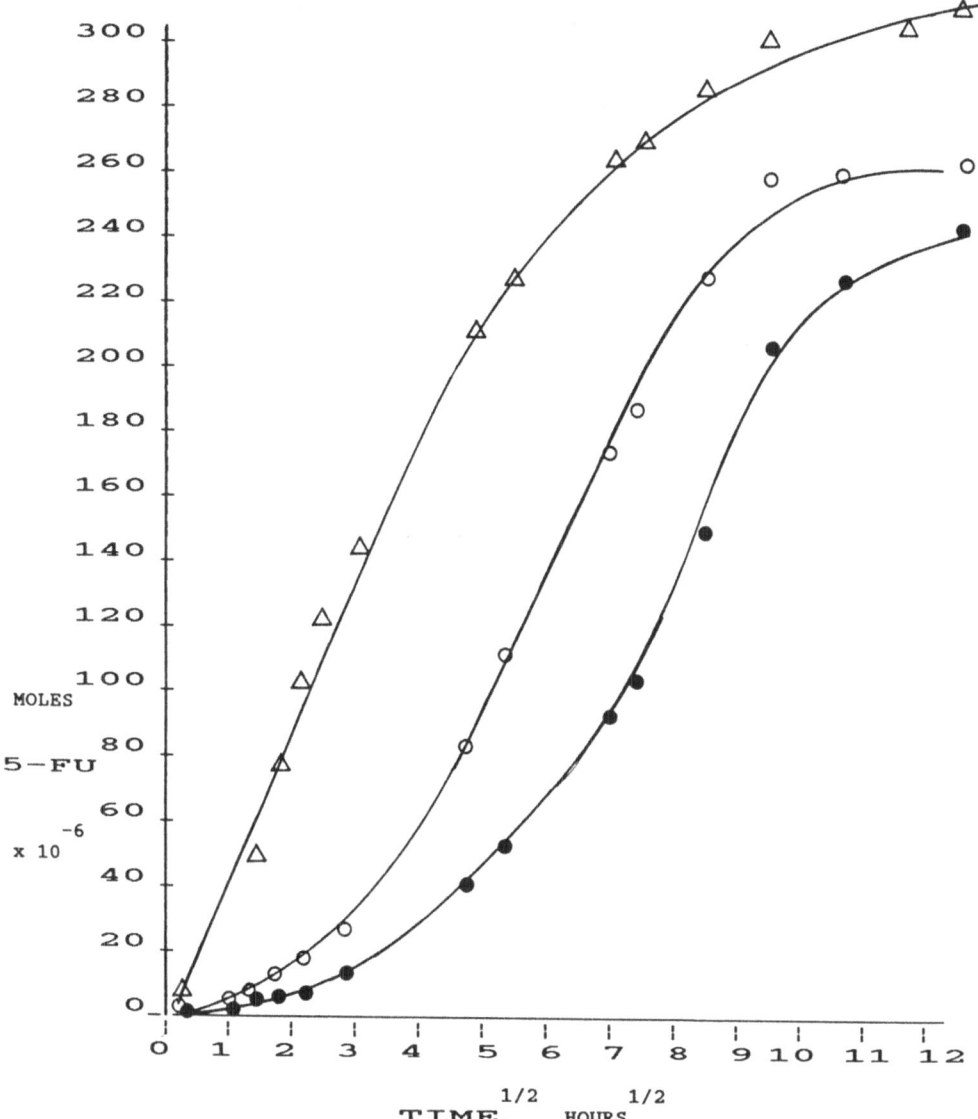

Figure 8. Higuchi kinetic plots of the release of 5-fluoro-
uracil from EMCF:MMA = 50:50 copolymers and monolithic dispersions in poly(caprolactone). The individual runs are: (symbol, sample type); o ,
EMCF:MMA powdered material; ● , EMCF:MMA pellet
form; △, FU:PC 25:75, pellets.

ever, completely different. Here this release requires several steps, as
illustrated in Figure 9. In Step 1 the water diffuses into the polymer
sample. The rate of this diffusion would probably be similar to that
obtained in the [FUPC] systems, and should be fairly rapid. In Step 2 the
5-FU must become hydrolyzed from the polymer chain by the water that has
diffused into the sample. In a homogeneous system, this would be a second
order reaction with moderate rates of reaction. In the present case,
however, the reaction is heterogeneous and would likely become slower.

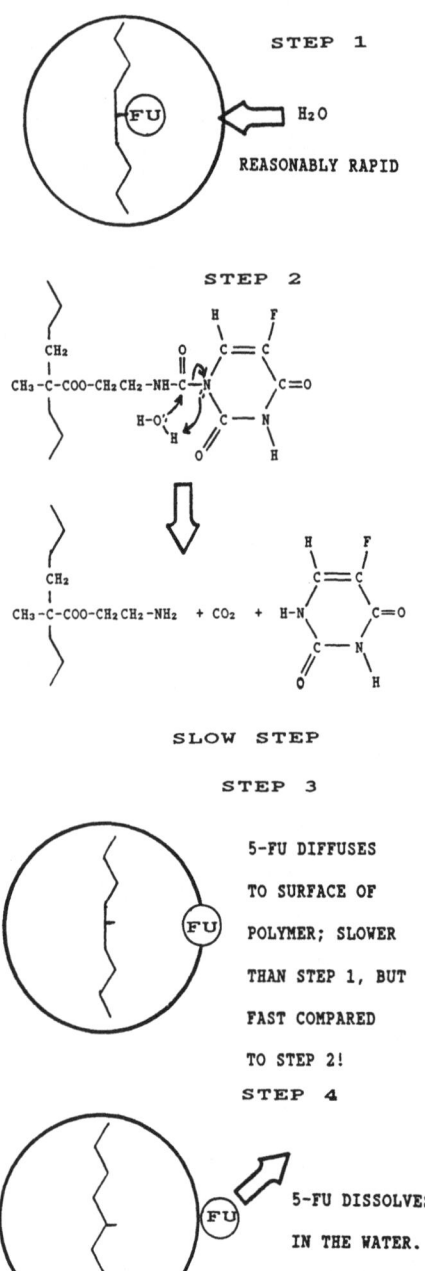

Figure 9. The mechanism of the release of 5-fluorouracil from the copolymers. Step 1 shows the rapid diffusion of water into the sample. Step 2 shows the rate-determining hydrolysis of the 5-fluorouracil off from the polymeric backbone. Step 3 shows the diffusion of the 5-fluorouracil molecules to the surface of the copolymer particles where it is released into the solution in step 4.

After this hydrolysis, the 5-FU must diffuse to the polymer surface in Step 3, where it would be released into the aqueous phase in Step 4. While the rate of diffusion of the 5-FU out of the polymer might be expected to be slightly slower that the rate of diffusion of water into the sample, both should be reasonably rapid, and both should be Fickian. The fourth step would be expected to be of comparable speed to the rate of solution of 5-FU, which is slow compared to the release of the 5-FU from either the monomeric [EMCF] or its copolymers.[4-6]

The Fickian diffusion rates in the first or third steps should not result in zero-order kinetics. Likewise, we might expect these rates to be relatively rapid and somewhat comparable to the rates observed with the [FUPC] systems, but this is definitely not the case.

The third step of the release from the copolymers would involve the hydrolysis of the drug unit from the polymer chain. As noted earlier, this would be a second order reaction in a homogeneous system and would exhibit second order kinetics. The reaction should be first order in both polymer and in water. In these heterogeneous systems, however, the polymer is an isolated solid and would not appear in the kinetic expression. Likewise, the water is present in swamping quantities and would either be absorbed into the rate constant or show no apparent effect on the rate of reaction.

This hydrolysis reaction does, however, still occur and must still depend upon the interactions of the diffusing water on the covalent bonds between the 5-FU and the polymer chain. Unless the diffusion rates for the water become slower than the actual rates of this heterogeneous hydrolysis, an unlikely event, the rate expression would become independent of the concentrations of both the water and the polymer. This would default to a pseudo-zero-order kinetic expression, which agrees with the data actually observed with these copolymer drugs.

The actual difference in the rates for individual samples or shapes of a specific copolymer would become almost completely dependent upon the surface area of these samples. Thus, the powdered samples hydrolyze faster and release the 5-FU more rapidly that the pellets, but both forms still observe the zero-order kinetic pattern that is the result of the heterogeneous hydrolysis reaction.

The [FUPC] systems do not have any such hydrolysis step and therefore follow the Higuchi kinetic pattern. The "fit" for this Higuchi equation pattern is much better for those [FUPC] samples that contain less than 25% 5-FU. This problem arises because the 25:75 [FUPC] sample is probably at or slightly beyond the physical limit of containment for the 5-FU within the poly(caprolactone). This is a "mechanical" problem common to all monolithic systems in which a drug, etc. is admixed (or dissolved) in a polymeric matrix. At some concentration level the drug is no longer truly homogeneously dispersed, even if it might appear to be so under visual inspection. The isolated pockets of the drug begin to interconnect with each other and departures from the "typical Higuchi" kinetic pattern would be observed. Eventually, the true heterogeneous nature of the dispersion would become evident visually as the amount of the internal phase increases. In the present system, the initial onset of this lack of uniformity, as detected by the departure from the Higuchi kinetic pattern, appears to occur at about the 25% 5-FU level.

The covalently bound drugs do not suffer from this difficulty, however, and can maintain a uniform dispersion at much higher levels. The upper limit is normally set by the maximum amount of the drug that can be incorporated into the copolymer. For those materials such as [EMCF], which polymerize via a chain-growth, addition process this limit is the same as the concentration of the drug in the monomer. In the present case, the maximum amount of 5-FU in the [EMCF] monomer or homopolymer would be 45.6%. and the 50:50 EMCF:MMA copolymer would contain 22.8% 5-FU. It is usually not possible to maintain a uniform dispersion with this amount of internal phase in a typical monolithic system. The only reasonable deviation from this completely uniform pattern shown in the copolymer systems would be where the drug unit tends to segregate into micelle-like clusters. Even there, the dispersion would remain uniform on the gross scale of the samples themselves. Unless these clusters became large, these systems should still exhibit the zero-order kinetic pattern.

CONCLUSIONS

The release of 5-fluorouracil from the [EMCF] copolymers follows a different mechanism than the release of 5-FU from a monolithic dispersion in poly(caprolactone). The copolymers consistently exhibit zero-order kinetics while the [FUPC] systems never show this pattern. In addition, much higher levels of the 5-FU can be incorporated into the polymeric system than into the monolithic dispersion system. In the present case, this was 45+% compared to less than 25%. For therapeutic use, the zero-order kinetics would offer the additional advantage of a completely controlled dose rate that could be maintained constant for long periods of time. The exact release rate can be controlled through the concentration of the drug monomer in the copolymer and the nature of the comonomer(s). This combination of properties can not be readily obtained in any other system without the use of complex membranes and the like.[14] In short, the polymeric drug approach does offer many distinct advantages over the usual controlled release systems and should prove to be the more desirable system for use in medication.

ACKNOWLEDGEMENTS

This research is abstracted, in part, from the Thesis of TM which was submitted to Youngstown State University in partial fulfillment of the requirements for the Master of Science degree in Chemistry, August, 1987. The research was partially supported by grants from PPG, Inc. and the YSU Research Council.

REFERENCES

1. C. G. Gebelein, R. M. Morgan, R. Glowacky & W. Baig in: "*Biomedical & Dental Applications of Polymers*", C. G. Gebelein & F. F. Koblitz, Eds., Plenum Publ. Corp., New York, 1981, p. 191.
2. C. G. Gebelein in: "*Biological Activities of Polymers*", C. E. Carraher, Jr. & C. G. Gebelein, Eds., American Chemical Society, Washington, DC, 1982, p. 193.
3. C. G. Gebelein, Proc. Polym. Mat. Sci. Eng., 51, 127-131 (1984).
4. R. R. Hartsough & C. G. Gebelein, Proc. Polym. Mat. Sci. Eng., 51, 131-135 (1984).
5. R. R. Hartsough & C. G. Gebelein in: "*Polymeric Materials in Medication*", C. G. Gebelein & C. E. Carraher, Jr., Eds., Plenum Publ. Corp., New York, 1985, pp. 115-124.

6. C. G. Gebelein & R. R. Hartsough in: *"Controlled Release of Bioactive Materials, 11th International Symposium"*, W. E. Meyers & R. C. Dunn, Eds., Controlled Release Society, Lincolnshire, IL, 1984, pp. 65-66.

7. M. Yoshida, M. Kumakura & I. Kaetsu, Polymer, **19**, 1375 (1978).

8. M. Yoshida, M. Kumakura & I. Kaetsu, Polymer, **11**, 775 (1979).

9. I. Kaetsu, M. Yoshida, M. Kumakura, A. Yamada & Y. Sakurai, Biomaterials, **1**, 17 (1980).

10. I. Kaetsu, M. Yoshida & A. Yamada, J. Biomed. Mater. Res., **14**, 185 (1980).

11. C. G. Gebelein, R. R. Hartsough & T. Mirza in: *"Controlled Release of Bioactive Materials, 13th International Symposium"*, I. A. Chaudry & C. Thies, Eds., Controlled Release Society, Lincolnshire, IL, 1986, pp. 188-189.

12. C. G. Gebelein, T. Mirza & R. R. Hartsough in: *"Controlled Release Technology, Pharmaceutical Applications"*, P. I. Lee & W. R. Good, Ed., American Chemical Society, Washington, DC, 1987, pp. 120-126.

13. T. Higuchi, J. Pharm. Sci., **59**, 353 (1961).

14. Y. W. Chien, Ed., *"Novel Drug Delivery Systems: Fundamentals, Developmental Concepts and Biomedical Assessments"*, Marcel Dekker, New York, 1982.

SYNTHESIS OF ANTITUMOR POLYSACCHARIDES

Kei Matsuzaki[a], Iwao Yamamoto[a], Koji Enomoto[a], Yutaro Kaneko[b], Tohru Mimura[b] & Tsuyoshi Shiio[b]

(a) Faculty of Textile Science & Technology
    Shinshu University
    Ueda 386, Japan
(b) Ajinomoto Co., Ltd.
    1-5-8, Kyobashi, Chuo-ku
    Tokyo 104, Japan

Previously, we have synthesized several antitumor polysaccharides having D-glucopyranose, D-mannopyranose, D-arabinofuranose, or its oligomer, as side chains of $(1\rightarrow3)-\beta$-
glucan, or $(1\rightarrow4)-\beta$-glucan by the orthoester method as models
of natural antitumor polysaccharides, such as lentinan, etc.
Some of these have indicated high antitumor activity against
Sarcoma 180 implanted into mice, to the same extent as the
natural polysaccharides. In this report, water soluble,
branched polysaccharides having L-arabinofuranose or its
oligomer, L-arabinopyranose, or D-galactopyranose as side
chains were synthesized, and their structures and antitumor
activities were determined, in order to investigate the effect of the kind of side chains on the antitumor activity.
These synthetic polysaccharides showed high antitumor
activity.

INTRODUCTION

In Japan, several polysaccharides, such as lentinan, krestin and
shizophyllan, which are extracted from mushrooms, are being used clinically as antitumor drugs in combination with chemotherapeutic agents, such
as Tegafur, or with irradiation. Their antitumor activity results from
their ability to enhance the immunity by stimulating the immune system of
living bodies.[1] Therefore, their antitumor activity is only exhibited in
living bodies. The extension of patient's lives by taking these polysaccharides together with chemotherapeutic agents has been established.

Lentinan is a polysaccharide extracted from shiitake (black mushroom), a popular mushroom widely used in Chinese foods, and shizophyllan
is a polysaccharide which is extracted from suehiro-take. Both are
branched polysaccharides; their main chain is a $(1\rightarrow3)-\beta$-glucan, and the
side chains are glucopyranosyl units attached at the 6th position of the
glucose units in the main chain. The other type of polysaccharide is

krestin or PSK, in which the main chain is a (1→4)-β-glucan and the side chains are also glucopyranosyl units attached at the 6th position of the glucose units in the main chain. These structures and features are summarized in Table 1.

We have synthesized several branched polysaccharides having D-glucopyranose or D-mannopyranose as side chains of (1→4)-β-glucan (cellulose), (1→3)-β-glucan (curdlan), (1→4)-β-mannan (ivorynut mannan, or konjak glucomannan. Some of these showed high antitumor activity against Sarcoma 180 implanted into mice (Table 2).[2-4]

Table 1. Summary of natural antitumor polysaccharides.

Lentinan or Shizophyllan:
(1→3)-β-glucans with (1→6)-β-D-glucopyranosyl branches for every 2.5-3.0 glucose units.
PSK or Krestin (polysaccharide component):
(1→4)-β-glucan with (1→6)-β-D-glucopyranosyl branches for every 5 glucose units.

Table 2. The synthesized branched polysaccharides[a] and their antitumor activity.

Main Chains	Side Chain	Degree of Branching	Solubility in water (%)	Molecular Weight	Antitumor[b] Activity (%)
Cellulose	D-glucose	30	100	125,000	53.7
Cellulose	D-glucose	47	100	290,000	94.2
Cellulose	Oligo-D-arabinose	67[c]	100	n.d.	29.4
Curdlan[d]	D-glucose	53	90	n.d.	47.0
Curdlan	D-glucose	n.d.	98	n.d.	100
Curdlan	D-arabinose	9	57	n.d.	75.2
Curdlan	Oligo-D-arabinose	27[c]	100	n.d.	100
Curdlan	D-mannose	12	89	n.d.	82.7
Ivorynut mannan	D-glucose	11	49	n.d.	41.9
Konjak[d] glucomannan	D-glucose	10	100	550,000	46.3

(a) Acetates of main chain polysaccharides were reacted with orthoesters, except (d).
(b) Dose level is 5-10 mg/kg mouse x 10. See Experimental Section.
(c) Ratio of Ara/Glc.
(d) Unsubstituted polysaccharide was reacted with acetyl glucose orthoester.

1) Arabinomannan

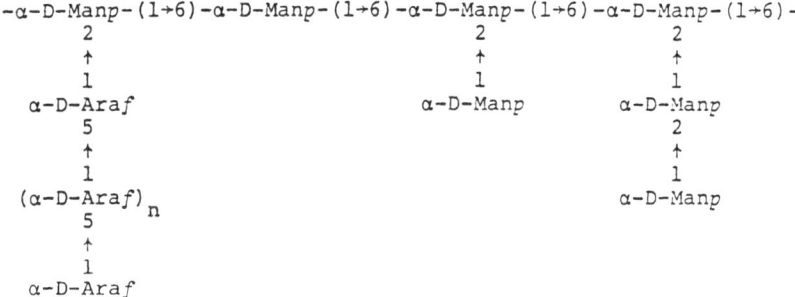

2) Arabinogalactan

```
-β-D-Galp-(1→6)-β-D-Galp-(1→4)-β-D-Galp-(1→6)-β-D-Galp-(1→4)-
                          3
                          ↑
                          1
                      α-D-Araf
                          2
                          ↑
                          1
                   (α-D-Araf)
                          5    n
                          ↑
                          1
                      α-D-Araf
```

Figure 1. The structure of the polysaccharide components of
the cell wall of *Mycobacteria tuberculosis*.

It is known that BCG vaccine has antitumor activity. Its polysaccharide components were isolated, the structures were investigated by
Misaki, and are shown in Figure 1.[5] Their main structural feature is the
presence of D-arabinofuranosyl side chains. Arabinose is widely distributed in the vegetable kingdom, but it is present in the L-form. We have
synthesized branched polysaccharides having D-arabinofuranose, or its
oligomer, as side chains and have found that they exhibited high antitumor activity as shown in Table 2.[6]

In this investigation, we have synthesized branched polysaccharides
having L-arabinofuranose, its oligomer, L-arabinopyranose, or D-galactopyranose as side chains in order to determine the effect of the nature of
the side chains on the antitumor activity. We were especially interested
in the effects of the optical isomers, that is D- and L-arabinose, on
this antitumor activity because compounds with different stereochemistry
often give quite different effects on living organisms.

EXPERIMENTAL

Main Chain Polysaccharides

Curdlan acetates or cellulose acetates were used as the main chain
polysaccharides. Cellulose acetates with a degree of substitution of

about 2.0 were obtained by the mild hydrolysis of cellulose triacetate. Curdlan acetates with a degree of substitution between 1.5 and 2.3 were obtained by acetylation of curdlan with acetic anhydride in pyridine.[2]

Orthoesters

For attaching L-arabinofuranose to the main chain polysaccharides, 3,5-di-O-benzoyl-(1,2-O-ethylorthobenzoyl)-β-L-aribinofuranose, (F-bicyclic orthoester), [1], was used. For the synthesis of oligo-L-arabinofuranose branched polysaccharides, 3-O-benzoyl-(1,2,5-O-orthobenzoyl)-β-L-arabinofuranose, (tricyclic orthoester), [2], was used. For the synthesis of L-arabinopyranose branched polysaccharides, 3,4-di-O-benzoyl-(1,2-O-ethylorthobenzoyl)-β-L-arabinopyranose, (P-bicyclic orthoester), [3], was used. For the synthesis of D-galactopyranose branched polysaccharides, 3,4,6-tri-O-acetyl-(1,2-O-ethylorthoacetyl)-β-D-galactopyranose, [4], was used. The orthoesters were synthesized by the methods shown in Schemes 1 and 2.[7].

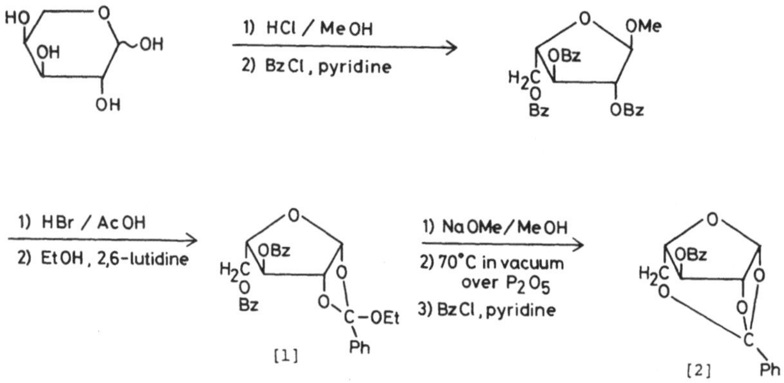

Scheme 1. The synthetic scheme for [1] and [2].

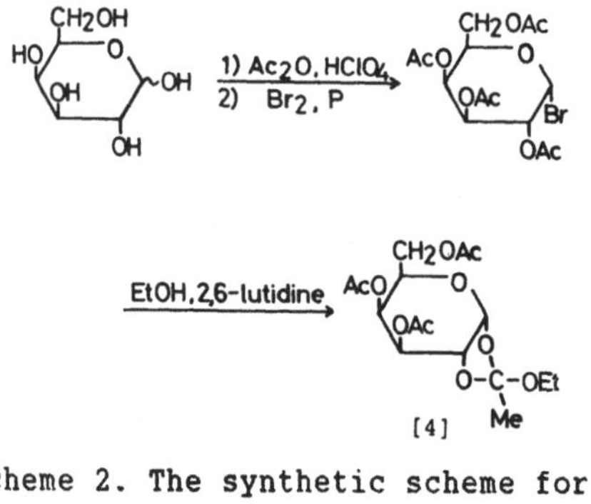

Scheme 2. The synthetic scheme for [4].

Reaction of Orthoesters with Main Chain Polysaccharides

The main chain polysaccharides were activated by solvent exchange before the reaction. The condensation reaction was carried out by refluxing the mixture of the acetates of the main chain polysaccharides and the orthoester in chlorobenzene for 2 hrs. with 2,6-dimethylpyridinium perchlorate as the catalyst. The reaction was repeated to obtain products with a high degree of branching.

Isolation of Free Polysaccharides

The reaction products were then de-esterified with 1 M sodium methoxide solution in methanol or with 0.5 M aqueous sodium hydroxide to give the free polysaccharides. The solution was dialyzed against water for 3-4 days, and the insoluble polymer was removed. The solution was concentrated and freeze-dried to give the water-soluble branched polysaccharides. This reaction scheme is illustrated in Figures 2 and 3.

Methylation Analysis

The free polysaccharides were permethylated by the Hakomori method,[8] hydrolyzed with 90% formic acid at 100-110°C for 8 hrs., and then with 2 M trifluoroacetic acid at 100-110°C for 3 hrs. The hydrolyzates were then reduced with sodium borohydride and acetylated with acetic anhydride in pyridine. The partially methylated alditol acetates thus obtained were analyzed with a Hewlett-Packard 5790 gas chromatograph.

Antitumor Activity

Ascites sarcoma 180 cells (10^6) were implanted in the armpit of ICR-JCL mice. The polysaccharide solution, with a concentration of 1-10 mg/kg mouse, was injected intraperitoneally for ten days, starting 24 hr after the implantation of the ascites tumor. All mice were kept under observation for 5 weeks and then sacrificed for the evaluation of the effect of the treatment on the tumor growth. The inhibition ratios were calculated by the following equation, where A is the average tumor weight of the control groups and B is that of the treated groups.

$$\text{Inhibition Ratio (\%)} = 100(A - B)/A$$

RESULTS AND DISCUSSION

Tables 3-4 indicate the reaction conditions, composition and water solubility of the synthesized branched polysaccharides. It can be observed from these Tables that the branched polysaccharides with more than a 30% ratio of Ara/Glc, or degree of branching (number of branches

Table 3. Synthesis of branched polysaccharides with L-arabinose or oligo-L-arabinose side chains.

Exp. No.	Monomer	Reaction Time (min.)	Ratio (%) (Ara/Glc)	Solubility in water (%)
Ara-1	F-bicyclic	120 + 120	8	20
Ara-2	F-bicyclic	120 + 120 + 120	8	40
Ara-3	F-bicyclic	100 + 100 + 100 100 + 100	21	84
Ara-4	P-bicyclic	100 + 100 + 100	8	11
Ara-5	P-bicyclic	100 + 100 + 100 100 + 100	7	56
Ara-6	Tricyclic	90 + 90	47	70
Ara-7	Tricyclic	100 + 100 + 100	68	98

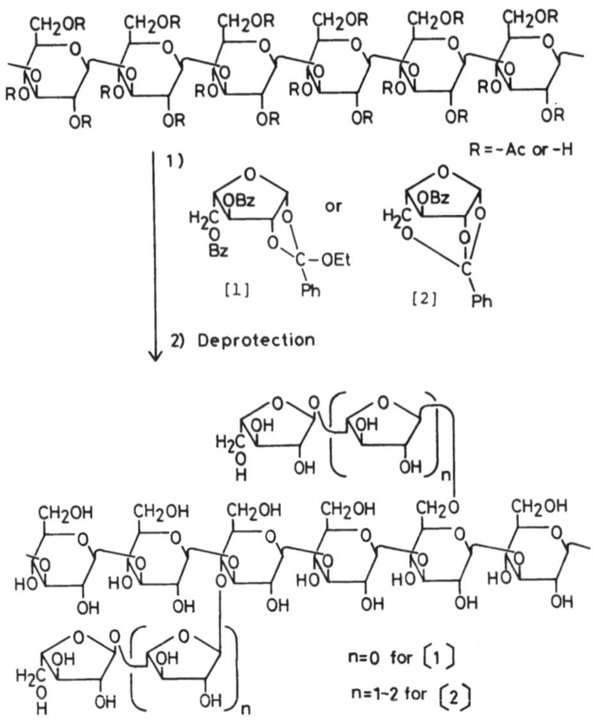

Figure 2. The synthesis of branched polysaccharides having
L-arabinofuranose and oligo-L-arabinofuranose as
side chains.

per 100 glucose units in the main chain), are almost (near 100%) water
soluble. From Table 3 it can be seen that the tricyclic orthoester is
more reactive than the bicyclic one, giving a higher ratio of Ara/Glc.

Table 5 shows the results on the arabinose-branched polysaccharides
tested for antitumor activity. The antitumor activity was 100% for a dose
level of 5 mg/kg mouse, indicating no difference in the activity between
branched polysaccharides having D-arabinofuranose or L-arabinofuranose
and their oligomers, or L-arabinopyranose as side chains.

Table 4. Synthesis of branched polysaccharides with D-galactopyranose side chains.

Exp. No.	Starting Polymer	Degree Subst.	Reaction time (min.)	D.R.[a]	Solubility in water (%)
Gal-1	Curdlan acetate	2.05	120 + 120 + 120	19	76
Gal-2	Curdlan acetate	1.89	120 + 120	79	35
Gal-3	Curdlan acetate	–	120 + 120 + 120	41	83
Gal-4	Cellulose acetate	2.05	120 + 120	97	97

(a). Degree of branching.

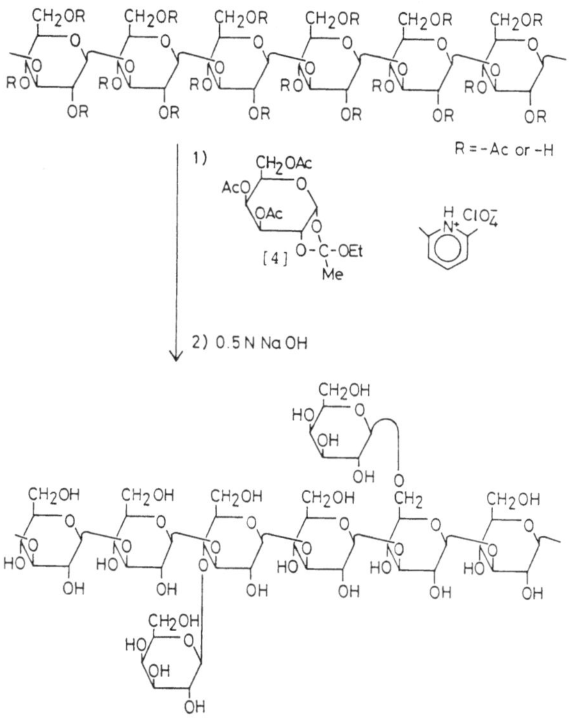

Figure 3. The synthesis of branched polysaccharides having
D-galactopyranose as side chains.

Table 6 shows the antitumor activity of the D-galactose-branched polysaccharides, synthesized as shown in Table 4. A branched $(1\rightarrow3)$-β-D-glucan having D-galactose side chains showed a much higher activity than a branched $(1\rightarrow4)$-β-D-glucan. One of the reasons for the low activity is due to the low molecular weight of the product.

Table 5. Antitumor activity of branched polysaccharides
having L-arabinose or oligo-L-arabinose as side
chains.

Sample No.[a]	Dose (mg/kg)	Tumor Inhibition	Complete Regression
Ara-1 (F)	5	100	7/7
Ara-2 (F)	5	100	7/7
Ara-4 (P)	1	88	5/7
	10	99	6/7
Ara-5 (P)	1	80	5/7
	10	95	4/7
Ara-6 (T)	5	100	7/7
Curdlan	5	10	0/7

(a) F means synthesized with F-bicyclic orthoester.
    P means synthesized with P-bicyclic orthoester.
    T means synthesized with tricyclic orthoester.

171

Table 6. Antitumor activity of branched polysaccharides
having D-galactopyranose as side chains.

Sample No.	Dose (mg/kg)	Tumor Inhibition	Complete Regression
Gal-1	1	95	5/7
	10	100	7/7
Gal-2	10	76	2/7
Gal-3	1	48	4/7
	10	100	7/7
Gal-4	10	11	1/7

The methylation analyses (Tables 7 and 8) reveals that the L-arabino-furanose side chains in the branched (1→3)-β-D-glucan are a mixture of branches occurring at both the C-6 and C-4 positions in the glucose units of the main chain. The reason for the higher branching at C-4 (secondary OH) than at the C-6 (primary OH) in L-arabinose-branched polysaccharides may be due to blocking of the condensation reaction by acetyl groups preferentially introduced at the C-6 position during the acetylation reaction.

Oligo-L-arabinose side chains substitute mainly at the C-6 OH groups, and the degree of polymerization of the side chains, calculated from the (2,3-Ara)/(2,3,5-Ara) + 1 is 2.0-2.5.

The methylation analyses and structure of the branched polysaccha-rides having D-galactopyranose side chains is shown in Tables 9 and 10. The side chains form at the C-6 and C-4 positions of the curdlan main chain, whereas for cellulose the branching occurs mainly at the C-6 posi-tion of the glucose units in the main chain.

In conclusion, the most important factor for high antitumor activity of the polysaccharides is the main chain structure and the molecular weight. In this sense, (1→3)-β-glucan showed high antitumor activity. The

Table 7. Methylation analysis of branched polysaccharides
having L-arabinofuranose or oligo-L-arabinofuranose
as side chains.

Partially methylated alditol acetates[a]	Ara-1	Ara-2	Ara-6	Ara-7
2,3,5-Ara	1.00	1.00	1.00	1.00
2,3-Ara	–	–	1.00	1.51
2,4,6-Glc	12.96	7.05	2.79	2.91
2,6-Glc	0.88	0.55	0.15	0.14
2,4-Glc	0.34	0.33	0.25	0.38

(a) 2,3,5-Ara = 2,3,5-Tri-O-methyl arabinitol acetate.
2,3-Ara = 2,3-Di-O-methyl arabinitol acetate.
2,4,6-Glc = 2,4,6-Tri-O-methyl glucitol acetate
2,6-Glc = 2,6-Di-O-methyl glucitol acetate.
2,4-Glc = 2,4-Di-O-methyl glucitol acetate.

Table 8. Structures of branched polysaccharides having L-arabinofuranose or oligo-L-arabinofuranose as side chains.

Exp. No.	Ratio (Ara/Glc)	Length of Branch	Branching Position C-4:C-6
Ara-1	8	1.00	72:28
Ara-2	8	1.00	62:38
Ara-6	47	2.00	38:62
Ara-7	68	2.51	27:73

Table 9. Methylation analysis of branched polysaccharides having D-galactopyranose as side chains.

Partially methylated alditol acetates[a]	Gal-3 (Curdlan)	Gal-4 (Cellulose)
2,3,4,6-Gal	1.00	1.00
2,4,6-Glc	1.93	–
2,3,6-Glc	–	0.75
2,6-Glc	0.33	0.08
3,6-Glc	–	0.10
2,3-Glc	–	0.40
2,4-Glc	0.11	–

(a) Abbreviations as in Table 7.

Table 10. Structure of branched polysaccharides having D-galactopyranose as side chains.

Sample No.	Main Chain	Ratio (Gal/Glc)	Percent Substitution at Branching Position			
			C-6	C-4	C-3	C-2
Gal-3	Curdlan	41	25	75	–	–
Gal-4	Cellulose	71	70	–	13	17

side chain structure also affects the activity. So far, the branched polysaccharides having D- or L-arabinose, their oligomers, or D-galactose have shown the highest antitumor activities. It may be possible that these polysaccharides may be effective to recover the lost immunity of AIDS patients.

Another possible application of these polysaccharides involves the sulfates. When helper T-cells are cultured with the AIDS virus, they are destroyed in 6 days. However, when the sulfates of the branched polysaccharides, for example, oligo-L-arabinose-branched $(1\rightarrow3)$-β-D-glucan, were added in the concentration of 10 microgram/mL, no destruction of the T-cells occurred. Additional experiments are under way in the laboratory of Professor Yamamoto, Faculty of Medicine, Yamaguchi University, Japan.

REFERENCES

1. G. Chihara, "*Gan to Men-ekizokyo*" ("*Cancer and Immunopotentiation*"), Kodansha, Tokyo, 1980.
2. K. Matsuzaki, I. Yamamoto, T. Sato & R. Oshima, Makromol. Chem., **186**, 449 (1985).
3. K. Matsuzaki, I. Yamamoto, T. Sato & R. Oshima, Makromol. Chem., **187**, 317 (1986).
4. K. Matsuzaki, I. Yamamoto, T. Sato & R. Oshima, Makromol. Chem., **187**, 325 (1985).
5. A. Misaki & I. Azuma, "*Annual Report of the Sciences of Living*", Osaka City University, 29, 33 (1981).
6. K. Matsuzaki, T. Sato, K. Enomoto, I. Yamamoto, R. Oshima, K. Hatanaka & T. Uryu, Carbohydrate Res., **157**, 171 (1986).
7. N. K. Kochetkov, A. Ya. Kohlin, A. F. Bochkov & I. G. Yazlovetskii, Izv. Akad. Nauk. SSSR, 15, 2030(1966).
8. S. Hakomori, J. Biochem. (Tokyo), 55, 205 (1964).

BIOLOGICAL ACTIVITIES OF TIN-CONTAINING SACCHARIDES AND POLYSACCHARIDES

Charles E. Carraher, Jr.[a], Cynthia Butler[b],
Yoshinobu Naoshima[c], Van R. Foster[d], David Giron[e], and
Philip D. Mykytiuk[f]

Florida Atlantic University
Departments of Chemistry[a] and Biological Sciences[b]
Boca Raton, FL 33431

Okayama University of Science[c]
Department of Chemistry
Ridaicho, Okayama 700 Japan

Wright State University
Departments of Chemistry[f] and Microbiology and Immunology[e]
Dayton, OH 45435

DAP[d]
P.O. Box 277
Dayton, OH 45431

A number of hydroxyl-containing natural products including sucrose, xylan, dextran and cellulose have been condensed to produce tin-containing materials. Many of these materials inhibit selected microorganisms in the bulk and as additives. Inhibition is generally in the order $CH_3 > C_2H_5 > C_3H_8 > C_4H_9$.

INTRODUCTION

The biological activity of organostannane-containing polymeric materials is well established.[1-7] These materials can be divided into two groupings with respect to the attachment of the stannane-moiety. The first has the tin connected to the polymer through relatively nonpolar bonding with carbon as shown in [1]. The second has tin bonded to the polymer through a more electronegative, non-carbon atom usually an oxygen or nitrogen as shown in [2] and [3]. As expected, the hydrolytic stabilities and concentration levels to achieve a desired level of biological activity are generally less for products containing the organostannane connected through the more polar linkages.

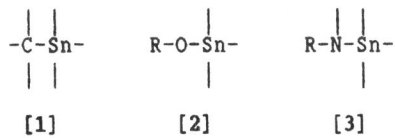

$$-\overset{|}{\underset{|}{C}}-\overset{|}{\underset{}{Sn}}- \qquad R-O-\overset{|}{\underset{|}{Sn}}- \qquad R-N-\overset{|}{\underset{|}{Sn}}-$$

[1]   [2]   [3]

We recently have been emphasizing the use of renewable resource materials as feed stocks for the production of non-petroleum based polymers containing metals. While the biological activities of some of these products has been reported, emphasis has generally been placed on the synthetic and structural characterization. Here the focus will be placed on the biological activities of some of these products, specifically those derived from monomeric and polymeric carbohydrates.

EXPERIMENTAL

Synthetic, physical and structural characterizations have been reported elsewhere.[1-6]

Bacterial studies were conducted in the usual manner. For instance, plates containing a suitable growth medium, such as triptic soy agar or Mueller Hinton agar, were seeded with suspensions of the test organism that would produce an acceptable lawn of test organism after 24 hours incubation at 37°C. Shortly after the plates were seeded, the test compounds were introduced as solids directly or as solids in an emulsion or in solution employing sterile disks (standard 5 mm). The plates were incubated and the inhibition noted. Compounding was accomplished through grinding the products into powders and then adding the powder to the latex paste with mixing and, finally, allowing the mixture to dry to a film.

RESULTS AND DISCUSSION

General structures for saccharides dealt with in this study are given as [4-7]. All can be considered as being composed of hydroxyl-containing units which contain varying amounts and condensation sites of the mono-halo (as shown in Figure 1 for xylan) and dihalo (as shown in Figure 2 for dextran and dibutyltin chloride) organostannanes. Some units may contain one, two or more moieties derived from the organostannane. The products derived from reaction with dihalostannanes and dextran and cellulose are crosslinked and insoluble in all attempted liquids. The

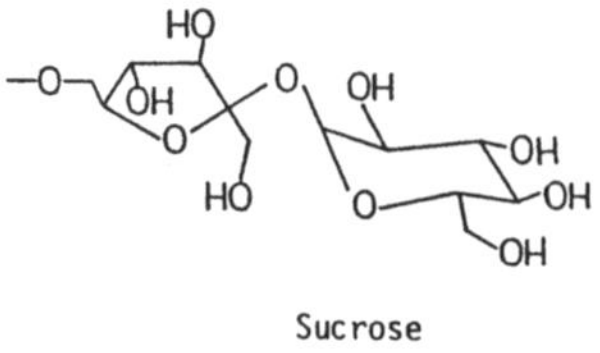

Sucrose

Structure [4].

Cellulose

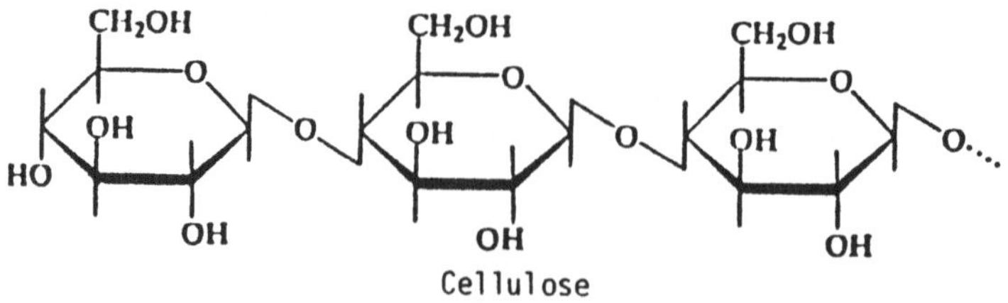

Structure [5].

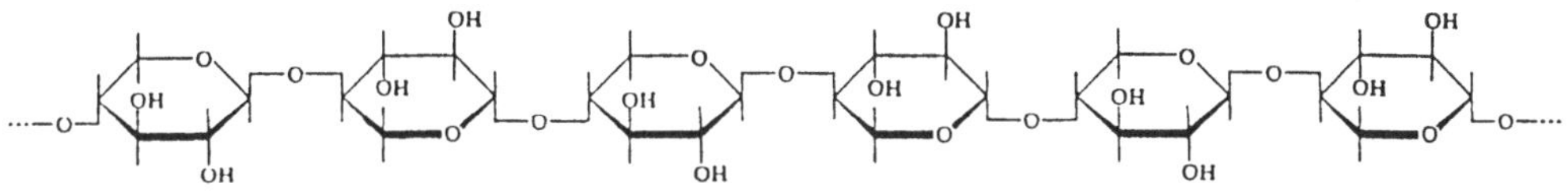

Xylan

Structure [6].

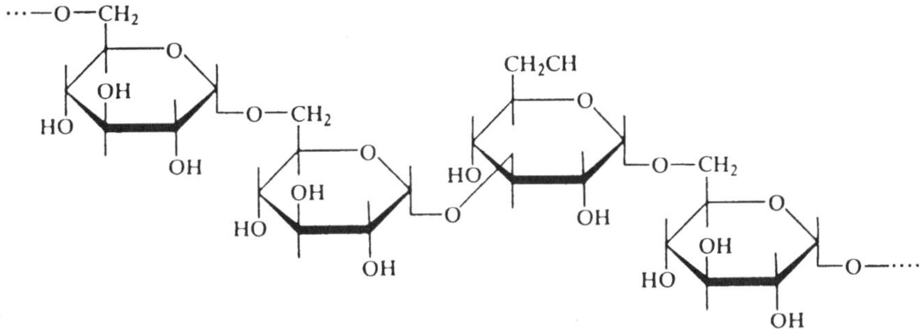

Structure [7], Dextrans.

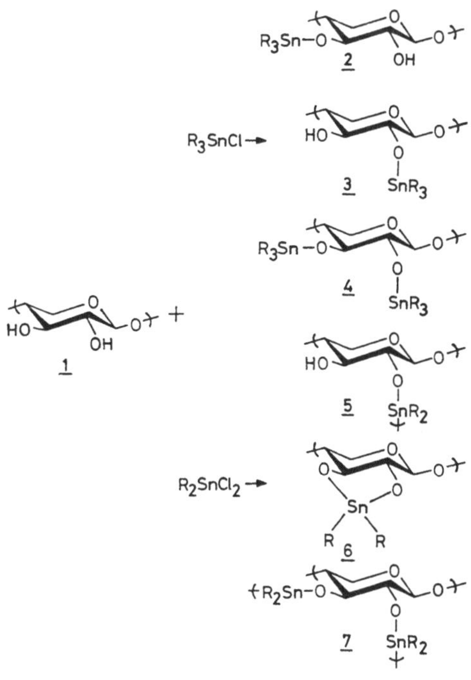

Figure 1. Possible repeat unit structures for the condensation of xylan with mono- and dichlororganostannanes.

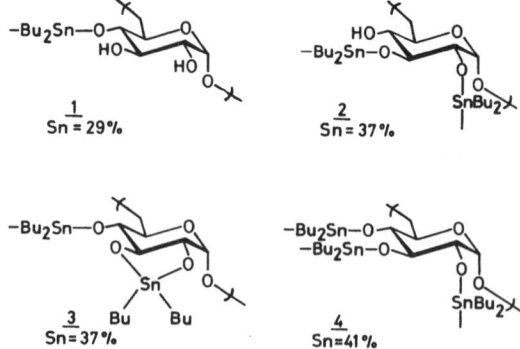

Figure 2. Possible structures for tin-containing units derived from dextran. Percentage tin values are noted for each structure.

products from dihalostannanes and sucrose and xylan contain varying fractions that are soluble in dipolar aprotic liquids such as DMF, DMA, DMSO, HMPA and TEP. Products derived from monohalostannanes are soluble in dipolar aprotic liquids. The products derived from dihalostannanes and xylan are believed to contain the stannane largely within five-membered rings as shown in Figure 1.

Table 1. Biological assays for organostannane containing products.

Reactants	% Sn	Zone of Inhibition (mm)		
		(a)	(b)	(c)
Dextran, Me_2SnCl_2	12	7	9	6
Dextran, Bu_2SnCl_2	26	0	7	3
Dextran, Bu_2SnCl_2	20	0	1.5	3
Dextran, Bu_2SnCl_2	10	0	1.7	3
Dextran, $(C_6H_5CH_2)_2SnCl_2$	14	0	4	2
Dextran, $(C_8H_{17})_2SnCl_2$	23	0	0	0
Dextran, $(C_{12}H_{25})SnCl_2$	15	0	0	0
Dextran, $(C_6H_5)_3SnCl$	14	0	6	0
Sucrose, Me_2SnCl_2	31	7	8	4
Sucrose, Et_2SnCl_2	31	8	6	4
Sucrose, Pr_2SnCl_2	33	4	6	6
Sucrose, Bu_2SnCl_2,	–	0	–	–
Sucrose, $(C_6H_5)_2SnCl_2$	34	0	4	2
Dextran-Control	0	0	0	0

(a) *P. aeruginosa*
(b) *S. aureus*
(c) *E. coli*

Table 2. Biological assays for condensation products derived from organostannane dihalides and sucrose.

	Organostannane (%Sn)		
Organism	Me_2SnCl_2 (31)	Pr_2SnCl_2 (32)	Bu_2SnCl_2 (21)
B. catarrhalis	I	I	I
E. coli	I	I	SI
S. epidermidis	I	I	SI
E. aerogenes	N	I	I
N. mucosa	I	I	N
K. pneumoniae	I	I	I
P. aeruginosa	I	I	N
A. calcoaceticus	I	I	I

where:
I = complete inhibition
SI = slight inhibition
N = no inhibition.

For purposes of expense and time only topical applications were considered, concentrating on mildew, rot, and selected disease-causing microorganisms, mainly bacteria. Tests were carried out on powdered forms of the products as solids, and where appropriate, in solution. The results are given in Tables 1-4. Brief descriptions of some of the bacteria tested are given in Table 5.

Table 3. Biological assays for organostannane containing products derived from xylan.

	Organostannane		
γ Concentration	Bu_2SnCl_2	Bu_3SnCl	$(C_6H_5)_3SnCl$
B. subtilis			
5000	I (13)	I (21)	I (21)
500	I (11)	I (20)	I (20)
50	N	I (11)	I (12)
P. coli			
5000	SI	SI	SI
500	N	N	N
50	N	N	N

I = inhibition
SI = slight inhibition
N = no inhibition
( ) = diameter of inhibition in mm.

Table 4. Biological assays for organostannane containing products derived for cellulose generated from cotton.

Organostannane	Sn (%)	A. flavus	A. niger	A. fumigatus
Pr_2SnCl_2	21	4	4	3
Bu_2SnCl_2	37	4	4	3
Bu_2SnCl_2 (itself)	39	4	4	4
$(C_8H_{17})_2SnCl_2$	18	3	0	0
Ph_2SnCl_2	21	4	4	3

4 = 100% inhibition
3 = 75%
2 = 25%
0 = 0%

Of particular note are the results with *Pseudomonas aeruginosa* since it is responsible for about one half of the deaths of burn patients. As seen in Tables 1 and 2, products derived from Me_2SnCl_2, Et_2SnCl_2 and Pr_2SnCl_2 generally inhibit *P. aeruginosa* and thus may be effective in its control when mixed as a salve, ointment, etc. for use with burn patients. This is significant because there currently does not exist a good general mode of control for this organism on burn patients.

The general trend of bacterial toxicities given in Tables 1-4 is in agreement with toxicity generally decreasing with increase in aliphatic chain length. This tendency is general for organometallics. While the tendency for decreased toxicity with increase in aliphatic chain length is a general tendency, the actual toxicity-structure relationships vary with the mode of delivery, organism, delivery form (solid, salt solution, DMSO solution, etc.), etc. Thus Bu-Sn moieties are especially effective at inhibiting select salt-water species, such as barnacles, compared to the methyl-tin and ethyl-tin organometallic moieties. It is relatively non-toxic to mammals and most fish (compared to Me-Sn, Et-Sn, Pr-Sn). Barnes and Magee found that dioctyltin was non-toxic to rats, mice and guinea pigs in oral doses up to 400 mg/kg given 3 or 4 successive days, or incorporated in the diet of rats for four months at 200 ppm.[8] Toxic effects were produced following a single dose of 920 mg/kg in rats and 690 mg/kg in mice. Interperitoneal toxicity was about tenfold compared to oral toxicity.[8] The dermal toxicity of dialkyltin dichlorides applied cutaneously to male rats follows the accepted general trend of decreasing toxicity with increase in alkyl chain length, with the toxicity being of the order Me>Et>Pr>Bu>pentyl>hexyl.[9] On the other hand, Seinen et al. found Bu_2SnCl_2 to be the most toxic of the organostannanes tested, causing mortality in six of twenty weaning rats at a dietary level of 150 ppm and severe liver,[10,11] and biliary changes along with abdominal edemas.[8] Thus, while the trend of bacterial toxicity with respect to stannane structure is fairly well known, the toxicity-structure trends with respect to internal application of organostannanes is not well known.

A number of tin-containing products derived from dextran and sucrose were tested as solid additives to a latex acrylic paste employing usual industrial mixing procedures. Products derived from dimethyl, diethyl and dipropylstannane dichlorides showed a 50-75% decrease in growth of *A. niger* compared with samples containing no added product. A typical culture plate is shown in Figure 3.

Table 5. Brief descriptions of selected bacteria employed in
the present study.

Actinobacter calcoaceticus: Gram-negative rod.
Can be an opportunistic pathogen but is part of the normal
flora of the skin and mouth.
Associated with conjunctivitis, keratitus, and chronic ear
infections.

Alcaligenes faecalis: Gram-negative rod.
Part of the normal intestinal flora.
Has been found to cause urinary tract infections and in de-
bilitated individuals septicemia or meningitis.

Branhamella catarrhalis: Gram-negative diploccus.
Part of the normal oral and nasopharyngeal flora.
Has been associated with mucous membrane inflammations,
venereal discharges, meningitis, and bacterial endocarditis.

Enterobacter aerogenes: Gram-negative rods.
Part of the normal flora of the intestinal tract.
Has caused urinary tract infections, endocarditis, pneumonia,
and bacteremia.

Escherichia coli: Gram-negative rod.
Part of the normal intestinal flora.
Most frequent cause of urinary tract infections.
May cause cholecystitus, appendicitis, peritonitis, sinu-
sitis, and summer diarrhea.

Klebsiella pneumoniae: Gram-negative rod.
Part of the normal flora of the nose, mouth, and intestines.
May cause lesions in various parts of the body, pneumonia,
chronic lung abscess, sinusitis, and upper respiratory infections.

Neisseria mucosa: Gram-negative cocci.
Part of normal flora of the oronasopharynx.
Generally non-pathogenic but has been found in rare cases of
meningitis.

Pseudomonas aeruginosa: Gram-negative rod.
Common inhabitant of soil.
Frequently found as part of the normal flora of the intestine
and skin.
Opportunistic pathogen, may infect wounds, contaminates
burns, draining sinuses and decubitus ulcers, cause urinary
tract infections, eye infections, and meningitis.

Staphylococcus cocci: Gram-positive cocci.
Generally causes mild infections but has caused septicemia,
bacterial endocarditis, and urinary tract infections.

Staphylococcus aureus: Gram-positive cocci.
Causes "pimples", abscesses, impetigo, wound infections,
pyelitis, cystitis "food poisoning", pneumonia, meningitis,
and enteritis.

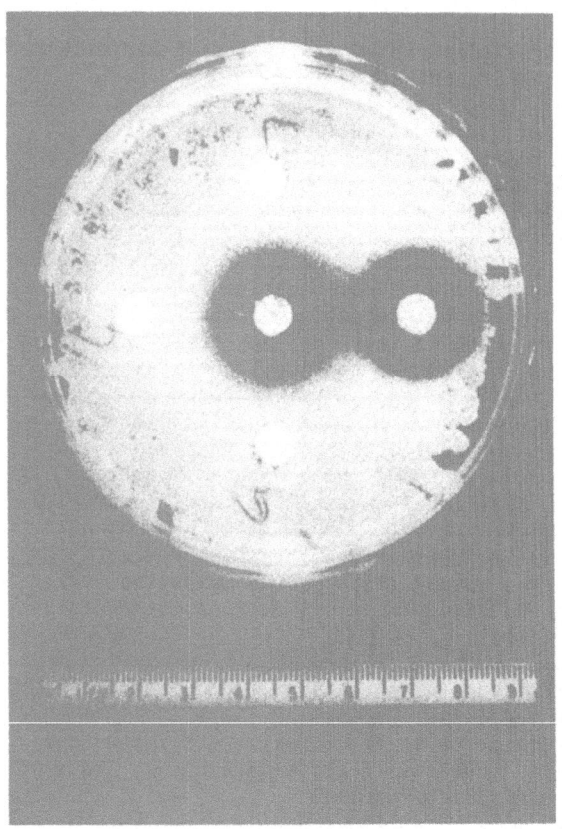

Figure 3. Culture plate results for inhibition of *P. aerugi-nosa*. Clockwise from top: (a), dextran, Bu_2Sn (20% Sn; (b), dextran, $(C_8H_{17})_2Sn$ (23% Sn); (c), sucrose, Et_2Sn (31% Sn); (d), sucrose, $(C_6H_5)_2Sn$ (34% Sn) and (e), (center) dextran, Me_2Sn (12% Sn).

ACKNOWLEDGMENT

We are pleased to acknowledge partial support from the American Chemical Society Petroleum Research Foundation Grant Number 19222-B7-C.

REFERENCES

1. C. Carraher, Jr., T. Gehrke, D. Giron, D. Cerutis and H. M. Molloy, J. Macromol. Sci-Chem., **A19**, 1121 (1983).
2. C. Carraher, Jr., W. Burt, D. Giron, J. Schroeder, M. L. Taylor, H. M. Molloy and T. O. Tiernan, J. Applied Polymer Sci., **28**, 1919 (1983).
3. Y. Noashima, C. Carraher, Jr., T. Gehrke, M. Kurokawa and D. Blair, J. Macromol. Sci-Chem., **A23**, 861 (1986).
4. Y. Naoshima, S. Hirono and C. Carraher, Polymeric Materials, **52**, 29 (1985).
5. C. Carraher, Jr., D. Giron, J. Schroeder and C. McNeely, U.S. Patent. 4,312,981, Jan. 26, 1982; Assignee: Wright State University.
6. C. Carraher, Jr., P. Mykytiuk, H. Blaxall, D. Cerutis, R. Linville, D. G. Giron, T. O. Tiernan and S. Coldiron, Organic Coatings and Plastics Chemistry, **45**, 564 (1981).
7. National Bureau of Standards, Communication with C. Carraher.

8. J. M. Barnes and P. M. Magee, J. Pathol. Bacteriol., **75**, 267 (1985).
9. J. B. Barnes and H. B. Stoner, Brit. J. Ind. Med., **15**, 15 (1985).
10. W. Seinen, Taxicol. Appl, Pharmacol., **42**, 197 (1977).
11. W. Seinen and M. I. Willems, Toxicol. Appl. Pharmacol., **35**, 63 (1970).

NUCLEIC ACID ANALOGS FOR HIGH PERFORMANCE LIQUID CHROMATOGRAPHY

Yoshiaki Inaki, Suguru Nagae, Takashi Miyamoto,
Yoshihiko Sugiura, and Kiichi Takemoto

Faculty of Engineering, Osaka University
Suita, Osaka 565, Japan

Nucleic acid base and nucleoside derivatives were bonded
to 3-aminopropyl-silanized silica (APS-silica) and silica
gel. These resins were useful as the columns of high performance liquid chromatography (HPLC) for the selective
separation of oligoethyleneimine derivatives having pendant
thymine or adenine bases. These column systems were also
found to be applicable to the separation of nucleosides,
nucleotide, and oligonucleotides.

INTRODUCTION

The synthetic nucleic acid analogs have recently much attention, and
numerous studies have been devoted to the preparation and the properties
of these analogs, which may find a number of application possibilities as
polymeric drugs, photosensitive polymers, and other valuable
materials.[1-5] The present paper concerns the preparation of the HPLC
resins containing nucleic acid derivatives which can be applied to HPLC
systems using specific interaction between nucleic acid bases.

In biochemical, medical, and biotechnological fields separation and
analysis of nucleic acids and their fragments are very important
problems. For nucleic acid fragments, the separation methods are column
chromatography and electrophoresis, and the analytical methods are electrophoresis, paper chromatography, and high performance liquid chromatography (HPLC). In biochemistry, the HPLC procedure has been developed for
analysis of nucleic acid fragments. Chemically bonded HPLC stationary
phases based on silica gel (such as reversed-phase liquid chromatography,
gel permeation chromatography, and ion-exchange chromatography) are commercially available and have been used widely.

It is known that nucleic acids form a polymer complex by a specific
interaction caused by stacking and hydrogen bonding interactions (Figure
1).[6,7] Therefore, application of the specific interaction between nucleic
acid bases for the HPLC system may give useful HPLC systems for the
analysis of the nucleic acid components. Applications of nucleic acid
base derivatives for column and HPLC systems have been reported.[8-14]

Similar to the HPLC systems, immobilization of nucleic acid base

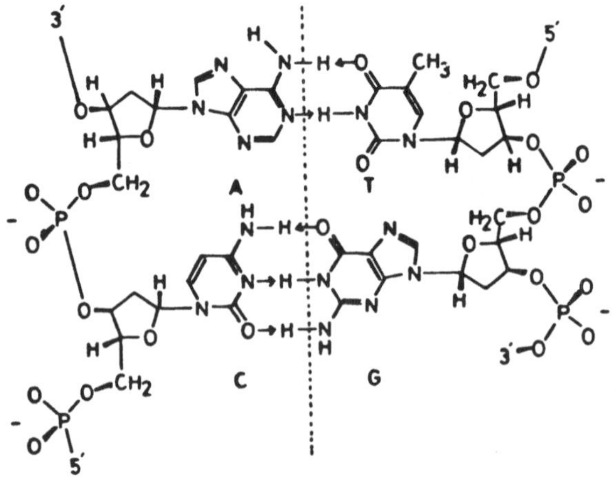

Figure 1. Specific base pairing of nucleic acid bases in DNA.

derivatives on silica gel and the separation of nucleosides and nucleic acid bases have been reported. In these systems, the separation of the nucleic acid base derivatives may be caused by base pairing but hydrophobic interactions may still remain. On the other hand, for column chromatography, polynucleotides and the fragments are immobilized on cellulose, Sepharose, and DEAE derivatives. In these systems, specific separation by base-pairing may be possible as in the case of biological systems. Such systems are known as affinity chromatography or template chromatography. These systems, however, can not be applied to HLPC systems because chemical, thermal, and physical stabilities are too low.

In the present paper, chemically and thermally stable nucleic acid derivatives are chemically bonded on silica gel for HPLC systems and specific separations of nucleic acid moieties are reported on.

EXPERIMENTAL

1. Preparation of HPLC Resins

Three types of HPLC resins were prepared: (1) nucleic acid base bonded silica gels: Si-Thy (1), Si-Ura (2), Si-Cyt (3), Si-Ade (4), Si-Hyp (5), and Si-Gua (6) (Figure 2); (2) poly-L-lysine derivatives bonded silica gels:Si-PLL-Cbz (7), Si-PLL-Thy (8), and Si-PLL-Ade (9) (Figure 3); and (3) nucleoside bonded silica gels: Si-Thd (10) and Si-Urd (11) (Figure 4). The detailed preparation methods of these silica gel derivatives will be shown elsewhere.[15-18]

1.1 Nucleic acid base bonded silica gel:[16-17] The hypoxanthine bonded silica gel (Si-Hyp; 5) was prepared by the reaction of the nucleic acid base derivatives with an 3-aminopropyl-silanized silica (APS-silica) Li-Chrosorb NH₂, Merck) according to Scheme 1, and free silanol groups and amino groups were blocked by trimethylsilyl and acetyl groups, respectively. The carboxyethyl derivative of hypoxanthine (13) was prepared from the carboxyethyl derivative of adenine (12) according to the literature.[19] The pentachlorophenyl activated ester (14) was reacted with the APS-silica to give the hypoxanthine bonded silica gel (Si-Hyp; 5). The same method was applied to the preparation of nucleic acid base

Si-Thy 1 Si-Ura 2 Si-Cyt 3

Si-Ade 4 Si-Hyp 5 Si-Gua 6

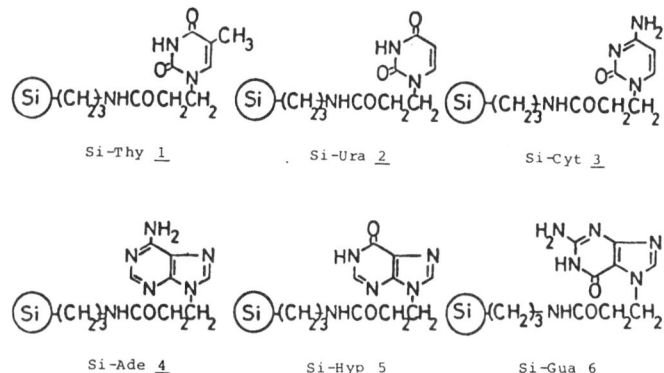

Figure 2. Nucleic acid base bonded silica gels.

bonded silica gels containing thymine (Si-Thy; **1**), uracil (Si-Ura; **2**), cytosine (Si-Cyt; **3**), adenine (Si-Ade; **4**), and guanine (Si-Gua; **6**).

Immobilization of the nucleic acid base derivatives on silica gel was confirmed by IR spectra and elementary analysis, and hydrolysis followed by measurement of UV spectra. The IR spectra for Si-Hyp suggested the presence of hypoxanthine units in the silica gel derivative. Quantitative determination of the content of hypoxanthine units in Si-Hyp was done by hydrolysis of the silica gel derivative followed by measurement of UV spectra bases on the spectra of the carboxyethyl derivative of hypoxanthine (**14**). The content of the hypoxanthine units in the silica gel derivative was about 1.5×10^{-4} mol/g.

1.2 Poly-L-lysine derivative bonded silica gel:[15] The poly-L-lysine derivative bonded silica gels having carbobenzyloxy (Si-PLL-Cbz; **7**), thymine (Si-PLL-Thy; **8**), and adenine (Si-PLL-Ade; **9**), were prepared as shown in Scheme 2 for Si-PLL-Thy (**8**). The nucleic acid base derivatives were grafted onto the poly-L-lysine having terminal carboxyl group, and were reacted with the APS-silica.

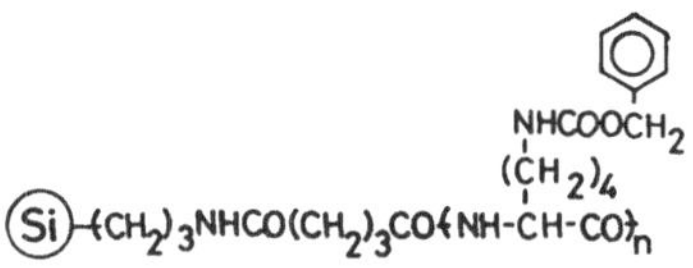

Si-PLL-Cbz 7

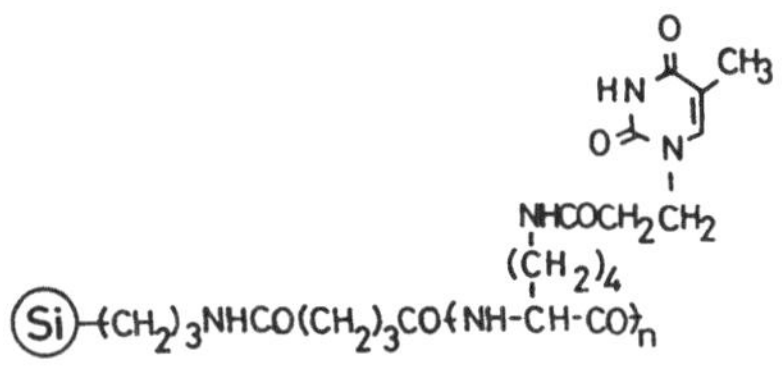

Si-PLL-Thy 8

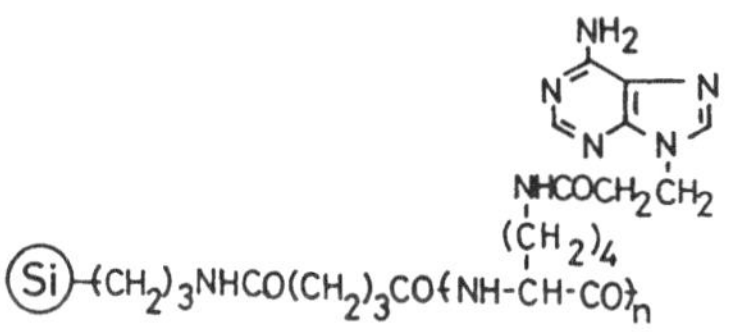

Si-PLL-Ade 9

Figure 3. Poly-L-lysine derivative bonded silica gels.

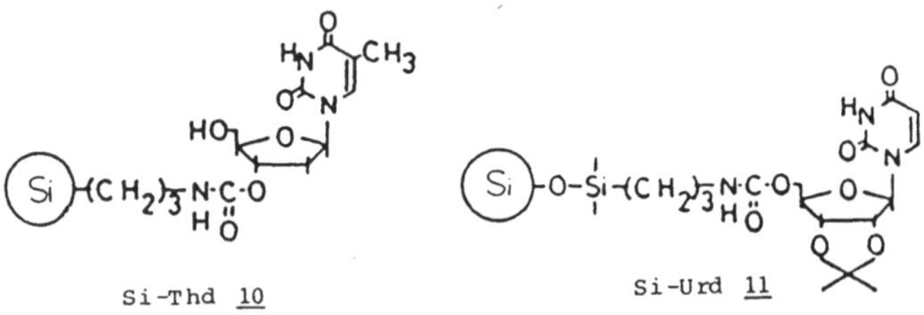

Figure 4. Nucleoside bonded silica gels.

At first, poly-L-lysine contains terminal carboxyl group and N[6]-carbobenzyloxy protecting group (PLL-Cbz-COOH; 16) was prepared. PLL-Cbz (15), which had a terminal amino group, was obtained by polymerization of the corresponding N-carbobenzyloxy amino acid (NCA) initiated by n-propylamine. The reaction of glutaric anhydride with the terminal amino group in the polymer (15) gave its PLL-Cbz derivative having a carboxyl group at the polymer end; PLL-Cbz-COOH (16). The degree of polymerization of this polymer (16) was determined to be 80 by viscometry ([η] = 7.75 x 10⁻², in DMF at 25°C).²⁰ The protecting groups of the side chains in the polymer (16) were removed by HBr gas in acetic acid, giving the polymer HBr·PLL-COOH (17).

The PLL derivatives containing nucleic acid bases were prepared according to reference 21. Polymer (18) (PLL-Thy-COOH) containing pendent thymine base was obtained from the reaction of (17) reacted with activated ester of thymine derivative. In the case of the adenine derivative, the amino group in adenine base was protected by a diphenylphosphynothioyl (Ppt) group, because the activated ester derivative was unstable. The molar ratios of the thymine and the adenine units to PLL in the polymers were 0.94 and 0.73, respectively, determined by NMR spectroscopy.

The terminal carboxyl groups of these polymers (for example) were allowed to react with pentachlorophenyl trichloroacetate to give the corresponding activated esters. The reaction of the amino group on APS-silica with the activated esters gave the desired silica gel derivatives Si-PLL-Cbz (7), Si-PLL-Thy (8), and Si-PLL-Ade (9). In these resins, the Cbz-group and nucleic acid bases were assumed to be in a regular arrangement on helix of poly-L-lysine.

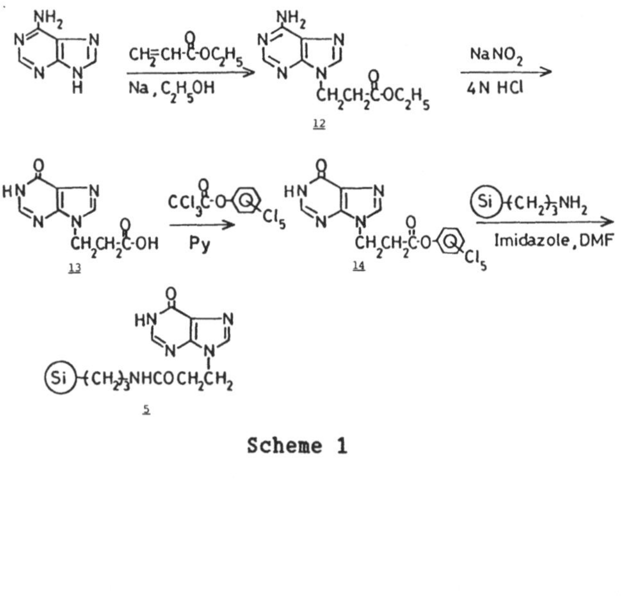

Scheme 1

188

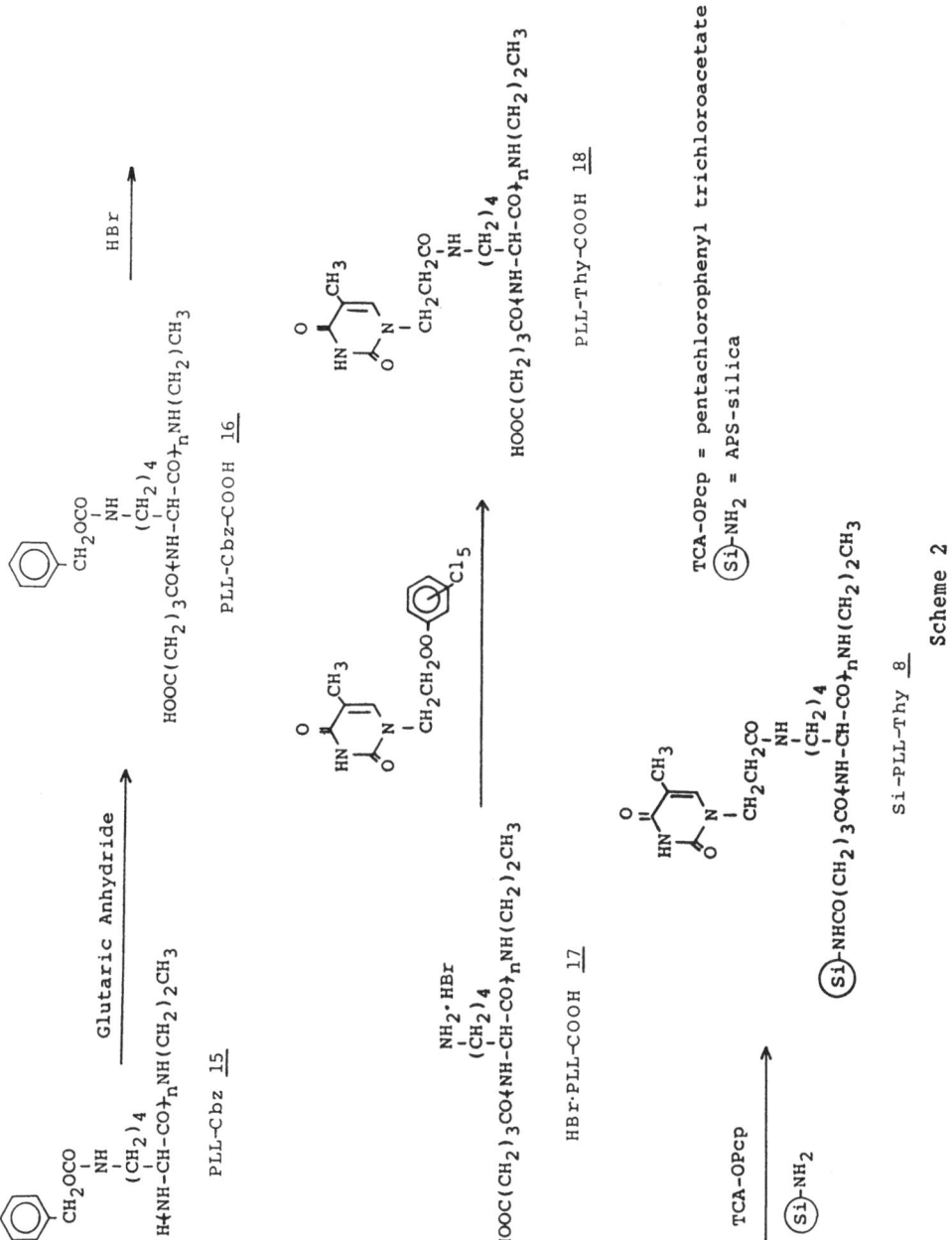

Scheme 2

Alternatively, a resin having adenine derivatives bonded by silanol bonding (Si-O-Si-PLL-Ade; 9') was prepared as follows: The terminal carboxyl group of the polymer (HBr·PLL-Ade-COOH) was silanized by the treatment with 3-aminopropyltriethoxysilane, followed by reaction with silica gel (LiChrosorb Si 1000, Merck). Immobilization of the PLL derivatives on silica gel was confirmed by IR spectroscopy and the content of the polymer in the silica gel derivatives were determined by elementary analysis.

1.3 Nucleoside bonded silica gel:[18]

The nucleoside bonded silica gels, Si-Thd (10) and Si-Urd (11) were prepared by the reaction of the protected nucleosides with the isocyanate derivative, followed by direct reaction with silica gel (Li-Chrosorb Si 100, Merck) as shown in Scheme 3. The protected uridine (2',3'-isopropyrideneurine; 19) was reacted with 3-isocyanatopropyltriethoxysilane to give the silane derivative of uridine (20). The uridine derivative (20) was, then reacted with silica gel under reflux of toluene to give Si-Urd (11). For the preparation of Si-Thd (10), 5-tritylthymidine was reacted with the isocyanate derivative followed by reaction with silica gel.

1.4 Samples:

Three kinds of oligoethyleneimine derivatives containing pendent thymine or adenine bases (Figure 5) were prepared as described in reference 22-24. EI-T-n and EI-A-n have thymine and adenine bases (n units in a molecule) and have no amino acid spacer groups. Another kind of compound, abbreviated as EI-A-βAla-n and EI-A-αAla-n for the adenine derivatives, have a spacer group of β-alanine and α-alanine, respectively. Nucleosides, nucleotides, and oligonucleotides were commercially available reagent grade.

1.5 Chromatographic Procedure:

All HPLC resins were packed into stainless steel tube (150 x 4.6 mm i.d.) under constant flow (3-4 ml/min, 100-130 kg/cm² of 50% (v/v) methanol-water solvent, respectively. The experiments were performed with a Toyo Soda HPLC 8000 equipped with a thermostatic column oven (30°C) and a UV detector operating at 254 nm.

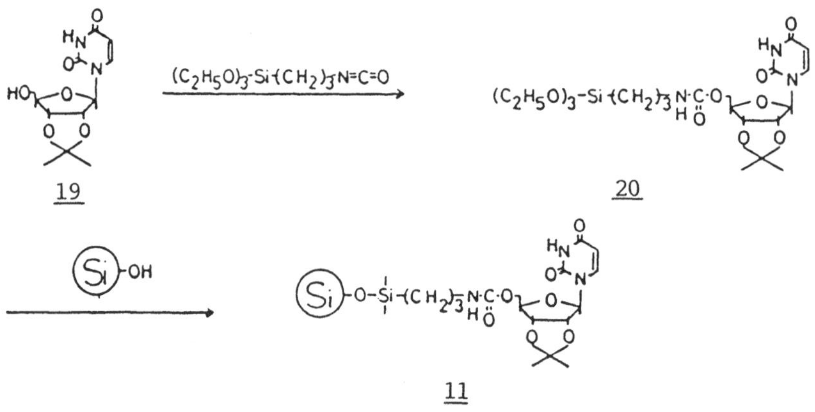

Scheme 3

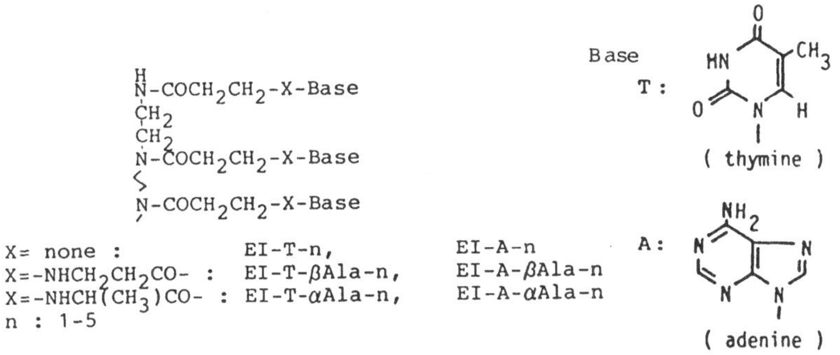

H
|
N-COCH$_2$CH$_2$-X-Base
|
CH$_2$
|
CH$_2$
|
N-$\overset{\text{C}}{C}$OCH$_2$CH$_2$-X-Base
\
N-COCH$_2$CH$_2$-X-Base
/

X= none :   EI-T-n,   EI-A-n
X=-NHCH$_2$CH$_2$CO- : EI-T-βAla-n,   EI-A-βAla-n
X=-NHCH(CH$_3$)CO- : EI-T-αAla-n,   EI-A-αAla-n
n : 1-5

Base   T :

(thymine)

A :

(adenine)

Figure 5. Oligoethyleneimines containing nucleic acid bases
          with and/or without spacer groups.

RESULTS

2. Separations of Nucleic Acid Base Derivatives by HPLC Systems

2.1 On the nucleic acid base bonded stationary phase (Si-Ade, 4), Si-Thy, 1): The specific separation of the nucleic acid oligomer models were studied using nucleic acid base bonded silica gels (Si-Ade and Si-Thy), poly-L-lysine derivatives bonded silica gels (Si-PLL-Cbz, Si-PLL-Ade and Si-PLL-Thy), and a commercially available reverse-phase column (ODS column). The oligomers investigated were oligoethyleneimine derivatives containing adenine (EI-A-n) and (EI-T-n) as shown in Figure 5, where n means the number of nucleic acid base units in the oligomer.

Figure 6 shows chromatograms of EI-T-n and EI-A-n with water-methanol (1/1, v/v) as the mobile phase at 40°C. For EI-T-n, the oligomers can be separated according to the degree of polymerization on the Si-Ade column, while the separation was negligible with the ODS and the Si-Thy columns. For EI-A-n, on the other hand, the oligomers were separated on the Si-Thy column, while the separation was negligible with the ODS and the Si-Ade columns. The results suggest that the separation of the oligomers occurred by the specific hydrogen bonding interaction between adenine and thymine. Similar results were obtained for the poly-L-lysine derivative bonded silica gel columns. It is useful to study the difference of the separation behaviors between the monomeric nucleic acid base bonded columns (such as Si-Ade) and the polymeric nucleic acid base bonded columns (such as Si-PLL-Ade). The detailed study will be reported in the future. In this paper, the separation of oligomer models are reported in detail using the Si-PLL-Ade and the Si-PLL-Thy columns.

2.2 On the poly-L-lysine derivative bonded stationary phase; Si-PLL-Cbz (7), Si-PLL-Thy (8), and Si-PLL-Ade (9): At first, separation of the oligoethyleneimine derivatives containing adenine or thymine was investigated with a controlled HPLC system consisting of a PLL-Cbz-bonded stationary phase and three kinds of mobile phases. From the chromatograms of EI-T-n and EI-A-n on Si-PLL-Cbz (7), retention data was obtained, and summarized in Figures 7 and 8. EI-T-n and EI-A-n can be separated with this system only by using water as the mobile phase, where as oligomers having nucleic acid bases were clearly separated by hydrophobic interaction with PLL-Cbz on the stationary phase.

The chromatograms obtained employing the PLL-Thy bonded stationary phase (Si-PLL-Thy; 8) gave the retention data for EI-T-n and EI-A-n (Figures 7 and 8). In the case of EI-T-n, separation of the oligomers

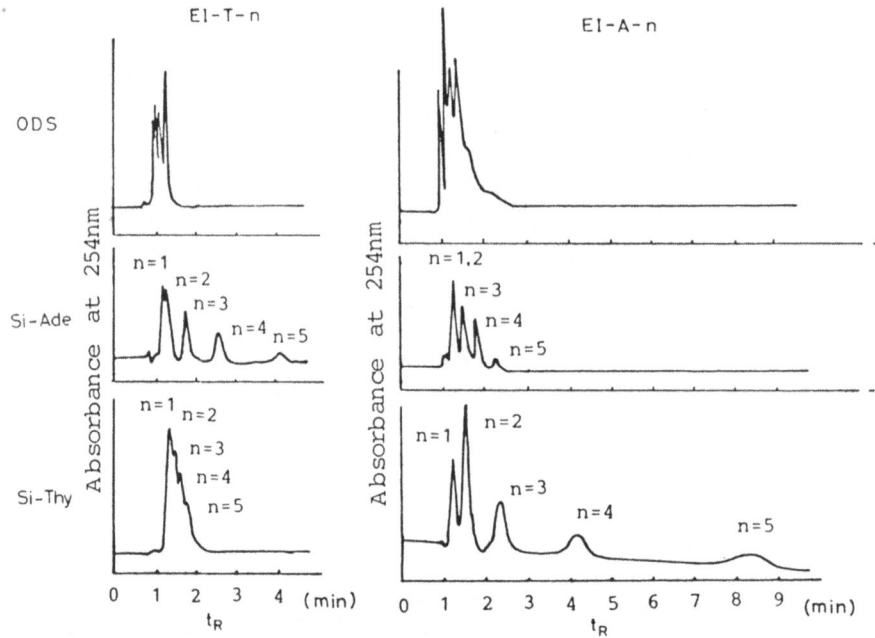

Figure 6. Chromatograms of EI-T-n and EI-A-n on Si-Ade and Si-Thy columns with water/methanol (1/1, v/v) mobile phase. Flow rate: 1.0 mL/min. Temperature: 40°C. Detector: 254 nm.

occurred for each eluent system. However resolution values (Rs) were low, suggesting insufficient separation. On the other hand, the oligomers EI-A-n were separated completely according to molecular weight with all mobile phase systems used.

Results for the separation of EI-T-n and EI-A-n using Si-PLL-Ade HPLC system (9) are also shown in Figures 7 and 8. The oligomer EI-T-n, which contained the complementary thymine bases, were completely separated on

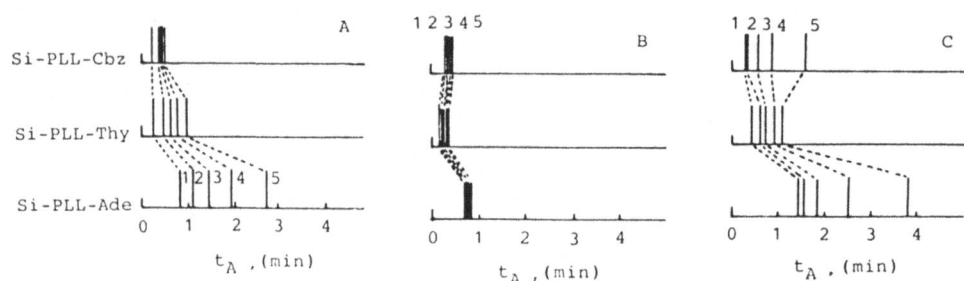

Figure 7. Adjusted retention time (t_A) of EI-T-n on Si-PLL- Cbz, Si-PLL-Thy, and Si-PLL-Ade. Mobile phase: A), methanol; B), water-methanol (1/1, v/v); C), water. Flow rate: 1.0 mL/min. Temperature: 30°C. Detector: 254 nm. Peaks: (1), EI-T-1; (2), EI-T-2; (3), EI-T-3; (4), EI-T-4; and (5), EI-T-5.

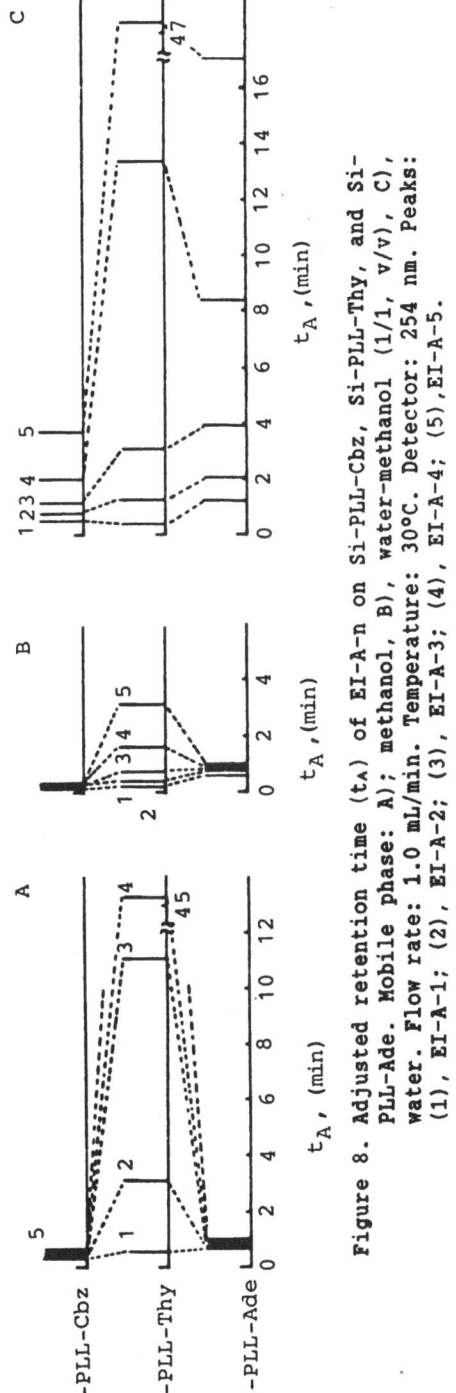

Figure 8. Adjusted retention time (t_A) of EI-A-n on Si-PLL-Cbz, Si-PLL-Thy, and Si-PLL-Ade. Mobile phase: A); methanol, B), water-methanol (1/1, v/v), C), water. Flow rate: 1.0 mL/min. Temperature: 30°C. Detector: 254 nm. Peaks: (1), EI-A-1; (2), EI-A-2; (3), EI-A-3; (4), EI-A-4; (5), EI-A-5.

the Si-PLL-Ade stationary phase with both methanol and water as the mobile phase. Dependence of the retention times on the mobile phase for the EI-T-n/Si-PLL-Ade system resembles those for the EI-A-n/Si-PLL-Thy system. In the case of EI-A-n, however, separation employing the Si-PLL-Ade system was observed only with water as the mobile phase.

3. Specific Separation of Nucleic Acid base Derivatives

3.1 Specific Interaction of the Synthetic Nucleic Acid Analogs: A variety of synthetic nucleic acid analogs have been prepared. The interaction of these synthetic analogs with polynucleotides, and the interaction between these nucleic acid analogs have been studied. Nucleic acids are formed from chains which have backbones composed of alternative phosphodiester and sugar units and carry nucleic acid bases. There is one electronegative charge per monomer unit. Consequently, strong columbic repulsion between chains exist. Nevertheless, two or more chains associate through the formation of hydrogen bonding between the nucleic acid bases in aqueous solution. On the other hand, the backbone polymers of these analogs are synthetic polymers and the nucleic acid bases are presented in the side chains. The synthetic analogs of nucleic acids have neutral, less flexible, chemically and thermally stable, and sterically inhomogeneous backbones. Therefore, the interaction behavior of the synthetic analogs are different from that of polynucleotides. For example, selected specific interactions are stable at high temperature, in organic solvent, and high and low pH values.

The interaction of nucleic acid bases is affected by three main factors; hydrophobic, hydrogen bonding, and electrostatic interactions. For the neutral nucleic acid analogs, the electrostatic interaction may be neglected. The hydrophobic interaction is the main factor in aqueous solution. Therefore, slow elusion of a adenine derivatives on the thymine containing column should be explained by the hydrophobic interaction instead of specific base pairing. In order to elucidate the importance of specific base pairing in the HPLC system, exclusion of the hydrophobic interaction is necessary.

3.2 Selective Separation of Thymine and Adenine Derivatives: As shown in Figures 7 and 8, EI-T-n and EI-A-n were separated employing a Si-PLL-Cbz column which contained no nucleic acid bases. The nucleic acid bases are known to be hydrophobic and are separated by reverse-phase chromatography.[25-27] It is also known that the hydrophobicity of purine bases is higher than that of pyrimidine bases, and that the retention of purine derivatives is longer than that of pyrimidine derivatives when measurement was made by reversed-phase chromatography. Therefore, the separation of EI-T-n and EI-A-n on Si-PLL-Cbz with water mobile phase may be explained by the hydrophobic interaction between the nucleic acid base derivatives and PLL-Cbz polymer on silica gel, because the retention times of purine derivatives (EI-A-n) are longer than those of pyrimidine derivatives (EI-T-n).

Figure 9 shows chromatograms for the mixture of dimer models (EI-T-2 and EI-A-2) on three kinds of silica gels; Si-PLL-Cbz (7), Si-PLL-Thy (8), and Si-PLL-Ade (9) with methanol as the mobile phase. The dimers could not be separated on Si-PLL-Cbz column with methanol as the mobile phase, suggesting that hydrophobic interaction was negligible between the dimer models and the PLL-Cbz polymer in methanol. The Si-PLL-Thy column, however, gave good separation of the dimer models by using methanol as the mobile phase, where the retention time for EI-A-2 was longer than that for EI-T-2. In this system, hydrogen bonding interaction should be principally responsible for the separation instead of hydrophobic inter-

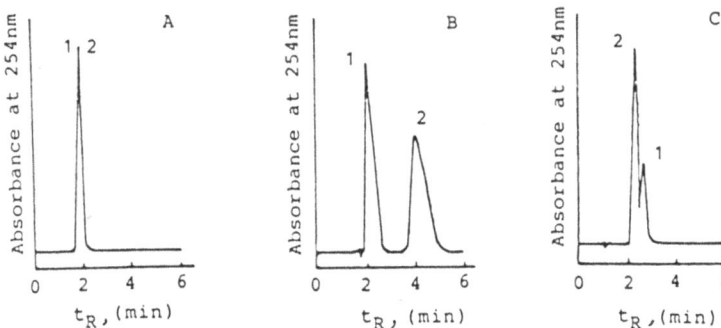

Figure 9. Chromatograms of EI-T-2 and EI-A-2 mixture. Column:
A), Si-PLL-Cbz; B), SiPLL-Thy; C), Si-PLL-Ade.
Mobile phase: methanol. Flow rate: 1.0 mL/min.
Temperature: 30°C. Detector: 254 nm. Peaks: (1),
EI-T-2; (2), EI-A-2.

action. Also for the Si-PLL-Ade column, the retention time for EI-T-2 was
longer than that for the EI-A-2 dimer. From these results, the separation
of the dimer models on Si-PLL-Ade or on Si-PLL-Thy can be concluded to be
caused by the specific hydrogen bonded base pairing between adenine and
thymine bases, which was observed in hypochromicity data for the polymer
complex formation in solution.[5]

3.3 Effects of Mobile Phase on the Specific Separation: Figure 10
shows chromatograms of EI-T-n on a nucleic acid analog HPLC system,
consisting of a PLL-Ade-bonded stationary phase (Si-O-Si-PLL-Ade; 9')
with three kinds of mobile phases; water, water-methanol (1/1, v/v), and
methanol. It is clearly shown in Figure 10 that in addition to the interaction of nucleic acid base, more than two other factors should have an
effect on the separation of the oligoethyleneimine derivatives containing

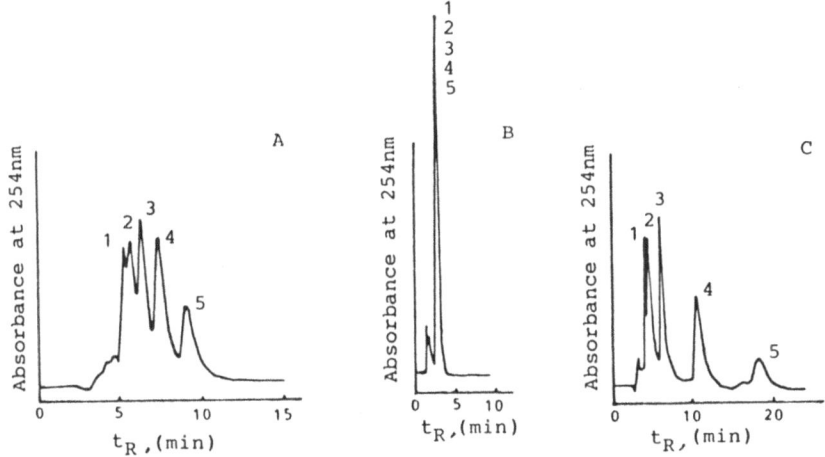

Figure 10. Chromatograms of EI-T-n. Column: Si-O-Si-PLL-Ade.
Mobile phase: A), methanol; B), water-methanol
(1/1, v/v); C), water. Flow rate: A), 0.5 mL/min;
B), 1.0 mL/min; C), 1.0 mL/min. Temperature: 30°C.
Detector: 254nm. Peaks:(1), EI-T-1; (2), EI-T-2;
(3), EI-T-3; (4), EI-T-4; (5), EI-T-5.

adenine and thymine; that is, effects of the mobile phase and the degree of polymerization of the oligomers. For the water and the methanol mobile phases, the oligomers can be separated according to the degree of polymerization, while the separation was negligible with a water-methanol (1/1, v/v) mobile phase.

Separation of the oligomers with an aqueous mobile phase may be explained by a hydrophobic interaction as shown in the case of the PLL-Cbz system. However, with water-methanol (1/1, v/v) as the mobile phase, separation of the oligomer was not observed, and the retention time (t_R) was the shortest for all three kinds of mobile phase systems. This may be caused by the decrease in hydrophobic interaction, brought about by addition of methanol. On the other hand, the methanol mobile phase system showed good separation of EI-A-n and the longest retention times. For the latter case the possibility of hydrophobic interactions in methanol may be negligible. It is assumed, therefore, that the specific base pairing by hydrogen bonding between complimentary nucleic acid bases should be present between PLL-Thy in the stationary phase and EI-A-n in the methanol mobile phase. I.e., the specific base pairing by hydrogen bonding between complimentary nucleic acid bases.

In the case of EI-T-n (Figure 7), effects of the mobile phase on the separation of the oligomers with the Si-PLL-Ade column system were clearly observed to be similar to those shown in Figure 10. The oligomer EI-T-n, which contained the complimentary thymine base, were completely separated on the Si-PLL-Ade stationary phase with methanol because of the specific hydrogen bonding interactions between complimentary nucleic acid bases. On the contrary, the oligomers were not separated employing either Si-PLL-Cbz or Si-PLL-Thy with methanol as the mobile phase, and were separated only with water as the mobile phase because of hydrophobic interactions. However, separation of thymine oligomers on the Si-PLL-Thy stationary phase was minimal even with methanol as the mobile phase. This may also be explained by considering a hydrogen bond interaction between thymine bases. Further this was observed in polymers containing thymine base as an intramolecular interaction.[5]

On the other hand, the oligomers EI-A-n were separated completely on Si-PLL-Thy with all the mobile phase systems (Figure 8). The oligomers (EI-A-n) were separated with a aqueous mobile phase because of hydrophobic interactions such as shown in the case of Si-PLL-Cbz systems. The separation with methanol as the mobile phase was the result of specific hydrogen bonding. In the case of EI-A-n, however, separation on the Si-PLL-Ade system was observed only with water as the mobile phase. In this case it can be assumed that the separation was caused by hydrophobic interactions. It is difficult to assume that there exists stacking interaction between adenine bases, because the oligomers having adenine bases were only minimally separated in a water-methanol mixture and methanol systems.

3.4 Polymer Effects on the HPLC System: Polymer effects on the interaction of nucleic acid bases in oligomer models were studied employing oligomers of polyethyleneimine derivatives containing nucleic acid bases.[5,22-24] The intermolecular interactions between these nucleic acid analogs in solution were particularly studied by UV spectra to give hypochromicity values which have been widely used as a measure of the degree of intermolecular interaction between nucleic acid analogs.

There are various factors influencing both intramolecular and intermolecular interactions of polymers. One of these factors is the degree of polymerization. The intramolecular interaction of the nucleic acid bases in a polymer chain increases with increased degree of polymerization.

196

This trend was found to be caused by the nearest neighboring units, and to be independent of remote units. The hypochromicity values for the 1/1 mixture of adenine and thymine derivatives are tabulated in Table 1.[5] The results suggest the affect of the molecular weight dependency of the intermolecular interaction. It can be seen from the Table that the interaction between the oligomers is fairly small, while interaction between the oligomers and the polymer are remarkable. The polymer effect observed for the intermolecular interaction may be caused by an entropy factor, because the polymer has a number of nucleic acid bases in one molecular chain as the interaction sites.

The polymer effects observed here in the HPLC system are the same as the effects observed for the intermolecular interaction of the polymers in solution. Therefore, it can be concluded that a similar factor affects the interactions both in solution and in HPLC systems i.e., the specific hydrogen bond interactions between complimentary nucleic acid bases.

3.5 Effect of Spacer Units in the Oligomer Models: This article is also concerned with the further study of the separation of oligomer models of polyethyleneimine derivatives with spacer-separated thymine and adenine bases in which β-alanine or α-alanine was used as the spacer. The intramolecular and the intermolecular interactions have been studied. Intramolecular and intermolecular interactions between nucleic acid bases in oligomers and in polymers appear to be largely affected by the position of the bases and the distance between them (Figure 11). For the oligomers and polymers, two factors should be considered: the distance between neighboring pendent groups along the main chain and that between pendent base and main chain, namely the length of the side chain. Hence, amino acids were incorporated into the side chains of the polyethyleneimine derivatives.

The effects of spacers on the intermolecular and the intramolecular interactions are summarized in Table 2. For the thymine derivatives, the intermolecular interaction is decreased both by the β-alanine and α-alanine spacer, and the intramolecular interaction is increased by the β-alanine spacer and decreased by the α-alanine spacer. For the adenine derivatives, the intermolecular interaction is increased by the β-alanine spacer and decreased by the α-alanine spacer, and the intramolecular interaction is decreased both by the β-alanine and the α-alanine spacers. Therefore, the intermolecular interaction of the synthetic nucleic acid analogs is concluded to be affected by the intermolecular interaction of the nucleic acid bases in the side chain, and the nature of the side chain.[5,22-24]

Table 1. Hypochromicity values (%) for 1/1 mixture.*

	EI-A-5	EI-A-6	PEI-A
EI-T-5	1.1	0.6	6.2
EI-T-6	0.5	0.5	8.6
PEI-T	15.8	18.8	26.0

* At 265 nm, in water/EG = 2/1, at 25°C , 10 days after mixing.

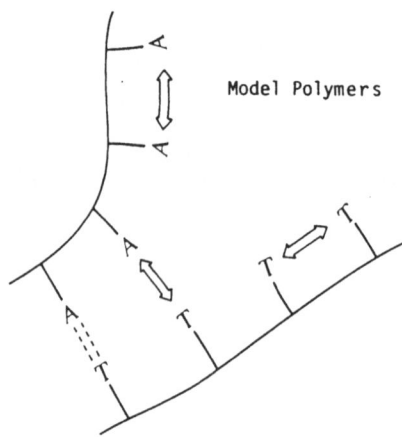

Model Polymers

Figure 11. Interactions between nucleic acid analogs.

Figure 12 shows the retention times for three kinds of tetramers which have different spacer groups using five kinds of column systems in methanol as the mobile phase. The separation of the tetramers was excellent with Si-Ade under these conditions. The data correlates with the ability of intermolecular interactions of the thymine derivatives to occur with the adenine derivative as shown in Table 2. The same results were obtained for the separation of the adenine oligomers as shown in Figure 13, where the retention times for the adenine dimer models were used because the longer oligomer eluted too slowly. For the adenine derivatives, the α-alanine spacer decreases the intermolecular interaction, and the β-alanine spacer increases the intermolecular interaction as shown in Table 2. Therefore the separation behavior of the nucleic acid base oligomers on the nucleic acid base bonded silica gels can be concluded to be same as the intermolecular interactions of the oligomers with the polymers in solution.

Table 2. Effect of spacers on intermolecular (and intra molecular) interactions.*

Compound	Spacer	
	β-Ala	α-Ala
Thymine derivs.	- (+)	- (-)
Adenine derivs.	+ (-)	- (-)

* + and - signify positive and negative effects, respectively; ( ) signifies intramolecular effects.

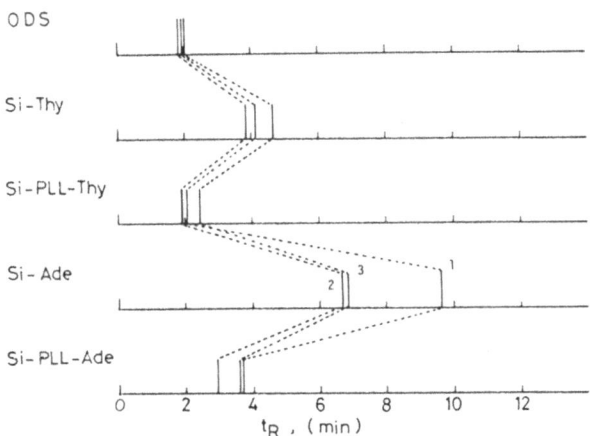

Figure 12. Retention times of the tetramer models containing thymine. Mobile phase: methanol. Flow rate: 1.0 mL/min. Temperature: 30°C. Peaks: (1), EI-T-4; (2), EI-T-αAla-4; (3), EI-T-βAla-4.

4. Separation of Nucleosides, Nucleotides, and Oligonucleotides

4.1 Nucleosides: The HPLC columns containing nucleic acid base derivatives were found to be effective not only for the oligomer models of nucleic acid but also for naturally derived nucleosides, nucleotides and oligonucleotides. Figure 14 shows the chromatograms of nucleosides on Si-Hyp with (A) water and with (B) ethanol mobile phases. In Figure 14(A), adenosine and guanosine eluted slowly in water as the mobile phase, because of the hydrophobic interaction between purine bases, adenine or guanine, and purine base hypoxanthine. A similar chromatogram was obtained using the commercial ODS column which is the reverse-phase column containing long alkyl chain. In the ethanol mobile phase where the hydrophobic interactions should be small, the retention times of the complimentary nucleoside (cytidine and guanosine) were longer than that

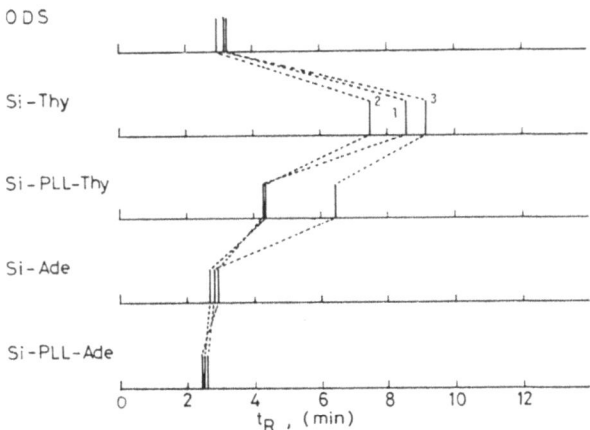

Figure 13. Retention times of the dimer models containing adenine. Mobile phase: methanol. Flow rate: 1.0 mL/min. Temperature: 30°C. Peaks: (1), EI-A-2; (2), EI-A-αAla-2; (3), EI-A-βAla-2.

199

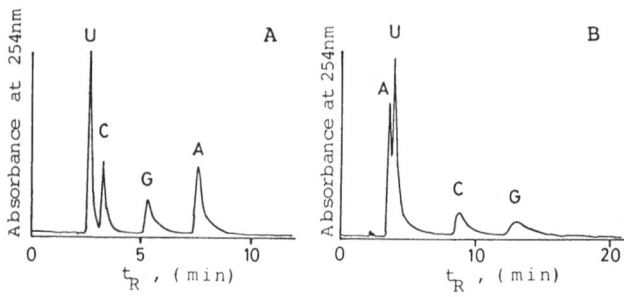

Figure 14. Chromatograms of nucleosides on Si-Hyp. Mobile
phase: (A), water; (B), ethanol. Flow rate: 1.0
mL/min. Temperature: 20°C. Detector: 254 nm.
Samples: (A), adenosine; (C), cytidine; (U),
uridine; (G), guanosine.

of other nucleosides. The separation in ethanol as the mobile phase may
be caused by the specific hydrogen bonding interaction between complimentary nucleic acid bases.

The results of the separations are summarized in Figure 15 (water
mobile phase) and Figure 16 (ethanol mobile phase) for six kinds of
nucleic acid bases bonded column systems. When the mobile phase is water,
as shown in Figure 15, two important factors should be considered; one is
hydrophobic interactions and the other is the hydrogen bonding interactions. In the case of the pyrimidine base bonded column systems (Si-
Thy, Si-Ura, and Si-Cyt), the specific hydrogen bonding interactions
between the complimentary nucleic acid bases seems to be the predominant
factor, so that the complimentary nucleoside (adenoside for Si-Thy and
Si-Ura, and guanosine for Si-Cyt) is eluted slower than other nucleosides. In the case of the purine base bonded column systems (Si-Ade, Si-
Hyp, and Si-Gua), on the other hand, the profile of the separation
resembles that of the ODS column with water as the mobile phase. Therefore, the predominant factor with respect to separation in the case of
the purine base bonded columns with water as the mobile phase is the
hydrophobic interaction between purine bases in the mobile phase and the
purine base on the silica gel.

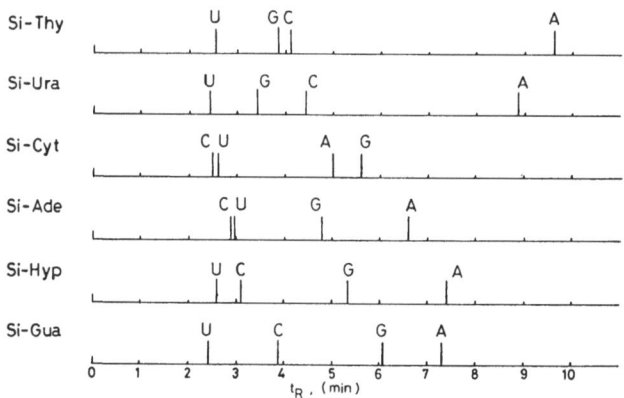

Figure 15. Retention times of nucleoside with water mobile
phase. Flow rate: 1.0 mL/min. Temperature: 20°C.
Detector: 254 nm. Samples: (A), adenosine; (C),
cytidine; (U), uridine; (G), guanosine.

200

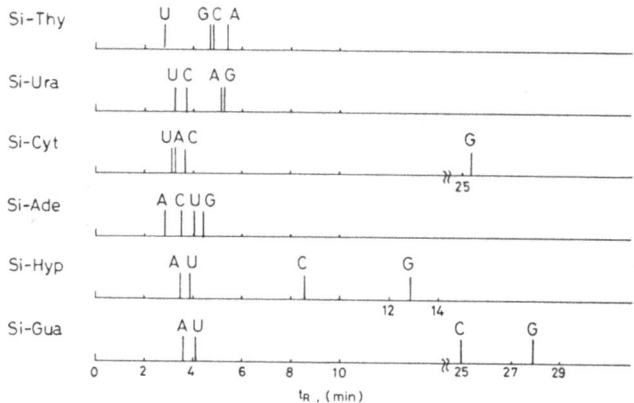

Figure 16. Retention times of nucleoside with ethanol mobile
phase. Flow rate: 1.0 mL/min. Temperature: 20°C
Detector: 254 nm. Samples: (A), adenosine; (C),
cytidine; (U), uridine (G), guanosine.

In ethanol mobile phases (Figure 16), the interaction between the
nucleic acid bases should be caused by specific hydrogen bonding instead,
of the hydrophobic interaction which is the predominant factor in water.
The separation behavior of the nucleosides in Figure 16 can be explained
by the specific interaction between complimentary nucleic acid bases;
adenosine for Si-Thy and Si-Ura, guanosine for Si-Cyt, Uridine for Si-
Ade, cytidine for Si-Hyp, and cytidine for Si-Gua. Slowest elusion of
guanosine for all the column systems may be caused by the highest ability
of guanine base for hydrogen bonding among the nucleic acid bases.

4.2 Nucleotides and Dinucleotides: Figure 17 shows the chromatogram
of the dinucleotides where adenosine is connected with another nucleoside
by diphosphate ester bond. The mobile phases used for the dinucleotides
were (A) water and (B) methanol with volatile buffer system of triethyl-
ammonium acetate. The clear separation of the dinucleotides as shown in
these figures shows that the separation of the dinucleotides depends on
the kind of nucleotide units, other than adenosine, in the dinucleotide.
Figures 18 (water mobile phase) and 19 (methanol mobile phase) show the
results for the six kinds of stationary phases. In both water and

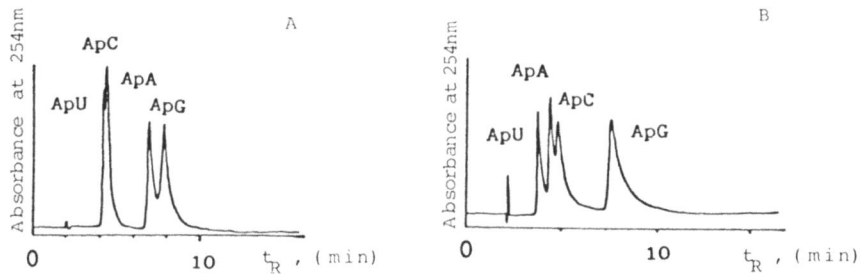

Figure 17. Chromatograms of dinucleotides on Si-Hyp. Mobile
phase: (A), 0.1M TEAA/water; (B), 0.1M TEAA/
methanol. Flow rate: 1.0 mL/min. Temperature: 30°C.
Detector: 254 nm. Samples: (ApA), adenyl (3'-5')
adenosine; (ApC), adenyl (3'-5') cytidine; (ApU),
adenyl (3'-5') uridine; (ApG), adenyl (3'-5')
guanosine.

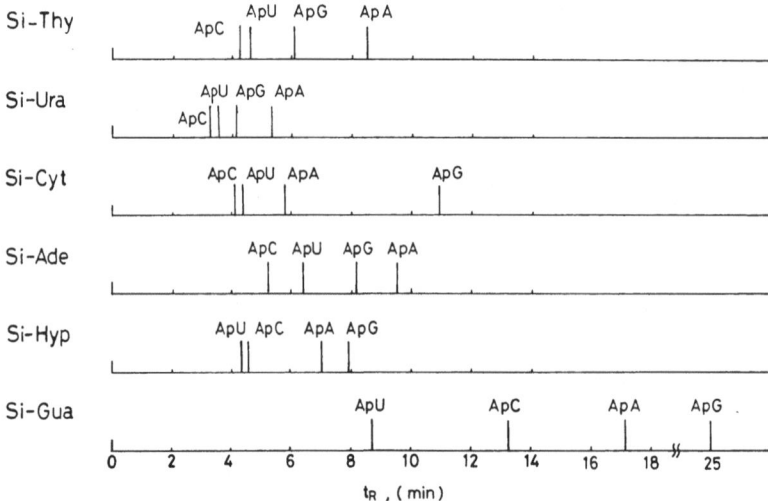

Figure 18. Retention times of dinucleotides. Mobile phase: 0.1M TEAA/water. Flow rate: 1.0 mL/min. Temperature: 30°C. Detector: 254 nm. Samples: (ApA), adenyl(3'-5') adenosine. (ApC), adenyl (3'-5') cytidine; (ApU), adenyl (3'-5') uridine; (ApG), adenyl (3'-5') guanosine.

methanol mobile phase systems, results were obtained that were similar to the results obtained for nucleosides. Therefore, the separations can be concluded to be caused by the interaction between nucleic acid bases in the mobile phase and in the stationary phase.

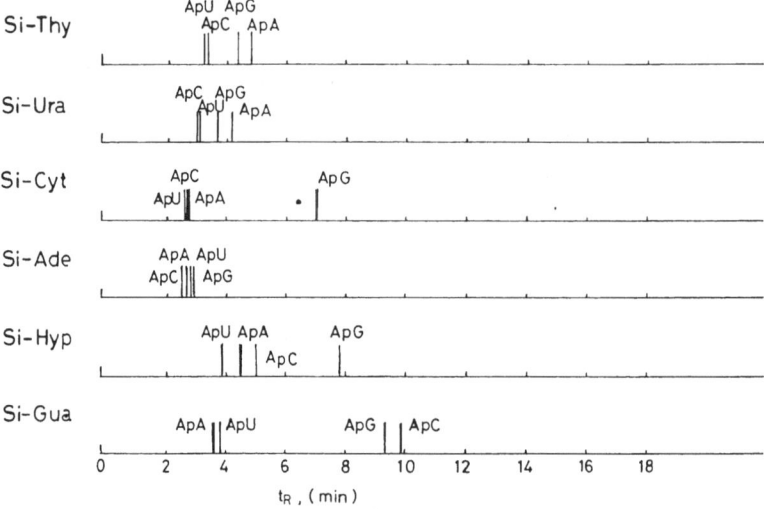

Figure 19. Retention times of dinucleotides. Mobile phase: 0.1M TEAA/methanol. Flow rate: 1.0 mL/min. Temperature: 30°C. Detector: 254 nm. Samples: (ApA), adenyl (3'-5') adenosine; (ApC), adenyl (3'-5') cytidine; (ApU), adenyl (3'-5') uridine; (ApG), adenyl (3'-5') guanosine.

202

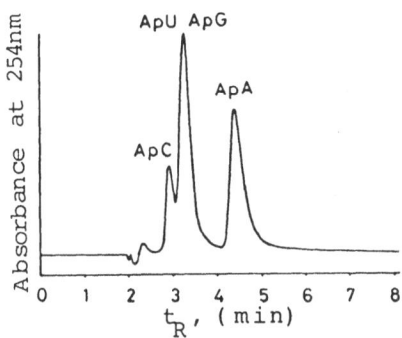

Figure 20. Chromatograms of dinucleotides on Si-Urd. Mobile
phase: 0.1M TEAA/water. Flow rate: 1.0 mL/min.
Temperature: 30°C. Detector: 254 nm. Samples:
(ApA), adenyl (3'-5')adenosine; (ApC), adenyl (3'-
5') cytidine; (ApU), adenyl (3'-5') uridine;
(ApG), adenyl (3'-5') guanosine.

The nucleoside bonded silica gel (Si-Urd, and Si-Thd) gave excellent
results for separation of dinucleotides. As shown in Figure 20, the
dinucleotides containing the complimentary adenine bases (ApA) were
selectively separated from the other dinucleotides on the Si-Urd column.
In this system, separation of mononucleotides was small, while adenosine
was separated completely from other nucleosides.

CONCLUSION

HPLC resins containing nucleic acid base derivatives were prepared.
These resins give excellent complimentary separation of nucleic acid base
derivatives, nucleosides, nucleotides, and oligonucleotides. These resins
may be useful for the separation of components of nucleic acids and polynucleotides as a specific separation system, while ion-exchange and
reverse-phase systems are non-specific separation systems.

REFERENCES

1. K. Takemoto and Y. Inaki, Adv. Polym. Sci., **41**, 1 (1981).
2. J. Pitha, Adv. Polym. Sci., 50, 1 (1983).
3. Y. Inaki and K. Takemoto in: "*Current Topics in Polymer Science.
   Vol. 1*", R. Ottenbrite, L. Utracki, and S. Inoue, Eds., Hanser
   Publisher, 1987, p. 79.
4. Y. Inaki and K. Takemoto, "*Functional Monomers and Polymers*",
   K. Takemoto, Y. Inaki, and R. Ottenbrite, Eds., Marcel Dekker (1987),
   p. 149.
5. Y. Inaki and K. Takemoto, Makromol. Chem., Suppl. **14**, 91 (1985).
6. J. D. Watson and F. H. C. Crick, Nature, **171**, 737 (1953).
7. P. O. P. Ts'o, Ed., "*Basic Principles in Nucleic Acid Chemistry*",
   Academic Press, New York, 1974, Vols. 1 and 2.
8. H. Tuppy and E. Kucheler, Biochem. Biophys. Acta., **80**, 669 (1964).
9. A. S. Jones, D. G. Parsons, and D. G. Roberts, Europ. Polymer J.,
   3, 187 (1967).
10. N. Ueda, K. Nakatani, K. Kondo, K. Takemoto, and M. Imoto,
    Makromolekulare Chem., **134**, 305 (1970).
11. H. Schott and G. Greber, Makromolekulare Chem., **145**, 11 (1971).
12. Y. Kato, T. Seita, T. Hashimoto, and A. Shimizu, J. Chromatogr.,
    134, 204 (1977).

13. K. Kondo, T. Horiike, and K. Takemoto, J. Macromol. Sci. Chem., **A16**, 793 (1981).
14. Y. S. Yu, K. Kondo, and K Takemoto, J. Macromol. Sci. Chem., **186**, 2311 (1985).
15. S. Nagae, Y. Suda, Y. Inaki and K. Takemoto, J. Polymer Sci. Polymer Chem. Ed., in press.
16. S. Nagae, Y. Inaki, and K. Takemoto, Polymer Preprints, Japan, **36**, 696 (1987); J. Polymer Sci. Polymer Chem. Ed., in preparation.
17. T. Miyamoto, S. Nagae, Y. Inaki, and K. Takemoto, Polymer Preprints, Japan, **36**, 697 (1987); J. Polymer Sci. Polymer Chem. Ed., in preparation.
18. Y. Inaki, Y. Sugiura, T. Miyamoto, and K. Takemoto, Polymer Preprints, Japan, **36**, 1955 (1987); J. Polymer Sci. Polymer Chem. Ed., in preparation.
19. Y. Inaki, S. Sugita, T. Takahara, and K. Takemoto, J. Polymer Sci., Polymer Chem. Ed., **24**, 3201 (1986).
20. Y. Suda, Y. Inaki, and K. Takemoto, J. Polym. Sci., Polym. Chem. Ed., **21**, 2813 (1983).
21. T. Ishikawa, Y. Inaki, and K. Takemoto, Polym. Bull., **1**, 85 (1978).
22. Y. Inaki, Y. Sakuma, Y. Suda, and K. Takemoto, J. Polym. Sci., Polym. Chem. Ed., **20**, 1917 (1982).
23. Y. Sakuma, Y. Inaki, and K. Takemoto, J. Polym. Sci., Polym. Chem. Ed., **20**, 3431 (1982).
24. Y. Sakuma, Y. Inaki & K. Takemoto, J. Polymer Sci., Polymer Chem. Ed., **22**, 2061 (1984).
25. M. Zakaria and P. R. Brown, J. Chromatogr., **226**, 267 (1981).
26. S. P. Assenza and P. R. Brown, Sep. Purif. Methods, **12** (2), 177 (1983).
27. H. Schott in: "*High Performance Liquid Chromatography in Biochemistry*", A. Henshen, Ed., Verlag Chemie, Weinheim, 1985, p. 413.

IMMUNE MODULATING EFFECTS OF POLY(ICLC) IN MICE, MONKEYS AND MAN

Hilton B. Levy[a] and Christopher Bever, Jr.[b]

(a) National Institutes of Allergy and Infectious Diseases
    Bethesda, Maryland
(b) Department of Neurology
    University of Maryland Hospital
    Baltimore, Maryland

The stabilized double stranded RNA, poly(ICLC), in addition to being an active interferon inducer, is able to modify a variety of humoral and cell associated immune activities in mice, monkeys and humans. In mice there is augmentation, *in vitro* and *in vivo* of macrophage activation and NK cell activity, as well as specific cytotoxic T cells. In primates, poly(ICLC) increases the amount and rapidity of formation of antibodies to a number of weak vaccines. In addition there is increased macrophage and 2'5' *A. synthetase* activities. At low doses there is an augmentation of NK cell action, but inhibition at higher doses. Increases in T4/T8 ratio were found. Lymphocyte subset populations are modified in different ways, depending on the dose. In general low doses augment the several immune actions much better than do the higher doses.

INTRODUCTION

This presentation will consist of two parts; the first will be a review of material that has been published and the second will summarize recent data dealing with cell associated hematological and immunological changes induced in monkeys and humans by poly(ICLC).

First a word about poly(ICLC). A number of years ago, interferon was thought of only in terms of a natural antiviral substance, with its effects on the immune system and as a cell growth inhibitor coming a good deal later. However, until recently, there was not enough IFN to do adequate antiviral trials in mice, let alone in humans, who would require much larger amounts. Investigators looked for non-replicating entities that would cause the host to produce large quantities of his own IFN. A number of such agents were found, the best of which was a ds-RNA containing one strand of poly(I) and one of poly(C). Poly(IC) is a good IFN inducer in mice, and is a good antiviral and antitumor agent in mice. However, when it was tried in primates, including humans, it induced very little interferon and had no antitumor action. It was shown that there is present in primate serum a high concentration of hydrolytic enzymes that

205

degrade and inactivate poly(IC), probably accounting for the lack of activity in monkeys, chimpanzees and people. A derivative of poly(IC) was prepared by adding poly l-lysine and carboxymethylcellulose, poly(ICLC), which partially resists this hydrolysis, and which is capable of inducing good qualities of IFN in primates.[1]

RESULTS

The activity of poly(ICLC) as an antiviral agent is shown in Table 1, which lists some of the virus diseases that have been treated with poly(ICLC).[1] It was soon realized that poly(ICLC) was not just a poor man's IFN, readily available and relatively inexpensive, but it also had a number of immune modifying effects, which often were not the same as those induced by IFN itself. One area of difference between IFN and poly-(ICLC) is the fact that, by and large, IFN inhibits antibody production to an antigen or vaccine, while poly(ICLC) is an effective immune adjuvant with many but not all antigens.

Table 1. Virus diseases of animals that have been treated with poly(ICLC).

Disease	Animal	Results
Simian hemorrhagic fever	Monkey	Complete protection if given before virus, none if given after virus
Venezuelan equine encephalitis	Monkey	No animals with light virus challenge died; poly(ICLC) reduced viremia by 50%
Yellow fever	Monkey	75% protection up to 8 hr. post-challenge
Japanese encephalitis	Monkey	50% protection up to 24 hr. post-challenge
Tacaribe virus	Monkey	No effect by poly(ICLC)
Rabies	Monkey & mouse	See text
Hepatitis	Chimpanzee	Virus controlled while on drug. Control ends when treatment stopped
Bolivian hemorrhagic fever	Monkey	Possible worsening of disease
Tick-borne encephalitis	Monkey	Strong protection
Vaccinia	Monkey	Strong protection
Vaccinia skin lesions (topical treatment)	Rabbit	Spread of lesions stopped

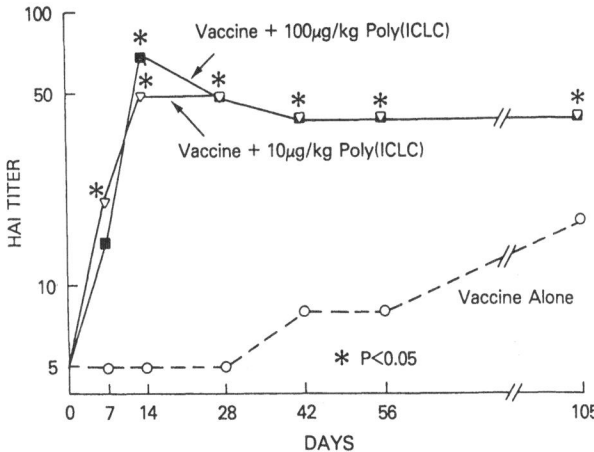

Figure 1. Hemaglutination inhibition antibody response of young monkeys given 200 CCA units of Swine Influenza Vaccine with poly(ICLC) as adjuvant. Number of monkeys = 4.

Three examples of this effect follow. A subunit vaccine vs. Swine Flu virus, is poorly effective in young people and in young monkeys. When this vaccine is given along with a small dose of poly(ICLC), the resultant antibody titer is elevated to the point where it would be expected to be effective in disease prevention.[2] See Figure 1.

Another example is the polysaccharide vaccine against *Hemophilus influenzae*. This agent causes serious disease in children, particularly young children, where the vaccine has poor effectiveness. The vaccine is also poorly effective in young monkeys. When low doses of poly(ICLC) is given along with the vaccine to young monkeys the antibody response is strongly augmented.[3] These results are summarized in Table 2.

The third example we will mention is the adjuvanticity of poly(ICLC) with a killed vaccine against *Venezuelan Equine encephalitis* virus, which is shown in Figure 2.[4] The upper part of this figure shows the production of antibody to the vaccine without poly(ICLC). The vaccine was given twice, as indicated. The lower part of the figure shows the increased,

Table 2. Effect of low doses of poly(ICLC) on antibody production by Rhesus monkeys in response to a polysaccharide vaccine for *hemophilus influenza* antibody levels.*

Treatment	Pre	Day 7	Day 14	Day 20	Day 28	Day 34	Day 42
Vaccine	100	590	348	286	225	187	113
Vaccine + poly(ICLC) 0.3 mg/kg	100	5643	5040	3340	2063	2182	780
Vaccine + poly(ICLC) 0.03mg/kg	100	6589	3904	1884	1132	839	721
* Normalized ng/ml.							

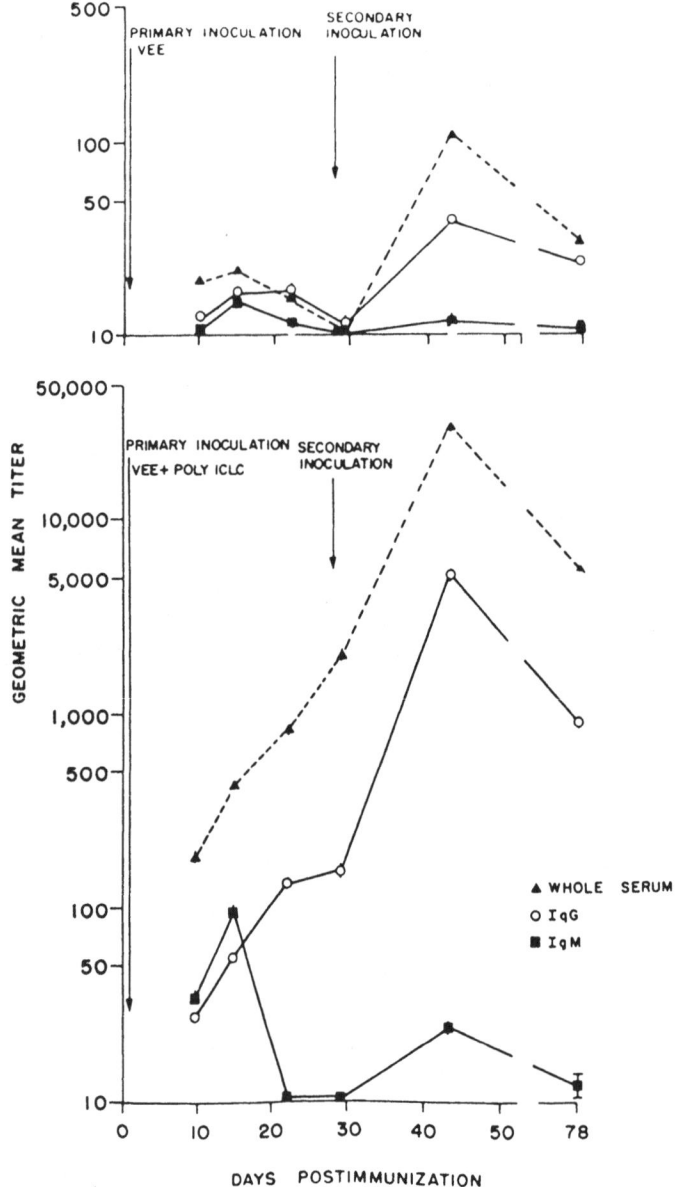

Figure 2. Adjuvant effect of poly(ICLC) in monkeys receiving
heat killed virus vaccine vs. *Venezuelan Equine
Encephalitis* Virus.

earlier response obtained when poly(ICLC) is given along with the
vaccine. A second dose of the vaccine, this time without poly(ICLC) leads
to the production of very high levels of antibody. The usual formation of
IgM followed by replacement with IgG, is not altered by poly(ICLC).

So far the data has dealt only with humoral immunity. Several
investigators have published observations about the effect of poly(ICLC)
on several cell-associated immune activities in mice.[5-7]

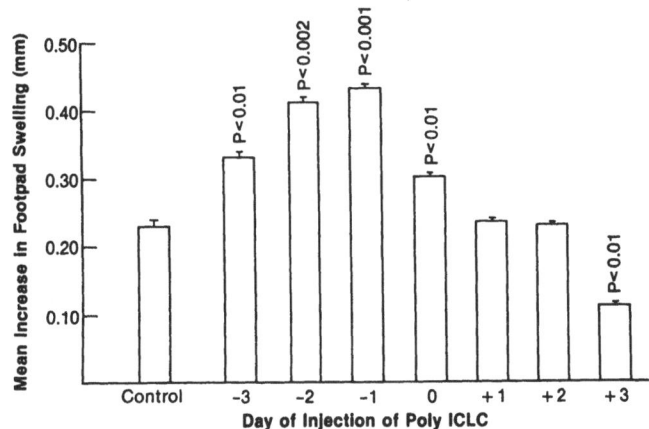

Figure 3. Effect of poly(ICLC) on delayed type hypersensitivity. Poly(ICLC) (10 micrograms) was
injected subcutaneously into mice previously
sensitized to sheep red blood cells (SRBC), on the
day indicated prior to rechallenge of mice with
SRBC. Four days after the rechallenge, footpad
swelling was measured.

Delayed Hypersensitivity (DTH)

When mice that have been sensitized to sheep red blood cells (SRBC)
are challenged in the foot pad with SRBC, there is a swelling of the
footpad. Figure 3 shows that poly(ICLC) given to mice already sensitized
to SRBC strongly enhanced foot pad swelling, when given any time between
3 days prior to the challenge up to the time of challenge.[5] This is a
strong contrast to what interferon does.[8] If IFN is given before the
challenge, a complete suppression of the DTH can occur. These differences
between IFN and poly(ICLC) may relate to the difference between the
effects of the two agents on colony forming cells and on production of
colony stimulating factor (CSF). Mouse granulocyte-macrophage precursor
cells can give rise to colonies if a glycoprotein, CSF is present. Poly-
(ICLC), both *in vivo* and *in vitro* augments colony formation, while IFN
either is inhibitory or has no effect.[5]

Table 3 shows that cultures of macrophages produce CSF when stimulated by poly(ICLC) and by IFN. To end the CSF story, Figure 4 shows the
effect of antibody to IFN on the production of CSF by IFN and by

Table 3. Effect of IFN and poly(ICLC) on production by
macrophage of soluble products.

Agent	IFN Units	CSF Units	Prostaglandin E
Control	0	30	70
Poly ICLC 10 µg/ml	50	ND	1400
50 µg/ml	1000	120	2000
IFN 500 IU/ml	NA	100	225

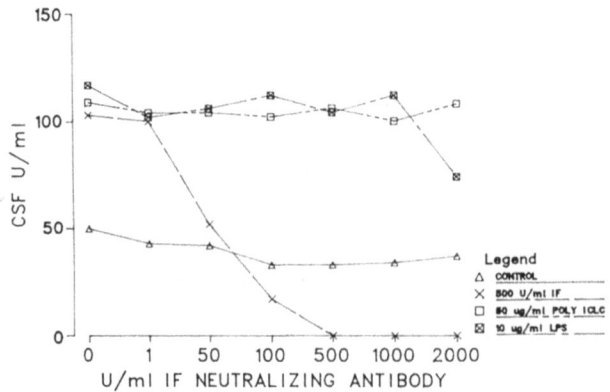

Figure 4. Effect of antibody to interferon on indication of
colony stimulating factor (CSF) in macrophage
cultures by interferon and by poly(ICLC).

poly(ICLC). When Ab to INF is added to the culture where CSF is being
induced by IFN the production of CSF is inhibited, but when Ab to IFN is
added to the cells being stimulated by poly(ICLC) there is no inhibition
of CSF production, suggesting that poly(ICLC) stimulates CSF production
independently of the IFN produced.[5]

Exposure of the macrophage to very low doses of the drug, *in vitro*
enhances peritoneal macrophage cytotoxicity vs. tumor cells, as shown in
Table 4. When the drug is given i.v. to mice at 8 or 16 µg/mouse peritoneal macrophage cytotoxicity is also increased, as shown in Table 5.[6]

When given i.v. to mice, poly(ICLC) augmented natural killer cell
activity in peritoneal cells, lungs and spleen. Figure 5 shows some
typical results.[6] There are many biological response modifiers that can
augment NK cell activity, after one or two treatments, but then they lose
their effectiveness. Mice do not develop this refractoriness after treat-

Table 4. *In vitro* activation of macrophage cytotoxicity.

Concentration µg/ml	Percent Cytotoxicity MBL-2	P815
0.001		2
0.005		21
0.05	62	
0.01		20
0.1	70	34
1.0	70	44
5.0	85	46
10.0	60	47

Ratio of macrophage to target cells; MBL-2 (10:1; P815 (10:1).
Control values subtracted from experimental.

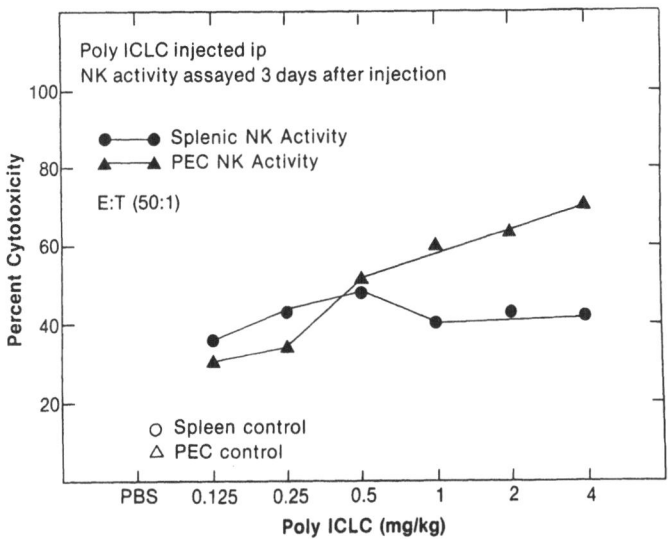

Figure 5. Effect of injection of poly(ICLC) into mice on
natural killer cell activity of peritoneal exudate
cells and of spleen cells.

ment with poly(ICLC). It can be given twice weekly for quite a few weeks
without a diminution in response. As mentioned later, they were boosted
at low doses but not at higher ones.

One other activity that is enhanced by the agent in mice is the mixed
lymphocyte reaction (MLR). If live spleen cells from C57B1 mice are co-
cultivated with irradiated cells from C3H mice the live cells respond by
increasing in growth rate, as measured by uptake of tritiated thymidine.
If poly(ICLC) is added to the cell mixture during the cocultivation, in
doses from 0.01 to 5 µg/ml., there is an increase in the MLR. At 10 µg/ml
there was inhibition (6). These results are summarized in Table 6.

It also has been shown that when mice are vaccinated with irradiated
tumor cells mixed with poly(ICLC), specific cytotoxic T cells are
developed. The vaccine of irradiated tumor cells alone has little or no
effect, as seen in Table 7.[7]

Table 5. *In vivo* activation of macrophage cytotoxicity.

Concentration Poly(ICLC) (mg/kg)	Percent Cytotoxicity Day of Observation		
	1	3	6
none	10	8	9
0.4	60	19	12
0.8	75	55	20

Mice received single i.p. treatment of either 0.4 or 0.8
mg/kg and peritoneal macrophages were harvested for assay 1,
3 or 6 days after treatment.

Table 6. Poly(ICLC) augmentation of spleen cell response in a mixed lymphocyte response (a).

µg/mL F5	C3H R(b) only	C3H+C57S(c)	S.I.(d)	S.I.(e)
Media	2,719	17,630	5.48	5.48
250.0	1,865	22,303	7.20	11.96
0.01	2,373	28,673	9.55	12.08
0.1	1,089	31,847	10.71	29.24
1.0	794	35,836	12.18	45.13
5.0	811	41,272	14.18	50.89
10.0	696	19,460	6.15	27.96

(a) Poly(ICLC) or Thymosin F5 was added to the culture at various concentrations. Media control was in the absence of BRM. The MLR was established using irradiated $C_{57}B1/6$ spleen cells as stimulator cell and C_3H spleen cells as responders at a suboptimal R:S ratio of 10:1. The cultures were pulsed on day 5 with 1 µCi ^{3}H-Thymidine for 24 hr. prior to harvest (N = 4).
(b) Responder C_3H spleen cells culture alone.
(c) C_3H spleen cells cultured with irradiated $C_{57}B1/6$ spleen cells.
(d) Stimulation index compared to media control.
(e) Stimulation index compared to drug control.

The net effect of these and possibly other immune modifications, is that poly(ICLC) can cause the regression and disappearance of small experimental tumors. However if the tumor is allowed to grow to a large size before initiation of treatment, the tumor mass must first be reduced by a cytocidal agent, like cytoxan, for the poly(ICLC) to be effective.[5]

Table 7. Immunoadjuvant activity of poly(ICLC) in a tumor challenge study (a).

Vaccine tumor cells	Adjuvant	µg/animal	Day 4, TB/total (Cm^3)		Day 63 TB/total (Cm^3)
–	HBSS	0.05	5/5	(0.082)	5/5
UV-2237	HBSS		4/5	(0.147)	4/5
UV-2237	Thymosin F5	500	0/5	–	0/5
UV-2237	Poly(ICLC)	50	1/5	(0.110)	0/4

(a) Mice were immunized intradermally with a vaccine composed of collagenase-DNase dissociated tumor cells (1 x 10^6) suspended in either HBSS, thymosin F5 or Poly(ICLC). Tumor challenge was 9 days later using 2 x 10^5 UV-2237 tissue culture propagated tumor cells injected into a posterior footpad.

Table 8. Effects of adjuvants on survival of mice immunized with vaccine to rift valley fever virus.*

Treatment		dose (µg/kg)	Percent survivors day 35 (N = 16)
Vaccine	Adjuvant		
Vaccine + Poly(ICLC)		20	50
		100	50
		200	13
Saline + Poly(ICLC)		200	6
Vaccine + Freund's complete adjuvant			6
Saline + Freund's complete adjuvant			6
Vaccine + Freund's incomplete adjuvant			6
Saline + Freund's incomplete adjuvant			0
Vaccine controls			19
Saline controls			0

In an experiment using a different type of endpoint, it was shown that poly(ICLC), given together with a killed vaccine vs. RVF virus, increases the survival of mice subsequently challenged with live RVF virus. Again the higher dose of the drug has less beneficial effect than does smaller doses, as summarized in Table 8.[9]

All the material presented so far has been a review of previously published work. The second part of this presentation deals with unpublished studies on hematological and cell associated immune modifications induced in monkeys and people by poly(ICLC). Table 9 lists the names of people who contributed to the work to be reported.

First, the data obtained in studies with monkeys will be given. Poly-(ICLC) was injected, i.v., into 2 monkeys at two different dose levels according to the following protocol. On day 0 blood was drawn for the determination of several hematological and immunological parameters. The first injection of poly(ICLC) was then given, i.v., at 0.2 mg/m². Then, 24 hours later (day 1) blood was drawn for the same battery of tests, and

Table 9. Names of people who were collaborators in the work to be reported.

C. Bever	NINCDS
A. Malluish	NCI
D. McFarlin	NINCDS
H. MacFarland	NINCDS
A. Salazar	Walter Reed
R. Tyndall	U. Texas Med. Ctr., Dallas

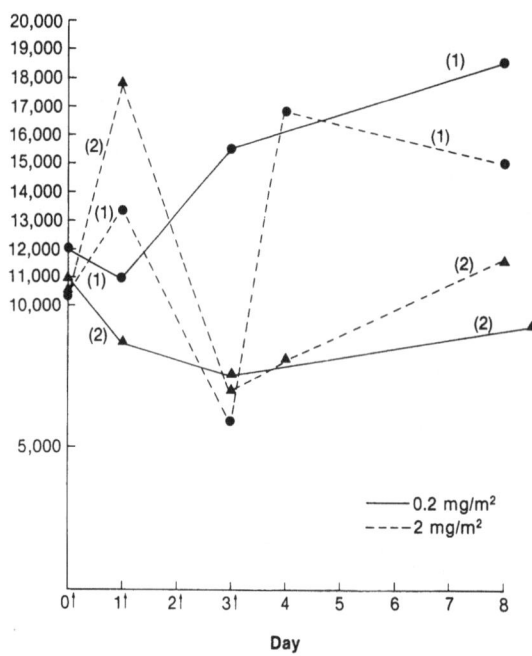

Figure 6. Effect of repeated injection of poly(ICLC) into
monkeys on total white blood cell numbers. Ordinate
is number of WBC/mm³ of blood, abscissa is the
numbers of days after injection. Arrows indicate
injection days.

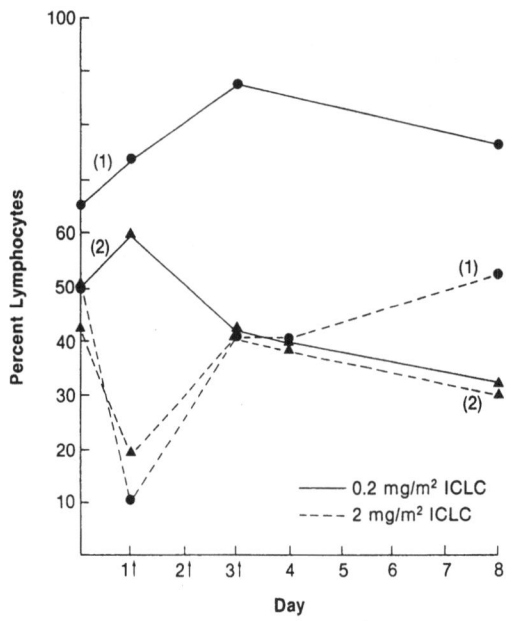

Figure 7. Effect of poly(ICLC) injection into monkeys on
percent of lymphocytes in peripheral blood.
Abscissa represents days after start. Arrows
indicate injection times.

another injection of the drug was given. The same procedure was done on days 2 and 3. On day 4 blood was drawn, but no drug was given. On day 8 blood was drawn again. The animals were not used again for 7 weeks and then the same procedure was repeated at a 10 fold higher drug level, 2.0 mg/m².

The data from the low dose of drug reveals that, while there is a large amount of fluctuation, there is a transient decrease in total wbc beginning on day 1, followed by a return to either normal or above by day 8. The higher dose leads to an increase on day 1, followed by a decrease to normal or slightly above by day 8, as shown in Figure 6.

The changes in composition of the different subsets of wbc are more informative than changes in total wbc. Figure 7 shows the changes in percent lymphocytes in the monkeys given the two levels of drug. At the lower level of drug, the % lymphocytes increased for a day or two, and then returned to normal, while at the higher level of drug, there was a transient (1.5 days) sharp lymphopenia, even though as shown in Figure 6 the total wbc increased, and then both returned to normal.

Since the great bulk of wbc consists of leukocytes and granulocytes, this means that with the high dose of drug there was a marked granulo-cytosis for 48 hours, with a return to normal, while at the lower dose there were only modest changes in granulocytes.

NK cell activity was modified differently at the two doses of drug. At the low dose there were either an initial drop or no change in NK activity, followed by a rise to above normal. At the higher dose there was a drop in NK activity, which remained down for the period of obser-vation. This lack of augmentation, or even inhibition at higher doses of immune modulators has been noted often. These results are summarized in Figure 8.

Table 10. Comparison of interferon titers in male and female Rhesus monkeys.

Sex	No.	Values are in I.U. per ml serum 8 Hour	24 hour
Male	1	3,200	200
	2	1,000	130
	3	4,000	200
	Geom. Mean	2,339	173
	Rel. S.E.	1.5	1.15
Female	1	250	5
	2	130	5
	3	630	10
	Geom. Mean	274	6.3
	Rel. S.E.	1.58	1.26
Male vs. Female		T = 3.72 d.f. = 4 p = 0.03	T = 12.2 d.f. = 4 p <0.001

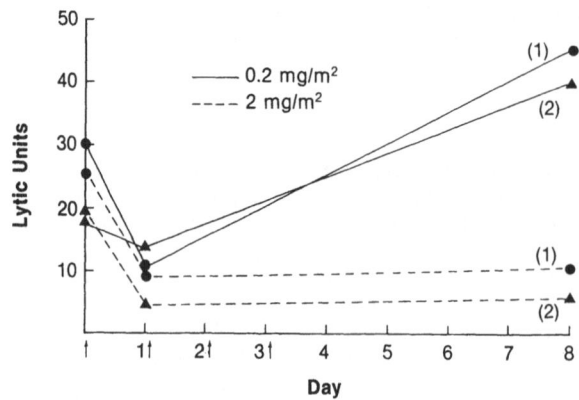

Figure 8. Effect of poly(ICLC) injection into monkeys on natural killer cell activity in peripheral white blood cells

Table 10 shows an interesting difference between male and female monkeys with regard to the production of interferon. It can be seen that male monkeys made significantly more interferon in response to a given dose of poly(ICLC) than did female monkeys.

Studies in people were done as part of therapeutic trials in 29 multiple sclerosis patients, at NIH, Walter Reed and the U. of Texas in Dallas (C. Bever, D. McFarlin, A. Salazar, R. Tyndall, H. MacFarland, and H. Levy, manuscript in preparation), and in 59 cancer patients studied at NIH and the Portsmouth Navel Hospital, (K. Foon, A. Malluish, J. Reed, and H. Levy, unpublished observations). Most of the M.S. patients stabilized for a while after the initiation of treatment.[10] Some declined,

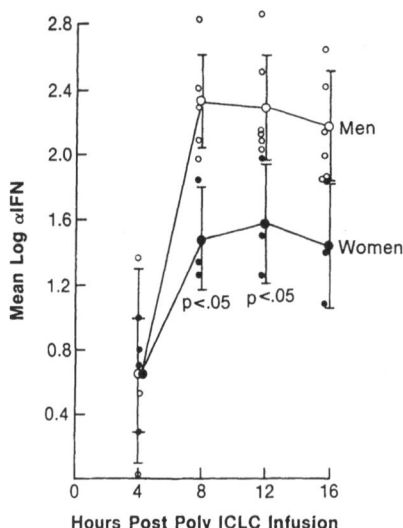

Figure 9. Difference between men and women in amount of interferon produced in response to injection of poly(ICLC) (100 µg/kg), intravenously.

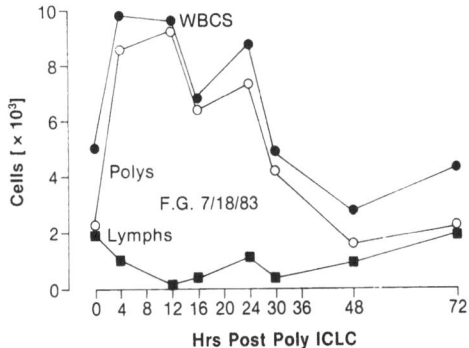

Figure 10. Typical response of injection of poly(ICLC) (100
μg/kg) into man on white blood cells and subsets.

perhaps half, after 6-8 months. The remainder remained stable during the
period of treatment and observation.

Figure 9 shows that as with monkeys, men made more interferon in
response to a given dose of poly(ICLC) than did women. Hematologic
studies in M.S. patients showed acute changes in total wbc, as well as in
lymphocytes and granulocytes. Within 4 hours after injection, total wbc
increased. As with the monkeys at the higher dose, there was a marked
decrease in lymphocytes and an increase in polymorphonuclear leukocytes.
Figure 10 shows a typical reaction.

Lymphocytes remained depressed for 48 hours before returning to
normal. The rapid decrease and rapid recovery suggest strongly that the
changes are due to sequestering of the cells rather than destruction. All
these data resemble those just reported in monkeys.

Table 11. Changes in % monocytes in patients receiving
poly(ICLC).

Patient	Date	0 hours	24 hours	% Increase after 24 hours
F. G.	3/13/83	9.54	15.22	89
	6/22/83	9.44	8.95	- 5
	7/19/83	7.95	6.39	- 20
	2/06/84	13.1	17.8	36
V. T.	2/17/83	7.29	32.3	349
	3/09/83	8.29	31.5	280
A. P.	2/16/83	6.07	26.0	328
	3/15/83	19.8	24.7	25
	4/13/83	7.48	26.5	254
	12/06/83	3.30	14.7	354
C. W.	1/09/84	3.70	15.0	305
R. R.	7/12/83	13.2	22.9	73
T. B.	7/06/83	15.1	46.2	206

Table 12. NK activity in M.S. patients.

| | | 40:1 E:T Ratio % Specific Lysis | | | |
		0	24 Hrs	48 Hrs	%Change
AP	7/13	29	–	52	+79
TP	12/06	27	15	38	+30
FG	2/06	45	25	37	–18
TB	2/27	28	18	46	+64
AP	12/06	26	15	37	+42
FG	10/18	40	–	49	+23
TB	11/18	40	–	41	+ 3
TB	7/13	31	–	72	+132
Averages		33.3		46.5	

$$p < 0.01$$

There was an increase in monocyte antitumor activity and in the percent monocytes in the blood in all patient groups examined. Table 11 shows the changes in the %monocytes. Monocytes in blood are, of course, the analog of macrophages in tissues which, as seen earlier, were also

Table 13. Changes in OKT[3+] cells in patients receiving poly(ICLC).

Patient	Date	0 hours	24 hours
F.G.	3/30/83	68.2	56.9
	6/22/83	65.3	56.1
	7/19/83	62.7	57.7
	2/06/84	62.6	41.3
V.T.	2/17/83	65.1	58.8
	3/09/83	70.2	60.6
	3/06/84	75.3	55.1
A.P.	2/16/83	74.7	66.6
	3/15/83	63.4	33.6
	4/13/83	77.9	51.8
	11/01/83	78.0	66.5
	12/06/83	78.6	53.9
	1/10/84	76.1	56.5
H.T.	5/02/83	58.8	43.2
C.W.	1/09/84	70.7	40.5
	2/15/84	53.2	51.4
R.R.	7/12/83	73.8	64.0
T.B.	7/06/83	66.4	39.0
	11/08/83	67.8	68.7
	2/27/84	66.8	47.8

Table 14. Effect of poly(ICLC) on DR expression in M.S. patients.

Patient	Date	%Cells Showing DR Time in Hrs. Post-treatment 0 hours	24 hours
FG	3/30	24.4	26.4
	6/22	26.7	28.6
	7/19	27.1	29.8
VT	2/17	17.7	46.4
	3/09	26.5	39.7
AP	2/16	16.5	36.8
	3/15	20.7	27.5
	4/13	15.2	33.9
HT	5/02	19.6	38.7
RR	7/12	25.1	29.9
TB	7/06	31.4	31.4
Averages		22.8	33.5
		$p < 0.001$	

elevated in the mouse. Natural killer cell activity in the peripheral wbc, in the M.S. patients was depressed 24 hours after injection but became elevated above the preinjection level by 48 hours, as shown in Table 12. In the cancer patients, at the low dose of $1mg/m^2$ there was some suggestion of elevation of NK cell activity, but there was a clear cut depression at the higher ($4mg/m^2$) dose.

Table 15. Effect of poly(ICLC) on helper/suppresser ratios.

	Treatment Date	0 Time	24 Hrs.	% Increase
F.G.	3/30/83	2.66	7.28	174
	6/22/83	3.12	4.32	39
	7/19/83	2.78	4.89	76
V.T.	3/09/83	2.36	2.50	6
A.P.	2/16/83	2.05	3.10	51
	3/15/83	3.26	2.54	-22
	4/13/83	2.01	2.19	9
H.T.	5/02/83	1.46	2.26	55
R.R.	7/12/83	2.81	3.35	19
T.B.	7/06/83	1.65	3.61	119

There was also a transient decline in cells responding positively to the OKT3 reagent in the FACS assay. This is taken to be a measure of T cells. (Table 13) Changes were seen in a protein of the major histocompatability locus, the DR antigen (Table 14) and also in Leu 11+ cells. Increased 2'5'*A. synthetase* activity was seen in all patients examined (Figure 11), even in those where no measurable interferon was found. Of particular interest in these days of concern with AIDS is the observation that the ratio of T helper cells (the T4 cells) to T suppresser (T8) cells, a measure that is depressed in AIDS patients, is elevated after injection with poly(ICLC). Table 15 shows some data to this effect in a group of multiple sclerosis patients. Table 16 shows the same phenomenon in one patient who was reportedly tested for this effect.

A number of the changes seen may reflect, at least in part, transient removal of specific wbc subsets from the blood stream, with sequestration into lymph nodes. This sequestration has been examined in greater detail in rats where the accumulation of lymphocytes into nodes after poly(ICLC) injection has been visualized. The extent of accumulation is proportional to the dose of poly(ICLC) given. As reported elsewhere, poly(ICLC) induces the production of increased levels of cortisol in people.[10] Some of the changes mentioned above are consistent with the effects that cortisol can bring about.

A few words about toxicity in humans should be inserted here. The original phase-1 toxicity study,[11] used the approach that was then standard with oncologists, namely determine what is the maximum tolerated dose (mTD), and then treat patients with that dose. In that study, 12 mg/m^2 i.v. was found to be the mTD. Subsequent trials, particularly with very ill patients found this dose to be excessively toxic. Fevers up to 104°F, severe myalgia and arthralgia were experienced. At this time it was determined from the mouse, monkey and human studies just summarized that high doses do not maximize immune enhancement and may actually be inhibitory. These earlier studies inadvertently were using doses that maximized toxicity and minimized effectiveness. Current studies range from 0.250 mg/m^2 i.v. in cancer patients to 3 mg/m^2 intramuscularly in M.S. patients. Side effects consist of a mild myalgia, with fever up to 99.5°F. The M.S. patients are being treated on an outpatient basis.

Table 16. Changes in OKT4/OKT8 ratio with repeat tests in one patient.

Date	0 hours	24 hours	% Increase
2/16/83	2.05	3.10	51
3/09/83	2.36	2.50	6
3/15/83	3.26	2.54	-22
3/30/83	2.66	7.28	174
4/13/83	2.01	2.19	9
5/02/83	1.46	2.26	55
6/22/83	3.12	4.32	39
7/06/83	1.65	3.61	119
7/12/83	2.81	3.35	19
7/19/83	2.78	4.89	76

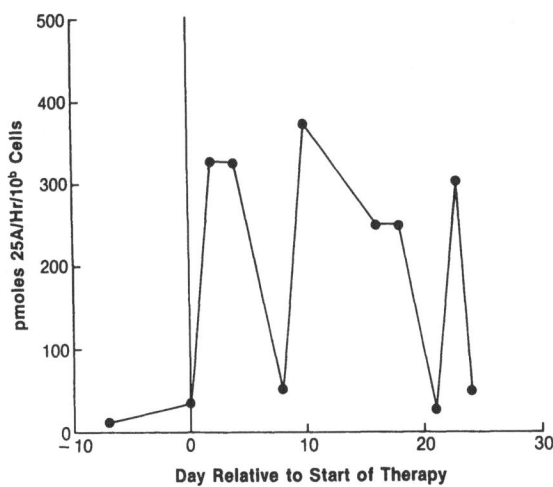

Figure 11. Effect of poly(ICLC) (100 µg/kg) injection to humans on 2'5' *A. synthetase*.

In summary, the injection of poly(ICLC) into primates, both monkeys and people, produces a number of changes in hematology and in immune reactivity, most of which are enhanced at low doses. Higher doses may actually lead to inhibition in some cases. Of particular interest is the observation that there is an elevation in the ratio of T-helper to T-suppresser cells. This poly(ICLC)-induced change plus its enhancement of monocyte and NK cell activity, and its antiviral activity, suggest that it should be considered for trial as a therapeutic agent in AIDS. The ability to elicit specific cytotoxic T cells might indicate potential usefulness as an adjuvant with AIDS vaccine.

REFERENCES

1. H. B. Levy, F. L. Riley in: "*Polymers in Medicine*", E. Chiellini & P. Giusti, Eds., Plenum Pub. Co., New York, 1983, pp. 33-35,
2. E. L. Stephen, D. E. Hilmas, J. A. Marigrafico & H. B. Levy, Science, **197**, 1289-1290 (1977).
3. H. B. Levy, J. Bioactive and Compatible Polymers, **1**, 348-385 (1986).
4. D. L. Harrington, C. L. Crabbs, D. E. Hilmas, J. R. Brown, C. A. Higbee, F. E. Cole & H. B. Levy, Infect. Immun., **24**, 160-166 (1979).
5. M. A. Chirigos, V. Papademetriou, A. Bartocci, E. Read, & H. B. Levy, Int. J. Immunpharmac. **3**, 329-337 (1981).
6. J. A. Talmadge, J. Adams, H. Philips, M. Collins, B. Lenz, M. Snyder, & M. Chirigos, Cancer Research, **45**, 1058-1065 (1985).
7. J. E. Talmadge & D. Hartmann, J. Biol. Resp. Mod., **4**, 484-489 (1985).
8. E. DeMaeyer & J. DeMaeyer-Guignard, Ann. N.Y. Acad. Sci., **350**, 1-11 (1980).
9. H. B. Levy & F. Riley in: "*The Lymphokines*", E. Pick, ed., Academic Press, New York, 1983.
10. C. T. Bever, Jr., H. F. MacFarland, D. E. MaFarlin, & H. B, Levy, J. Int. Res., in press.
11. A. S. Levine, M. Sivalich, P. H. Viernick, & H. B. Levy, Cancer Research, **39**, 1645, 1979.

EFFECT OF TETRAMISOLE AND ITS PLATINUM POLYAMINE ON MICE INFECTED WITH ENCEPHALOMYOCARDITIS-VARIANT-D VIRUS

Mary Trombley, Nancy J. Biegley, Charles E. Carraher, Jr. and David J. Giron

Wright State University
Department of Microbiology and Immunology
Dayton, Oh 45435

Florida Atlantic University
Department of Chemistry
Boca Raton, FL 33431

The effects of tetramisole and its platinum polyamine on the diabetogenesis of the diabetogenic D variant of encephalomyocarditis virus (EMC-D) was studied in nine-week old male ICR Swiss mice. These compounds are interferon inducers as well as immune modulators. The effect of these drugs at seven days after infection on the incidence and severity of diabetes were evaluated in virus-infected mice using the one-hour glucose tolerance test. When tetramisole was administered to mice eight days prior to EMC-D infection, little difference was seen in the incidence of diabetes which occurred in the mice compared to that seen in virus-infected mice. When given one day prior to virus infection, enhancement of both incidence and severity of diabetes occurred compared to that observed in the virus-infected mice. When tetramisole was given four days after virus infection, the severity of diabetes increased over that seen in the virus-infected diabetic mice. These and other results are consistent with the mice being more susceptible when their immune system is stressed.

INTRODUCTION

Warchalowski and Strausser found that Levamisole enhanced the diabetogenesis of EMC virus in DBA/2 mice; this effect of levamisole was attributed to its action upon T suppresser (Ts) lymphocytes.[1,2] Masturbara et. al. found that levamisole induction of interferon (IFN) in mice was thymus-dependent.[3] Also, no induction of IFN was detected in thymus-defective nude mice.[3] Nude mice are not susceptible to diabetes mediated by the encephalomyocarditis (EMC) virus.[4,5] Using the purified diabetogenic D variant of the EMC virus, (EMC-D), Gould et. al. noted that when IFN or low doses of IFN or the interferon inducer, poly(I:C) was given 4 days after initiation of EMC-D infection in male ICR Swiss mice, the severity and incidence of virus-induced diabetes melitis was increased.[6]

Based upon these observations, the object of this study was to determine the effects of tetramisole, which is a mixture of levamisole and dextramisole, on the diabetogenesis of EMC-D virus in ICR Swiss male mice. Also, the effects upon the induction of EMC-D virus-mediated diabetes of platinum polymers of tetramisole was evaluated.

TETRAMISOLE

Tetramisole was developed in 1966. It is a derivative of imidazole, which is an agent known to act on cyclic nucleotide phosphodiesterases.[7] Cyclic nucleotide phosphodiesterases are presently used to promote the increased breakdown of c-AMP and the decreased breakdown of c-GMP.[8] Also, at low concentrations, imidazole seems to inhibit mammalian alkaline phosphatase.[7] Tetramisole was developed in attempts to obtain a non-toxic, but biologically active form of imidazole.[7] The compound, tetramisole, actually consists of two optical isomers, levamisole and dextramisole. The structures are shown below.

$S(-)$ (levamisole) $R(+)$ (dextramisole)

tetramisole

Structure 1.

When tested in many species of animals and birds, tetramisole was effective against a wide range of gastrointestinal nematodes and exhibits only mild side effects in most cases.[3,7] Most of the biological activity of the mixture of tetramisole resides in the levorotatory isomer, levamisole, which is several times more potent but no more toxic than the dextrorotatory isomer, dextramisole.[7]

Levamisole, also known as L-2,3,5,6-tetrahydro-6-phenylimidazo[2,1-b] thiazole monohydrochloride, was the first synthetic chemical that possesses immunomodulatory properties and it has been found to react as an antianergic drug.[8] It potentiates the development of humoral[9] and cell-mediated immune responses when injected into animals at the same time as the antigenic stimulus,[10,11] and inhibits the growth of tumors.[10] The antitumor effect of levamisole appears to result from enhanced immune responses as shown by an increase in the responsiveness of the lymphocytes to mitogens and specific antigens,[12] as well as an enhancement of phagocytic and chemotactic responses of the macrophages.[13,14] Levamisole appears to restore normal macrophage and T-lymphocyte (T-cell) functions where deficient.[5] The mechanisms of action of levamisole involves both humoral and cell-mediated immunity. The drug, *in vitro*, has been shown to be mitogenic and to stimulate blastogenesis in both normal and leukemic lymphocytes to mitogens or specific antigens, cytotoxicity reactions and the total number of circulating active T lymphocytes.[15] Churchill and David hypothesized that levamisole might stimulate the immune response by increasing the responsiveness of sensitized lymphocytes.[16] Levamisole restores to normal levels the nitrogen responsiveness of hypo-responsive lymphocytes and augments the production of soluble mediators by the peripheral lymphocytes *in vitro*, while exerting no effect on lymphocyte proliferation.[17] In this study, 25, 50, or 100 µg/well amounts of tetramisole or polymer were added to the lymphocyte cultures in microtiter plates. These doses were in the concentration range demonstrated to

stimulate optimal augmentation of the proliferative response to the mitogen concanavalin A (ConA).[17] Whitcomb demonstrated that levamisole augments mediator production by mitogen stimulated lymphocytes *in vitro* in a
dose dependent manner; these responses were measured as an increase in
migration inhibitory factor (MIF) and macrophage activating factor (MAF)
activity present in the supernatant solutions of the mitogen-stimulated
lymphocyte cultures containing levamisole.[17] Since T-cells are targets
for mitogenic stimulation by photoagglutinine (PHA), the results of
Whitcomb et al., suggest that levamisole is active in the splenic T-cell
compartments. However, no drug effect was noted when mitogens were not
present.[17] Several investigators have studied the effect of levamisole on
the proliferative response of human lymphocytes *in vitro*.[18] Again, levamisole exerted no effect on lymphocyte proliferation *in vitro*.[18] Also,
levamisole had no effect on the proliferative response of human lymphocytes to either PHA or Con-A over a broad concentration range.[17] Another
study showed that levamisole augmented DNA synthesis of mouse spleen
cells and thymocytes in response to mitogens and alloantigens as well as
in the absence of these stimuli.[19,20] Levamisole induced only small
increases in the proliferative response to mitogens.[19,21]

In contrast, a few investigators have shown that levamisole increases
lymphocyte proliferation.[13] Con-A induced lymphocyte proliferation is a
separate event from MIF production and may involve distinct populations
of cells.[22] Thus, an increase in mediator production, e.g. MIF production, clearly may occur in the absence of an increase in lymphocyte
proliferation. Levamisole seems to stimulate increased mediator production without increasing lymphocyte production.[17]

Fisher found that treatment of weaning rats with levamisole increased
their resistance to infections with herpes virus and staphylococci.[23]
Immunosuppressed individuals respond to a greater extent to levamisole
than do those with normal or near normal immune capability. In both
groups, the response to suboptimum antigenic stimuli is relatively
unaffected.[13]

The effects of levamisole are most obvious in a compromised immune
system. The dose of levamisole is also important. Anderson et al., evaluated certain neutrophil and lymphocyte functions following administration
of a 150 mg oral dose of levamisole.[24] Levamisole stimulated neutrophil
motility, increased post phagocytic hexose monophosphate shunt activity
and protein iodination capacity. Levamisole increased lymphocyte DNA
synthesis but not protein synthesis in mitogen (PHA) - stimulated lymphocytes.[24] This latter observation supports Whitcomb's contention that
levamisole does not induce lymphocyte proliferation. Cell stimulation was
detected almost immediately upon treatment; the augmented neutrophil and
lymphocyte functions were still evident 24 hours later but not at 48
hours. This study showed that a 150 mg oral dose of levamisole can
potentiate DNA but not protein synthesis in lymphocytes from normal
individuals.[24] At lower doses of levamisole (0.1-1.0 µg/mL), the drug
augmented antibody production while suppressing specific lymphocyte
mediated cytotoxicity of tumor cells.[25] Higher doses were needed to augment the specific lymphocyte-mediated cytotoxicity.[26] Levamisole was
stimulatory only in a narrow range of low concentrations, the optimal
dose being 0.1 to 1.0 µg/mL dose. *In vitro* levamisole exerted a slight
but consistent stimulatory effect on DNA synthesis by spleen cells with
concentrations of 10-100 ng/mL. In contract, Whitcomb et al. found that
supra-optimum concentrations of levamisole were inhibitory.[17] The mode of
action of levamisole is dose-dependent in that low doses seems to suppress specific lymphocyte mediated cytotoxicity against tumor cells;
supra-optimum concentrations inhibit both humoral and certain cell

mediated immune (CMI) reactions while augmenting the cytotoxicity response against tumor cells.

Levamisole also augments the chemotactic response of phagocytes (neutrophils and monocytes) from normal and immunodeficient patients.[27] *In vitro*, the drug promotes stimulation of random migration, chemotaxis and directional mobility of normal and abnormal human neutrophils.[28] Al-Ibrahim et al., showed that levamisole directly stimulated phagocytes in a lymphocyte free system.[13] Enhancement was optimal at a concentration that inhibited antigen or mitogen induced stimulation of sensitive lymphocyte. Lower concentrations of levamisole (0.6 µg/mL) enhanced the proliferative lymphocyte response.[29] These investigators also noted the augmenting effect of levamisole on DNA synthesis at doses of 10-100 ng/mL.[20] Using a higher dose of levamisole (50 µg/mL), they did not see enhanced lymphocyte proliferation.[17] Poly(I:C) in combination with levamisole stimulated DNA synthesis in spleen cell suspension cultures. Levamisole augmented the DNA synthetic response to a supra-optimal concentration of PHA.[20]

Treatment of mice with levamisole enhances reticular endothelial system (RES) activity with enhanced phagocytic and bactericidal activity of peritoneal macrophages.[30] In vitro, levamisole augments phagocytosis of opsonized sRBC by peritoneal macrophages of mice.[31] Levamisole enhances directly the phagocytosis by human macrophages. Depression of phagocytosis was not noted at higher concentrations of levamisole.

Levamisole causes an enhancement of phagocytosis by macrophages. Data suggests at least two mechanisms for the potentiation of CMI seen *in vitro* with levamisole, namely, direct stimulation of inflammatory cells (monocytes and macrophages) or immunologic activation of mononuclear cells, i.e., lymphocytes, brought about by enhanced lymphokine production.

Levamisole potentiates a wide spectrum of immunologic reactivity. It restores cutaneous delayed hypersensitivity in anergic patients with cancer.[11] Tripodi et al., reported that levamisole administration increased delayed hypersensitivity reactions in 14 out of 20 anergic patients with solid tumors.[11] This increased responsiveness suggests that the drug induced stimulation is not specific and may extend to include all CMI responses.[11] Levamisole is not generally effective against bacterial or viral infections in immunocompetent adult animals but may be of some benefits in the treatment of chronic or recurrent infections in immunodeficient patients or immature animals.[15] Since levamisole has no demonstrable intrinsic antibacterial or antiviral properties, these effects are mediated by its immunopotentiating activity.[15] DeCree et al., noted correction of depressed neutrophil function (chemotaxis, phagocytosis, and antimicrobial activity) and T lymphocyte (E resetting and transformation) functions in a child with recurrent infection by levamisole treatment.[32] It is clear that levamisole in certain doses augments phagocytic activity in both normal and deficient individuals, but normalizes certain T cell functions only in immunocompromised individuals.

Interferon-gamma (IFN) may be induced following the administration of levamisole. Matsubara et al. showed that an i.p. injection of an optimum dose of levamisole (5-10 mg/kg) produces marked antiviral activity in DDT mice.[3]

Interferon-gamma induction by levamisole was abrogated completely in DDT mice pretreated with either X-ray or hydrocortisone acetate. Levamisole did not induce the production of IFN in athymic nude mice.[14]

Both irradiation (500-700 R) and a treatment dose of 2.5 mg of hydrocortisone acetate are known to reduce the functions of lymphoid cells responsible for humoral and CMI reactions (32). The effect of levamisole on IFN induction was dose dependent. Significant IFN activity in the sera was detected only when mice were treated with drug doses ranging from 5 to 10 mg/kg.

Levamisole potentiates weakened immune systems by exerting an effect on lymphocytes,[19] and by boosting response of T cells to mitogenic and allogenic stimulation. When depressed, lymphocyte responses can be restored when levamisole is given at a critical time.[47] If given too early after cytostatic treatment, levamisole induces a further depression followed by a delayed recovery.[34] It has also been found to abolish the suppresser cell activity of non-T cells in breast cancer patients.[34]

Levamisole augmented monocyte chemotaxis in patients with metastatic colonrectal carcinoma significantly more than in non-carcinoma patients.[26] Administration of levamisole to animals following chemotherapy was most effective when immune responses were most depressed.[35]

Levamisole has little effect on antibody production in immune competent animals and human subjects,[15] but it does augment antibody production in mice that are immunodeficient because of genetic factors and old age.[32] The relatively weak response to antigen is augmented more than the relatively strong response to mitogens: the effects are demonstrable more easily with cells from immunosuppressed subjects than with cells from normal subjects. The accumulated evidence suggests that the thymus-dependent lymphocytes are preferentially responsive to levamisole. Levamisole seems to induce responses in different ways in several biological systems and each response can be beneficial to the host organism.

Cis-DICHLORODIAMINE PLATINUM II (cis-DDP)

Platinum compounds have been found to react against tumors in biological systems. Most of the research involving the use of platinum compounds as antitumoral agents has focused in the study of cis-dichlorodiamine platinum II (cis-DDP) itself or a structurally close derivative. In 1964, Rosenberg and co-workers discovered that bacteria failed to divide, but continued to grow giving filamentous cells in the presence of platinum electrodes.[36] A major cause of this inhibition to cell division was due to cis-DDP. Platinum derivatives must possess a certain structural characteristic for antitumoral activity. For tumoral activity these derivatives should be neutral, contain two inert NH groups and two labile Cl ligands with the ligands in the cis conformation to one another. The structure of cis-DDP is shown below and displays the needed structural characteristics.

One of the major side effects seen with cis-DDP and structurally similar molecules is nephrotoxicity. This is the major dose limiting side effect of cis-DDP and is cumulative and eventually irreversible. Platinum is a heavy metal; soon after administration, a large percentage of the drug is filtered from the blood by the kidneys and excreted in the urine.

Structure 2. Cis-DDP

Renal damage is usually observed by the elevation of blood, urea, nitrogen, and creatinine, or by a decreased creatinine clearance.[37] Histological studies have shown this to be due to local acute tubular necrosis effecting primarily the distal convoluted tubules and collecting ducts, dilation of convoluted tubules and the formation of casts.[38] Other side effects have also been noticed. Neurotoxicity, in the form of tinnitus, is often complicated with audiogram abnormalities. This causes cumulative and irreversible hearing loss in the high subclinical range of 4,000-8,000 Hz. Continued treatment with platinum causes loss in the spoken range of 1,000-4,000 Hz.[37] Total deafness usually indicates that death is imminent. Other problems can develop including sensory or motor difficulties, seizures, loss of taste, loss of memory, intention tremor, and postural hypotension.[39] Also gastrointestional, hematopoietic, and immunosuppressive side effects have been noted.[38]

Much work centered about the clinical use of cis-DDP leading to the licensing of it as an antineoplastic drug. It is currently used in conjunction with other drugs for treatment against a wide variety of tumors.[43] Cis-DDP is active against a wide range of tumors in animals and man including several which are particularly resistant to treatment by other techniques including ovarian and testicular carcinomas.[44]

Rosenberg has hypothesized that the platinum complex enhances the antigenicity of tumor cells. The tumor cells are then attacked by the body in an immunological response.[36] Other effects of platinum may be related to the distribution of the drug. The liver and kidney contained the highest levels of platinum. The highest percentage of the drug stays in these tissues and in the blood, skin, and muscle because of the high body mass. Platinum concentrations in tumor tissues are no higher when compared to normal cells.[40] Also, the tumor does not cause increased retention of the drug. When cis-DDP is retained in the kidney it causes nephrotoxicity and the excretion rate is fast, 50% in the first 4 hours and then the rate becomes much slower. This may be due to the binding to biological material. The use of a polymer form may cause restrictive biological movement, controlled release, and increased probability of critical attachment. These favor a decreased toxic effect for platinum polymers.

Several procedures have been tested related to cis-DDP usage. The method of chemically modifying cis-DDP has been used to reduce toxic effects. Modification can range from simple ligand substitutions to the incorporation of the drug into a complex high molecular weight polymer system.

Structural derivatives of cis-DDP which conform to the limits of structural requirements have been synthesized that show reduced toxicity and enhanced antitumoral activity.[41] Chain lengths seem to play a roll in toxicity with lengths of about 100 or greater somewhat restricted in movement in comparison to the drug cis-DDP.[15] Areas of the body which are normally prone to high concentrations of cis-DDP are relatively protected when the drug is incorporated into a polymer. These are being tested for the reduction of toxic effects (for instance 40).

The majority of the polyamines alter the normal replication cycle of the poliovirus type 1 and EMC virus strain MM when tumor cells (mouse connective tissue, human cervical carcinoma, and human amnion cancer cells) where treated with virus without destruction of the cells themselves[42]

ENCEPHALOMYOCARDITIS-VARIANT-D

A murine model of insulin-dependent diabetes mellitus was developed by Craighead and colleagues in 1968, using the M variant of an encephalomyocarditis virus (EMC-M). EMC is a picornavirus which is a small lytic RNA virus in the cardiovirus family. The virus was recovered from swine that developed fatal myocarditis. This virus, passed once in mice, exhibited specific diabetogenic properties. These properties suggested that "wild" viruses which have specific beta-cell tropism and diabetogenic potential may be found in nature.[45] EMC-M was employed for infection, beta cell degranulation, coagulation necrosis, and alteration of the islet cells in susceptible mice.[46] The degree of beta cell damage correlated with the degree of hyperglycemia seen in mice.[47] In 1979, Yoon and colleagues discovered that EMC-M was a mixture of at least two viruses, the diabetogenic D variant, (known as EMC-D) and the non-diabetogenic B variant (EMC-B).[17] The induction of diabetes by EMC-D was inhibited by EMC-B during coinfection experiments. This demonstrated that the ratio of EMC-B: EMC-D in the inoculum determined the incidence of diabetes in the susceptible SJL/J mouse strain.[17]

The two variants of EMC-M exhibit different characteristics. The D variant of EMC-M produces large diffuse plaques on mouse L929 cells and does not induce interferon (INF); in contrast, the B variant produces small distinct plaques on mouse L929 cells and induces large amount of interferon.[48] Yoon noted that the passage history of EMC-M influenced its diabetogenicity.[48] After passage in mouse kidney cell cultures, the diabetogenic of the virus was markedly diminished, but was restored after one passage in mice.[49] No demonstrable time difference was seen in the appearance of neutralizing antibody to either the B or D variants.[10] It was further noted, that antibody action against one variant neutralized the infectivity of the other variant to the same extent.[17]

Differences in the two variants were also identified by Ray et al., who analyzed the two genomes by nucleic acid hybridization and RNA fingerprinting.[50] The ribonuclease T-digested RNA's, fingerprinted on two-dimensional poly(acrylamide) gels, revealed at least one oligonucleotides (20 to 25 nucleotides in length) present in the EMC-D RNA which was not present in EMC-B RNA.[50] Gould and colleagues demonstrated differences in tissue tropism and replication of the two variants in ICR Swiss mice.[48] EMC-D replicated in the spleen, pancreas, heart, lung and intestines while EMC-replication was limited to the spleen and pancreas.

EXPERIMENTAL

Polymer Synthesis

The synthesis of each polymer was performed in a glass Kimax flask. An aqueous solution of tetramisole was mixed with an aqueous solution of K_2PtCl_4 and allowed to stir for 24-36 hours. The resulting compound (polymer form of the inducer) was filtered and air dried in a glass petri dish.

Chemical Characterization of the Polymer

Elemental analysis was performed using a Perkin-Elmer 240 Elemental Analyzer for C, H and N and thermal analysis.

Infrared spectra were obtained using potassium bromide pellets employing a Perkin-Elmer 1330 Infrared Spectrophotometer and Digilab FTIR model FTS-20C/D.

Mass spectral analysis were obtained using a direct probe connected to a Kratos MS-50 Mass Spectrometer, operating in the El mode, 8 KV acceleration and 10 sec/decade scan rate with a probe temperature of 350° to 550°C.

Administration Time

Various times of administrating the drugs in monomer form and in polymer form relative to injection of EMC-D virus were used in this study to determine whether exacerbation of virus-induced diabetes occurred as described by Warchalowski and Strausser.[1] The drugs were injected i.p. before or after i.p. injection of 800 PFU of EMC-D virus.

EMC-D Virus

The D variant of encephalomyocarditis virus (EMC-D) was obtained from J. Yoon, NIH, Bethesda, MD. EMC-D was found to have mixed morphology in mouse L929 cells and to induce the production of interferon.[4] After passage of EMC-D through L929 cells 5 times, BHK21 cells (baby hamster kidney cells) two times, and one additional passage through L929 cells, the resulting virus stock was diabetogenic, produces large diffuse plaques in L929 cells, and does not induce the production of interferon in cell culture. The EMC-D variant was propagated and titered by methods previously described. The virus was diluted in HBSS containing 2% fetal calf serum. Mice were given a single i.p. injection of the diluted virus. An EMC-D dose of 800 PFU was used.

Animals

Male ICR Swiss were purchased from Harlan Laboratories, Indianapolis, IN. The animals were housed in groups of 10, and at the time of infection were 9 weeks of age.

Glucose Tolerance Test (GTT)

At specific times, a non-fasting GTT was done on each of the animals. Each mouse received an i.p. injection of glucose at a concentration of 2 mg/gm body weight. After 1 hour the animals were bled and the serum glucose levels were determined using a USI Model 23A glucose analyzer. It has been shown that non-fasting glucose levels demonstrate a greater sensitivity to reduction of insulin secretion than does fasting glucose.[51]

Glucose values lower than mean control values by more than three standard deviations (sd) were considered to be hypoglycemic, while glucose levels greater then 3 sd above the mean control values were considered hyperglycemic. The student T test was used to analyze the glucose tolerance test data in the various experiments.

RESULTS

Structural Characterization

Structural characterization will be reported elsewhere and is consistent with a polymer (weight average degree of polymerization of 280 in DMSO) containing a repeat unit of form 3.

Structure 3. Tetramisol polymer [3]

The Effects of Tetramisole And Its Polymer on EMC-D Virus-Induced Diabetes

Three doses of tetramisole and its polymer were administered i.p. to ICR Swiss mice at different times before and after infection by EMC-D virus.

The data in Table 1 shows that when tetramisole, in doses of 1 mg/kg or 5 mg/kg was given eight days prior to virus, a decrease in the severity and incidence of virus-induced diabetes was seen compared to untreated control virus mice. In contrast, mice receiving a 10 mg/kg dose of tetramisole eight days before virus exhibited a higher incidence and greater severity of diabetes. The tetramisole polymer, in doses of 1, 5, and 10 mg/kg administered eight days before virus exerted no demonstrable effect upon either the incidence or severity of virus-induced diabetes.

However, when tetramisole was given in doses of 1 mg/kg and 10 mg/kg the day prior to virus infection, (Table 2) an increase in the severity and incidence of virus-induced diabetes was seen. The 5 mg/kg dose does not seem to exert much effect upon either the incidence or severity of virus-induced diabetes. When the polymer was given in doses of 0.1, 0.5, 1.5, and 10 mg/kg the incidence of virus-induced diabetes was increased at each dose except 5 mg/kg which increased the severity of the disease. The 5 mg/kg dose had no effect on the severity of virus-induced diabetes.

When tetramisole was given in doses of 0.1, 0.5, 1.5, and 10 mg/kg 4 days post (EMC-D) infection (Table 3), the severity of virus-induced diabetes was increased; 0.1 and 0.5 mg/kg doses also increased the incidence of diabetes.

CONCLUSIONS

Tetramisole and its platinum polyamine were examined for their effects on EMC-D virus-induced diabetes in outbred ICR Swiss male mice. Both tetramisole and its isomer levamisole are potent immunomodulators capable of restoring immune responsiveness to normal levels in certain immune deficient patients while exerting no demonstrable effect on normal individuals[23] The immunomodulatory effects of levamisole have been more

Table 1. The effects of tetramisole and its polymer upon
virus-induced diabetes 8 days before virus infection.

Material injected mg/kg	GTT (7 days after virus infection) mg%*	**	EMC-D GTT mg%*	**	Normal control mg%*
TETRAMISOLE					
1	264 ± 114 (1,A)	2/10	349 ± 187	5/10	210 ± 78
5	220 ± 49 (1,B)	1/10	349 ± 187	5/10	210 ± 78
10	455 ± 173 (5,A)	9/10	349 ± 187	5/10	210 ± 78
POLYMER					
1	308 ± 125 (3,A)	5/10	349 ± 187	5/10	210 ± 78
5	362 ± 125 (3,A)	6/10	349 ± 187	5/10	210 ± 78
10	359 ± 201 (3,A)	7/10	349 ± 187	5/10	210 ± 78

*   Mean ± sd.
** Ratio of diabetic to total.

A, 1 = Not statistically significant
B, 2 = 0.050 < T < 0.025   90% - 95% significant
C, 3 = 0.025 < T < 0.010   95% - 98% significant
D, 4 = 0.010 < T < 0.005   98% - 99% significant
E, 5 = 0.005 < T   99%   significant

The numbers 1-5 refer to statistical analysis between the
sham immunized control glucose tolerance test and the chemically treated groups.

The letters A-E refer to statistical analysis between the
EMC-D glucose tolerance test standard and the chemically
treated groups.

extensively studied. Levamisole increases the synthesis and release of
lymphokines, including gamma interferon (IFN), but does not appear to
stimulate lymphocyte proliferation. The drugs were administered to ICR
Swiss males eight days and one day prior to virus infection as well as
four days after infection by EMC-D virus. These results are summarized in
Tables 4-6.

The lower doses of tetramisole and its polymer, given eight days
prior to EMC-D, (Table 4), may have stimulated T cells and macrophages.
The enhanced lymphokine secretion by T cells may have activated macrophages i.e. INF is a potent activator of macrophages. Therefore, virus
was readily inactivated when injected into such animals. In contrast the
10 mg/kg dose of tetramisole may have been high enough to have activated
T suppresser cells (Ts cells). As a result, a greater immunosuppression
would have occurred, permitting the virus to replicate in these animals
resulting in an increase in the incidence and severity of diabetes. When
tetramisole was given at day one prior to EMC-D infection, (Table 5), the
inflammation induced by the injection (i.p.) may have stimulated the
influx into the peritoneal cavity of circulating blood elements,
especially Ts cells and macrophages. As a result, tetramisole-activated
Ts cells (Ts cells are present in relatively high numbers in the circul-
ation) may have accumulated at the site of virus infection. The one day
interval between drug administration and virus infection may not have
been adequate for production of viral inhibitory concentrations of INF.

Table 2. The effect of tetramisole and its polymer upon virus-
induced diabetes when given 1 day prior to virus
infection.

Material injected mg/kg	GTT (7 days after virus infection) mg%*	**	EMC-D GTT mg%*	**	Normal control mg%*
TETRAMISOLE					
1	591 ± 172 (5,C)	9/9	378 ± 135	6/7	214 ± 27
5	404 ± 156 (5,A)	6/7	378 ± 135	6/7	214 ± 27
10	450 ± 120 (5,A)	8/8	378 ± 135	6/7	214 ± 27
POLYMER					
0.1	360 ± 144 (5,A)	7/10	301 ± 139	4/10	195 ± 59
0.5	321 ± 205 (2,A)	5/10	301 ± 139	4/10	195 ± 59
1.0	391 ± 157 (3,A)	5/10	301 ± 139	4/10	159 ± 59
5.0	388 ± 137 (5,A)	8/10	391 ± 246	6/10	200 ± 55
10.0	352 ± 139 (4,A)	7/10	301 ± 139	4/10	195 ± 59

* Mean ± sd.
** Ratio of diabetic to total.

A, 1 = Not statistically significant
B, 2 = $0.050 < T < 0.025$ 90% – 95% significant
C, 3 = $0.025 < T < 0.010$ 95% – 98% significant
D, 4 = $0.010 < T < 0.005$ 98% – 99% significant
E, 5 = $0.005 < T$ 99%   significant

The numbers 1-5 refer to statistical analysis between the
sham immunized control glucose tolerance test and the chemically treated groups.

The letters A-E refer to statistical analysis between the
EMC-D glucose tolerance test standard and the chemically
treated groups.

Since diabetes was evaluated seven days after virus infection, the
enhanced diabetes seen may reflect more the immunomodulatory effects of
INF, stimulated by tetramisole over a period of several days than the
antiviral effect of IFN-Gamma especially with the polymer forms. Due to
the insolubility of the polymer forms, a slow release of the compound is
suggested. The suppressive activity produced by tetramisole in this set
of experiments did not prevent formation of neutralizing antibodies
measured seven days after virus infection.

As seen in Table 6, when tetramisole and its polymers were given to
mice four days after the initiation of virus infection, marked inhibition
of neutralizing antibodies was seen three days later (i.e. seven days
after virus infection).

The animals given tetramisole at four days after infection have
already initiated an immune response against the virus. Tetramisole and
its polymer were able to stop this process possibly through enhanced
secretion of modulatory lymphokines by Ts cells. Also this enhanced stimulation of lymphokine secretions by suppressive T lymphocytes as well as
enhanced Ts activity by secreted IFN may have diminished destruction of

Table 3. The effects of tetramisole and its polymer upon virus-induced diabetes when given 4 days after virus infection.

Material injected mg/kg	GTT (7 days after virus infection) mg%*	**	EMC-D GTT mg%*	**	Normal control mg%*
TETRAMISOLE					
0.1	586 ± 155 (5,E)	10/10	273 ± 89	4/7	205 ± 41
0.5	409 ± 156 (5,B)	7/8	273 ± 89	4/7	205 ± 41
1	382 ± 168 (3,A)	3/6	273 ± 89	4/7	205 ± 41
5	386 ± 162 (5,A)	3/5	273 ± 89	4/7	205 ± 41
10	378 ± 163 (5,A)	4/8	273 ± 89	4/7	205 ± 41
POLYMER					
0.1	357 ± 168 (5,A)	6/10	301 ± 139	4/10	196 ± 59
0.5	215 ± 47 (1,B)	2/9	301 ± 139	4/10	196 ± 59
1	278 ± 144 (2,A)	3/9	301 ± 139	4/10	196 ± 59
5	399 ± 110 (5,A)	10/10	391 ± 246	6/10	200 ± 55
10	299 ± 119 (4,A)	6/10	301 ± 139	4/10	196 ± 59

* Mean ± sd.
** Ratio of diabetic to total.

A, 1 = Not statistically significant
B, 2 = 0.050 < T < 0.025   90% - 95% significant
C, 3 = 0.025 < T < 0.010   95% - 98% significant
D, 4 = 0.010 < T < 0.005   98% - 99% significant
E, 5 = 0.005 < T   99%   significant

The numbers 1-5 refer to statistical analysis between the sham immunized control glucose tolerance test and the chemically treated groups.

The letters A-E refer to statistical analysis between the EMC-D glucose tolerance test standard and the chemically treated groups.

virus-infected target cells (e.g. pancreatic beta cells, brain cells). Gould has shown that a small amount of virus is present in the spleen, pancreas, and heart four days after infection.[48]

Since the polymer would be releasing the drug over a long period of time the results in polymer-treated mice are more difficult to interpret. The 0.1 mg/kg polymer dose was the only polymer form to enhance both severity and incidence of diabetes when given four days after virus. The amount of tetramisole released from the polymers cannot be determined since the polymers are not soluble in water or serum. Since Vailletes et al.,[52] as well as Gould,[53] have shown that immunosuppression by cyclosporin A enhances the diabetogenicity of either the EMC-M (mixture of B and D) variants,[52] or the EMC-D,[53] a role for activation of the Ts cell-macrophage regulatory circuit in the genesis of virus-induced diabetes was suggested. Warchalowski and Strausser attributed the enhancement of EMC virus-induced diabetes in mice by levamisole to its action of Ts cells.[45]. Aune and Pierce have shown that levamisole inhibits the ability

Table 4. Summary of the effects of tetramisole and its polymer given eight days prior to EMC-D virus infection.

Dosage mg/kg	Tetramisole incidence	severity	Polymer incidence	severity
1	-	-	0	0
5	-	-	0	0
10	+	+	0	0

+ denotes an increase in the effect, compared to the controls.
- denotes a decrease in the effect, compared to the controls.
0 means there was no difference was noted between the groups given the compound and the diabetic controls.

Table 5. Summary of the effects of tetramisole and its polymer given one day prior to EMC-D virus infection.

Dosage mg/kg	Tetramisole incidence	severity	Polymer incidence	severity
0.1	nd	nd	+	+
0.5	nd	nd	+	+
1	+	+	+	+
5	+	+	+	+
10	+	+	+	+

nd means that the sample was not tested.
+ denotes an increase in the effect, compared to the controls.
- denotes a decrease in the effect, compared to the controls.
0 means there was no difference was noted between the groups given the compound and the diabetic controls.

Table 6. Summary of the effects of tetramisole and its polymer given four days post EMC-D infection.

Dosage mg/kg	Tetramisole incidence	severity	Polymer incidence	severity
0.1	+	+	+	+
0.5	+	+	-	-
1	0	+	0	0
5	0	+	0	0
10	0	+	+	0

+ denotes an increase in the effect, compared to the controls.
- denotes a decrease in the effect, compared to the controls.
0 means there was no difference was noted between the groups given the compound and the diabetic controls.

of macrophages to oxidize soluble immune response suppresser (SIRS) to SIRSox, the actual inhibitor of lymphocyte proliferation.[2] In this study tetramisole, given eight days prior to virus, probably stimulated both helper (Th) and suppresser (Ts) lymphocytes to release lymphokines as shown by Whitcomb.[17]. Since animals possess much higher numbers of helper T cells, the effects of stimulated Th cells would outweigh the suppression mediated by Ts cells. Consequently, it is suggested that those animals receiving the 1 and 5 mg/kg doses of tetramisole were able to clear the virus infection more effectively by mobilizing effecter T cell-mediated immune mechanisms early in infection. In some virus infections, effecter T cell responses are demonstrable by day four.[19] The 10 mg/kg dose of tetramisole may have stimulated a more effective and /or prolonged release of suppresser T cells; the stimulation of IFN release would enhance the activation of Ts cells.

When tetramisole is given one day before virus, stimulation of Ts cells and the release of SIRS may well have outweighted the antiviral effects of IFN released by the levamisole. Consequently, early immune clearance of the virus infection was compromised even though IFN was present to stimulate increased natural killer cell activity.[52]

When tetramisole was administered four days after infection with the diabetogenic EMC-D virus, exacerbation of diabetes was usually seen. Since tetramisole causes release of lymphokines from activated T cells, these results suggest that EMC-D infection in animals developing diabetes also selectively activates Ts cells. The lymphokines released by activated Ts cells block the virus-specific antibody-producing B cells from receiving the helper signals from the Th cells. Consequently, antibody synthesis is blocked.

The low doses of tetramisole (0.1 or 0.5 mg/kg) may have selectively stimulated suppression of virus (antigen)-activated lymphocytes, e.g. any cytotoxic (Tc) or delayed type hypersensitivity (Ts) effecter T cell protective mechanisms, and in turn, B cell responses. The 0.5 mg/kg dose of levamisole was a more effective inhibitor of neutralizing antibody production than was the 0.1 mg/kg dose. The higher doses of tetramisole also decreased neutralizing antibody formation and increased the severity of the diabetes. These results suggest that T lymphocyte effecter mechanisms may be of prime importance during the first four days of virus infection in allaying or preventing virus-induced diabetes.

REFERENCES

1. G. Warchalowski & H. Strausser, Immunol. Comm., **8**, 33 (1979)
2. T. M. Aune & C. W. Pierce, Int. J. Immunopharmacol., **5**, 91 (1983).
3. S. Matsubara, F. Suzuki & N. Ishida, Cell Immunol., **43**, 214 (1979).
4. K. Buschard, N. Hastrup & J. Ryaard, Diabetologia, **24**, 42 (1983).
5. F. K. Jansen, O. Thurneyssen & H. Muntefering, Biomed., **31**, 1 (1979).
6. E. T.Blaz & M. Talas, Acta. Virol., **17**, 168 (1973).
7. M. E. Wolff, "*Burger's Medicinal Chemistry*", 4th Ed., Part II, John Wiley and Sons Inc., New York, 480, (1979).
8. C. F. Borden, T. E. Davis, J. J. Croutey, W. H. Wolberg, B. McKnight & M. A. Chirigos in: "*Immunotherapy of Human Cancer*", Section IV, Elsevier, New York, Terry Rosenberg, Ed., 1982, p. 187.
9. G. Renoux & M. Renoux, Infect. Immunol., **8**, 544 (1973).
10. G. Renoux, Nature New Biol., **240**, 217 (1972).
11. D. A. Tripodi, L. C. Parks & J. Grugmans, New Eng. J. Med., **289**, 354 (1973).

236

12. S. H. Chan, S. K. Lee & M. J. Simons, Proc. Soc. Exp. Biol. Med., **151**, 716 (1976).
13. M. S. Al-Ibrahim, R. S. Holzman & H. S. Lawrence, J. Infect. Dis., **135**, 517 (1978).
14. M. C. Pike & R. Snyderman, Cell Immunol., **32**, 234 (1977).
15. J. Symoens, Res. J. Reticuloindothelial Soc., **21**, 175 (1977).
16. W. H. Churchill & J. R. David, New Eng. J. Med., **289**, 375 (1973).
17. M. E. Whitcomb, V. J. Merluzzi & S. R. Cooperband, Cell. Immunol., **21**, 272 (1976).
18. H. Verhaegen, J. DeCree, W. DeCock & F. Verbruggen, New Eng. J. Med., **289**, 1148 (1973).
19. J. H. Hadden, R. C. Coffry & E. M. Hadden, Cell Immunol., **20**, 98 (1975).
20. A. Woods, M. J. Siegel & M. A. Chirigos, Cell Immunol., **14**, 327 (1974).
21. D. Lichtenfeld, Fed. Proc. Fed. Am. Soc. Exp. Biol., **59**, 790 (1974).
22. R. E. Rocklin, R. P. MacDermot, L. Chess, S. F. Schlossman & J. R. David, J. Exp. Med., **140**, 1303 (1974).
23. A. Faanes, Clin. Exp. Immunol., 33 (1977).
24. R. Anderson, R. Oosthuizen, A. Theron & A. Van Renberg, Clin. Exp. Immunol., **35**, 478 (1979).
25. Mantovani & Spreafico, Eur. J. Cancer, **11**, 537 (1975).
26. E. DeMaeyer, G. Galasso & H. Schellekens, "*Interferon and the Immune System. The Biology of the Interferon System*", Elsiever, New York, 1981, p. 203.
27. Wright., Prog. Cancer Res. Ther., **227** (1977).
28. R. Anderson, A. Glover, H. J. Koornaf & A. R. Rabson, J. Immunol., **117**, 428 (1976).
29. W. H. Wolberg, Cancer Res., **37**, 3711 (1977).
30. G. Renoux, Fed. Proc. Fed. Am. Soc. Exp. Biol., **35**, 336 (1976).
31. Oliveira-Lima, Experimentia, **30**, 945 (1974).
32. G. Renoux, J. Immunol., **113**, 779 (1974).
33. H. N. Claman, New Eng. J. Med., **287**, 388 (1972).
34. Y. Levo, V. Rotter & B. Pamot, Biomedicine, Ps23Ps, 198 (1975).
35. K. Perk, M. A. Chirigos, F. Fuhran & H. Pettigrew, J. Nat. Cancer Inst., **54**, 253 (1975).
36. B. Rosenberg, L. Van Camp & T.Krigas, Nature, **205**, 698 (1965).
37. M. Rozenweig, D. Van Hoff & M. Slavik, Ann. Int. Med., **86**, 803 (1977).
38. I. Krakoff, Cancer Treatment Rep., **63**,1523 (1979).
39. D. Van Hoff, R. Schilski & C. Reichert, Cancer Treat Rep., **63**, 1527 (1977).
40. W. Wolf & R. Manaka, J. Clin. Hemato. Oncol., **7**, 79 (1977).
41. J. Davidson, D. Faber & R. Fisher, Can Chemother. Rep., **59**, 287 (1975).
42. C. E. Carraher, W. J. Scott, I. Lopez, D. J. Giron, D. R. Cerutis, & T. Manek in: "*New Monomers and Polymers*", B. Culbertson and C. Pittman, Eds., Plenum, New York, 1983, Chapter 8.
43. D. Higby, H. Wallace D. Albert, J. Holland, J. Urology, **112**, 100 (1974).
44. B. Rosenberg, Cancer Chemother. Rep. Pt.1., **59**, 589 (1975).
45. J. Craighead, J. New Eng. J. Med., **299**, 1439 (1978).
46. E. Rayfield & Y. Seto, Diabetes, **27**, 1126 (1978).
47. K. Hayashi, D. Boucher & A. L. Notkins, Amer. J. Path., **75**, 91 (1974).
48. C. L. Gould, M. L. Trombley, N. J. Bigley, K. G. McMannama & D. J. Giron, Proc. Soc. Exp. Biol. Med., **175**, 449 (1984).
49. J. Yoon, T. Onodera & A. L. Notkins, J. Gen. Virol., **37**, 225 (1977).
50. U. Ray, G. Aulaakh, M. Schubert, P. McVlintock, J. Yoon & A. L. Notkins, J. Gen. Virol., **64**, 947 (1983).
51. R. Chairez, J. Yoon & A. L. Notkins, Virology, **85**, 606 (1978).

52. B. Vailletes, D. Baume, C. Charpin, R. DeMayer, J. Guignard & D. Vague, J. Clin. Lab. Immunol., **10**, 35 (1983).
53. C. L. Gould, "*Host Responses to Virus-Induced Murine Diabetes*", Ph.D. Dissertation, Wright State University, Dayton, OH, 1984.

INFLUENCE OF SHORT CHAIN PHOSPHOLIPID SPACERS ON THE PROPERTIES OF DIACETYLENIC PHOSPHATIDYLCHOLINE BILAYERS

Alok Singh and Bruce P. Gaber

Bio/Molecular Engineering Branch, Code 6190, Naval Research Laboratory, Washington, D.C. 20375-5000

Diacetylenes in phospholipid bilayers have been the subject of extensive studies in our laboratory, not only because of the highly conjugated polymers they form, but also because of their ability to transform bilayers into interesting microstructures. Consequent to our synthesis and characterization of several isomeric diacetylenic phospholipids, we have found that the polymerization in diacetylenic bilayers is not complete. In order to achieve participation of all diacetylenic lipid monomer in the polymerization process, diacetylenic phospholipid was mixed with a spacer' lipid, which contained similar number of methylenes as were between the ester linkage and the diacetylene of the polymerizable lipid. Depending upon the composition of the mixtures different morphologies, ranging from tubules to liposomes, have been observed. Polymerization efficiency has been found to be dependent on the composition of the two lipids and in all cases the polymerization was more rapid and efficient than the pure diacetylenic system. We present the results on the polymerization properties of the diacetylenic phosphatidylcholines in the presence of a spacer' lipid which is an acetylene-terminated phosphatidylcholine.

INTRODUCTION

Polymerized vesicles[1] represent a new class of organic polymers which may find broad application in areas of research and technology such as controlled release systems, drug carriers, biosensors, catalysis, microelectronics, and so forth.[2] Polymerization has provided durability to lipid bilayer systems, making them attractive for applications. Several polymerizable entities have been used in amphiphiles, such as methacryloyl,[3,7,8] diacetylene,[4-6] diene,[9,10] and vinyl.[11] Diacetylenes have been the subject of extensive studies in our laboratory not only because of their high degree of conjugation as polymers but also because of their ability to transform bilayers into interesting microstructures, i.e. tubules.[12,13]

The diacetylene containing alkyl chain has two sets of methylene segments; the first set which is present between the diacetylene and

239

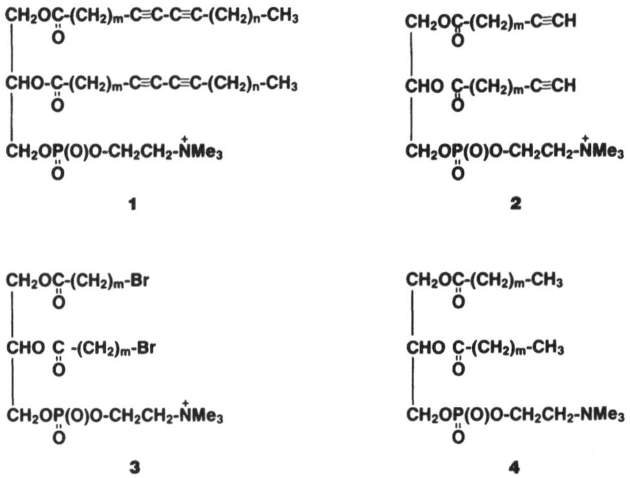

CH₂OC-(CH₂)ₘ-C≡C-C≡C-(CH₂)ₙ-CH₃ ... (structures as image)

$CH_2OC\text{-}(CH_2)_m\text{-}C{\equiv}C\text{-}C{\equiv}C\text{-}(CH_2)_n\text{-}CH_3$
$\quad \overset{\|}{O}$
$CHO\text{-}C\text{-}(CH_2)_m\text{-}C{\equiv}C\text{-}C{\equiv}C\text{-}(CH_2)_n\text{-}CH_3$
$\quad \overset{\|}{O}$
$CH_2OP(O)O\text{-}CH_2CH_2\text{-}\overset{+}{N}Me_3$
$\quad\overset{\|}{O}$

1

$CH_2OC\text{-}(CH_2)_m\text{-}C{\equiv}CH$
$\quad\overset{\|}{O}$
$CHO\ C\text{-}(CH_2)_m\text{-}C{\equiv}CH$
$\quad\overset{\|}{O}$
$CH_2OP(O)O\text{-}CH_2CH_2\text{-}\overset{+}{N}Me_3$
$\quad\overset{\|}{O}$

2

$CH_2OC\text{-}(CH_2)_m\text{-}Br$
$\quad\overset{\|}{O}$
$CHO\ C\ \text{-}(CH_2)_m\text{-}Br$
$\quad\overset{\|}{O}$
$CH_2OP(O)O\text{-}CH_2CH_2\text{-}\overset{+}{N}Me_3$
$\quad\overset{\|}{O}$

3

$CH_2OC\text{-}(CH_2)_m\text{-}CH_3$
$\quad\overset{\|}{O}$
$CHO\ C\text{-}(CH_2)_m\text{-}CH_3$
$\quad\overset{\|}{O}$
$CH_2OP(O)O\text{-}CH_2CH_2\text{-}NMe_3$
$\quad\overset{\|}{O}$

4

Figure 1. Structures of the Phosphatidylcholines; Diacetylenic PC [1] (**1a**, m = 8, n = 9; **1b**, m = 8, n = 11; **1c**, m = 10, n = 13); Acetylenic PC [2, m = 8]; Bromoalkanoyl PC [3, m = 10]; Dialkanoyl PC [4] (**4a**, m = 5; **4b**, m = 7; **4c**, m = 10; **4d**, m = 12).

carboxyl end is denoted by "m" and the second set, which lies between diacetylene and methyl end, is denoted by "n". Our synthesis and characterization of a series of isomeric diacetylenic phospholipids[14] revealed that the polymerization of the diacetylenic moiety in the bilayers was never complete. We attempted to improve polymerization efficiency by two approaches: first, other olefinic and methacrylate polymerizable moieties were introduced at the lipid chain termini;[15] and second, utilization of mixtures of the diacetylenic PC (Figure 1) [1] and various short chain PCs [2] containing analogus "m". As a result of the second approach efficient polymerization has been achieved. Depending upon the composition of the mixtures and their concentration in dispersion, different morphologies ranging from tubules to vesicles have been observed. In this report we present our results on the properties of dispersions obtained from such lipid mixtures.

EXPERIMENTAL

1. Materials

L-α Glycerophosphorylcholine cadmium chloride complex was prepared by hydrolyzing egg lecithin which was isolated from egg yolk. 1-Dodecyne, undecylenic acid, 11-bromo undecanoic acid, nonanoic acid, lithium acetylide ethylenediamine complex, dimethylaminopyridine (DMAP), and dicyclohexylcarbodiimide (DCC) were purchased from Aldrich Chemical Co. Milwaukee, WI. Tridecyne was obtained from Farchan Laboratories, Gainesville, FL, and 1,2-dihexanoyl and 1,2-dipalmitoyl PC were purchased from Avanti Polar Lipids, Birmingham, AL. Mixed bed resin AG 501-X8(D) was procured from Bio-Rad Laboratories, Richmond, CA. Chloroform was distilled freshly over phosphorus pentoxide just before the use. Other solvents were used as received. The water was triply distilled and deionized.

2A. Synthesis of phospholipids

The phospholipids, 1,2-bis-(tricosa-10,12-diynoyl) (Figure 1, [1a], m = 8, n = 9; DC 8,9 PC), 1,2-bis-(pentacosa-10,12-diynoyl) ([1], m = 8, n = 11; DC 8,11 PC), 1,2-bis-(nonacosa-10,12-diynoyl) ([1c], m = 10, n = 13; DC 10,13 PC), 1,2-bis-(10-undecynoyl) [2, m = 8], 1,2-bis-(11-bromo-undecanoyl) [3, m = 10] and 1,2-dinonanoyl [4b, m = 7] sn-glycero-3-phosphocholines were synthesized starting with appropriate alkadiynoic, alkynoic or alkanoic acids. These acids were converted into anhydrides by reacting with 0.55 mol eq. DCC in methylene chloride which in turn reacted with L-a glycerophosphorylcholine cadmium chloride complex.[16] The course of the reaction was monitored by thin layer chromatography on silica gel (Merck) and the plates were developed by using a chloroform, methanol, water (65:25:4) solvent system. After completion of the reaction (which usually takes 36 hours), the contents were filtered and solvent was removed under reduced pressure. The crude reaction mixture was redissolved in chloroform, methanol, water (5:4:1) and passed through a column of mixed bed resin to remove DMAP and $CdCl_2$. Lipids from the reaction mixtures were separated by column chromatography on silica gel and were characterized by their IR and NMR spectra. The final yields of the chromatographed phospholipids were in the range of 60-80 %. All of these lipids were further purified by acetone precipitation and their purity was routinely checked by TLC (on silica gel plates, Rf values were as follows: diacetylenic lipids = 0.4; other lipids = 0.35).

2B. Preparation of Dispersions from Mixed Lipids

Typically diacetylenic and spacer phospholipid mixtures of varying molar ratios were prepared as follows: Weighed amount of lipids (mole: mole) in chloroform solution were dispensed into a test tube and the solvent was evaporated under a gentle stream of argon to coat the walls of the tube with a thin film of lipid mixture. The film was then vacuum dried for 16 hours and dispersed in distilled water by hydrating it at 10°C above the Tm of the higher melting lipid (usually diacetylenic PC) followed by intermittent vortexing. The final mixed-lipid concentration in the aqueous dispersions was maintained at 2 mg/ml. Samples used for differential scanning calorimetry had concentrations ranging between 150 and 200 mg/ml.

2C. Characterization of Lipid Dispersions

a. Differential Scanning Calorimetry. DSC scans were recorded on a Perkin Elmer DSC-7 calorimeter on well hydrated and dispersed mixtures of the lipids. The heating or cooling rate for each cycle was 2°C per min. After completion of each cycle the samples were equilibrated for 10 min. at the final temperature.

b. Langmuir Blodgett Film Balance. A modified Joyce-Loebl Langmuir Trough 4 housed in a class 100 clean room was used for the present study. Phosphatidylcholine [1a] was spread on the water surface and the resulting monolayer was compressed to a steady pressure. To allow the lipid molecules to pack well, the monolayer films were annealed for 15 minutes and also for 15 hours maintaining the pressure constant. These films were then polymerized at 18°C by irradiating with 254 nm UV light at the air-water interface and the increase in pressure was recorded against the UV exposure time.

c. Optical and Electron Microscopy. Microstructures from the DSC pans and dispersions of low lipid concentration (2 mg/ml), were examined employing optical and transmission electron microscopy. To observe the microstructures we use the cryo-TEM technique which utilizes instant freezing of the dispersion from a given starting temperature, allowing observation of microstructure morphology without staining.

2.D. Polymerization of Dispersions

For the polymerization studies, multilamellar vesicular dispersions were prepared by vortexing the hydrated lipid dispersions. These dispersions were gel filtered on a Sephadex G 50-150 column and were polymerized at 5°C by 254 nm irradiation in a Rayonette Photoreactor. The course of the polymerization was monitored by thin layer chromatography on silica gel using a chloroform:methanol:water (65:25:4) solvent system. The monomer participation was measured in polymerized and freeze dried samples by dissolving the monomers in chloroform and spotting on the TLC plate, developing in lipid solvent and measuring the phosphorus content under monomer and polymer spots.

RESULTS AND DISCUSSION

Polymerization of diacetylenes has been achieved in the solid state and studied extensively in non-lipid systems.[17] Polymerization in those systems proceeds quite efficiently. However, the diacetylenic moiety, once incorporated into the alkyl chain of phospholipid molecules, does not participate in polymerization process at high efficiency. One reason for this behavior may be the difference in packing of diacetylene groups in lipid bilayers as compared to solid crystals. Alkyl chain conformation in vesicles is sensitive to temperature variation. Below the chain melting temperature the vesicles are in a gel state and the hydrocarbon region is well ordered. This ordered packing of hydrocarbon in the gel state brings the diacetylene moieties closer, and facilitates polymerization. Figure 2 represents a simplified depiction of the lipid bilayers before and after intermolecular polymerization. In the process of polymerization new bond formation occurs which may cause a misalignment in the molecular packing of the phospholipids in the bilayer system, causing inefficiency in further polymerization. Raman data on aqueous dispersions of diacetylenic lipids revealed that these lipids pack much more tightly than the saturated analog of naturally occurring phosphatidylcholines, such as dipalmitoyl phosphatidylcholine.[18]

Mono- or bilayer films of DC 8,9 PC were spread on the air/water interface of a Langmuir/Blodgett film balance, and the effect of polymerizing such films was studied. Figure 3 shows that polymerization causes an increase in pressure in a compressed monolayer of DC 8,9 PC [1a]. The monolayer films were annealed for 15 minutes and also for 15 hours, keeping the pressure constant to allow the molecules to pack tightly. The films were then polymerized at the air water interface by exposing to 254 nm UV light. In both the cases, an increase in pressure was observed to accompany the new bond formation during the course of polymerization, suggesting that polymerized lipid has different molecular packing than the monomer. To assist in this molecular rearrangement we decided to utilize, along with diacetylenic lipid, a short chain lipid containing a matching 'm' segment as a spacer to accommodate the newly formed bond.

For the present study on the mixed-lipid systems, the lipids [1a] and [1b] were mixed with the lipid [2] in 1:1, 1:2, 1:3, 3:1 and 2:1 molar ratios (diacetylenic PC:acetylenic PC). These mixtures were found to disperse in water quite easily as compared with the pure diacetylenic PC's.

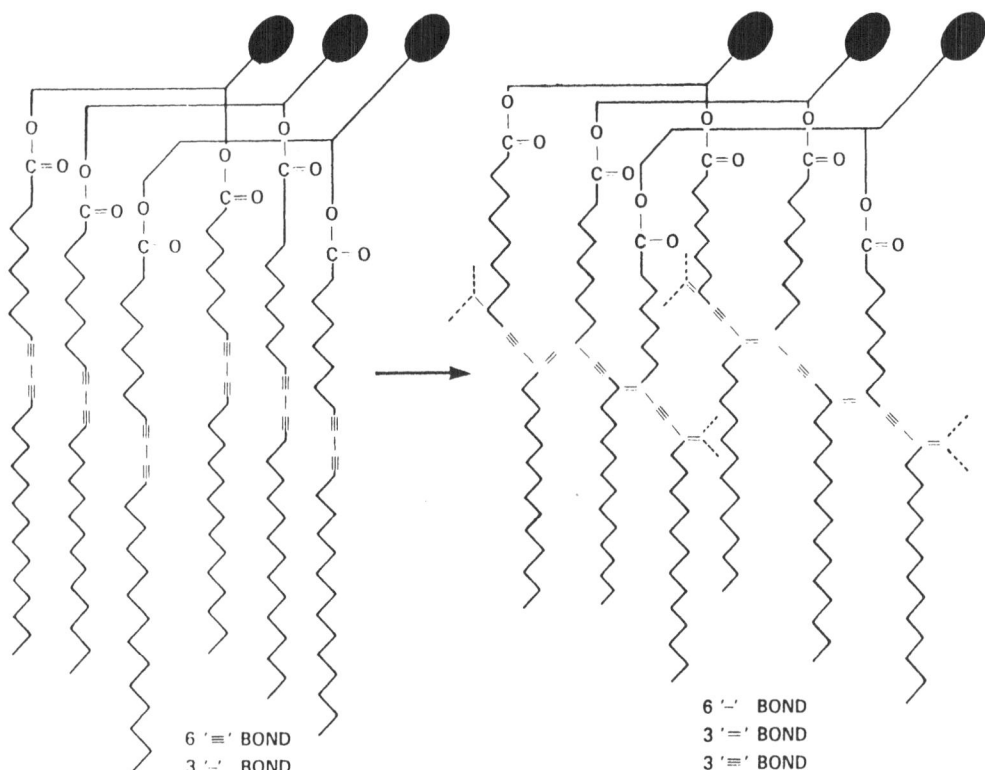

6 '≡' BOND
3 '-' BOND

6 '-' BOND
3 '=' BOND
3 '≡' BOND

Figure 2. Simplified illustration of the diacetylenic lipid
monolayers before and after polymerization. Note
that upon polymerization new bond formation occurs.

Polymerization studies were performed on multilamellar dispersions
prepared at low concentration, 2 mg/ml. The dispersions were gel filtered
on Sephadex G 50-150 column, so that any of the short chain lipid component that might be present in micelle form would be separated from the
mixed lipid vesicles. The vesicle preparations from the 1:1, 1:2 and 2:1
DC 8,9 PC mixtures were used in the polymerization study. The UV irradiated samples showed no evidence of participation by the acetylenic lipid
in the polymerization reaction, as indicated by measuring the phosphorus
content after separation of monomer by TLC. Diacetylenes polymerize when
they are aligned,[4-6] and in bilayer systems this situation arises only
below the lipid phase transition temperature. Thus, temperature may be
expected to play an important role in polymerization. Indeed, after UV
irradiation at room temperature brown or yellow dispersions resulted
which contained a substantial fraction of unreacted monomer. However,
polymerization of the mixtures for 1 minute at -5°C resulted in extensive
polymerization (more than 90% elimination of monomer). Figure 4 shows
that visible spectra of both the samples at 1 minute irradiation contained two major peaks at 532 and 494 nm. In contrast, pure DC 8,9 PC
dispersion, prepared and irradiated under identical conditions, showed no
clear signature of a polymer spectrum (defined peak around 500 nm) and
very little monomer participation. Schoen and Yager, on the other hand,
have demonstrated that the diacetylene lipid in tubular morphology shows
a defined spectrum, but that the participation of monomers in polymerization process is low.[19]

The monomer:polymer ratio for the lipid systems has been compiled in
Table 1. The mixed lipid system in which short chain lipid has served as

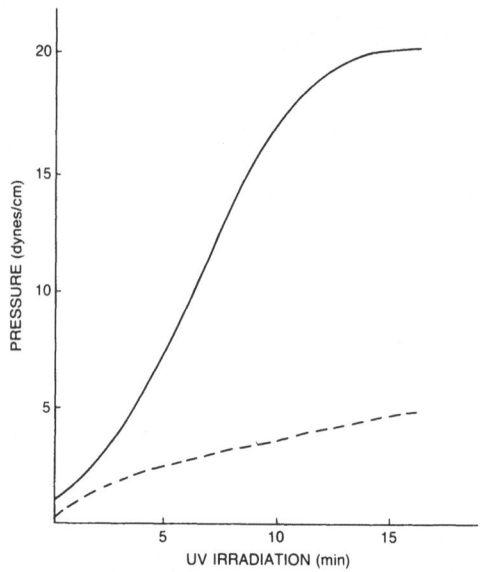

Figure 3. Effect of polymerization on the compressed diacetylenic PC [1a] monolayers. solid line represents 15
hour annealing and broken line represents 15
minutes annealing of the monolayers.

spacer, showed a clear advantage over the single component DC 8,9 PC
system in terms of efficiency and rapidity of the polymerization process.
Further irradiation of the mixed lipid samples for 5 minutes did not
produce any noticeable change in the visible spectrum, although TLC
results indicated a small decrease in monomer concentration.

These observations of the effect of spacers in mixed lipid systems
led to the synthesis of an unsymmetrical lipid, in which the alkyl chain
at sn-1 position contained a diacetylenic moiety and sn-2 position
contained the spacer chain (see Figure 5). This lipid was dispersed in
water to form vesicles, but did not show any polymerization enhancement.
This result suggests that symmetric short chain PCs are required for any
enhancement in polymerization.

Figure 6 summarizes the effect of the chain length of the spacer
lipid on polymerization. It is observed that the nature of the terminal
group on a spacer lipid did not produce any noticeable effect on polymer-

Table 1. Effect of short chain phosphatidylcholine (spacer)
on the diacetylenic phosphatidylcholine polymerization. Samples were polymerized at -5°C for 120
seconds. Monomer polymer ratio remain unchanged
after 5 minute of UV irradiation.

Lipid:Spacer	Monomer:Polymer
1:0	80:20
1:1	25:75
1:2	9:91
2:1	70:30

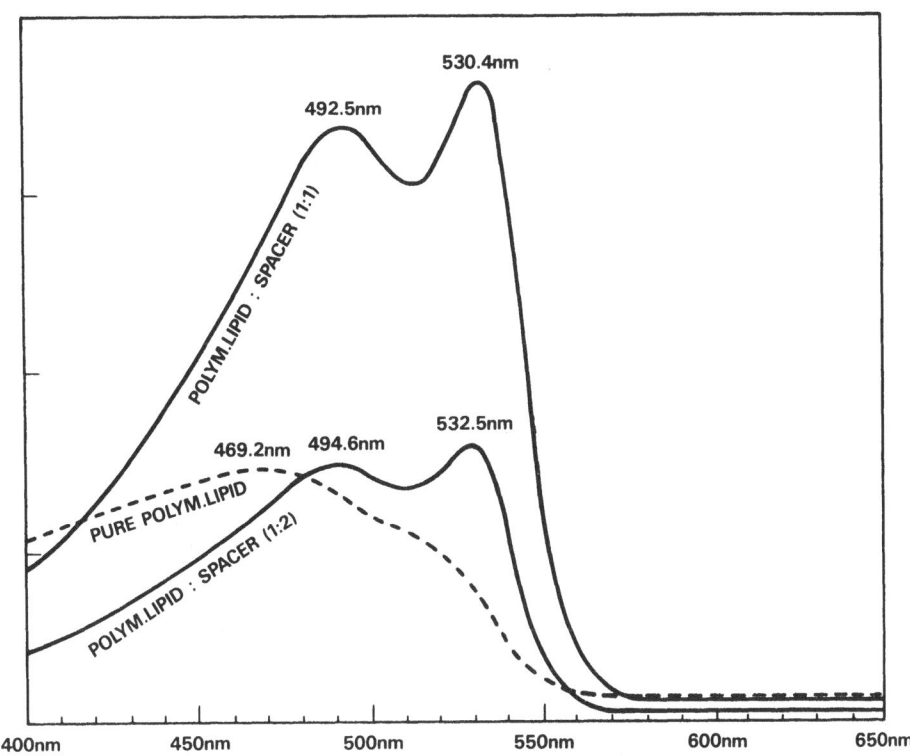

Figure 4. Visible spectra of polymerized diacetylenic lipid
dispersions. The samples were gel filtered and
polymerized at -5°C for 300 seconds.

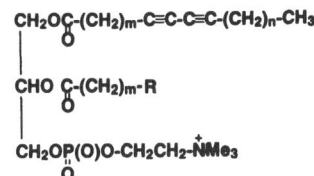

Figure 5. Structure formula of unsymmetric phosphatidylcholine. R= -C≡CH, m = 8, n = 9.

ization efficiency. Both acetylene and methyl terminated acyl chains
produced similar effects. However the length of the acyl chain is crucial
for inducing polymerization. The 'm' segment of spacer lipid must match
closely with 'm' segment of the diacetylenic PC. In addition to the [1a]
and [2 or 4b] systems, the [1c] and [3 or 4c] systems also showed positive results.

To understand the effect of mixing on the bilayers properties,
calorimetric studies were carried out. The heating scan of the pure diacetylenic lipids gave single endotherms at 43.4°C [1a] and 54°C [1b]. No
phase transition (T_m) was observed down to -10°C, for lipid [2]. The
mixtures showed unusual behavior. The heating scans on the mixtures
involving DC 8,9 PC showed multiple small peaks together with two major
peaks several degrees apart, suggestive of phase separation in the gel
state. Cooling scans provided only one exothermic peak in most cases,

245

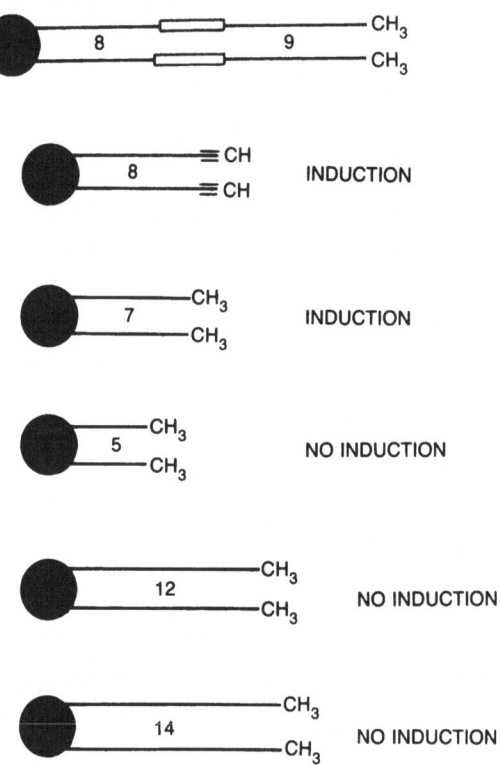

Figure 6. Effect of Acyl Chain length in short chain PC on
the polymerization.

suggesting improved mixing of the two lipids in the fluid phase. In one
case, the mixture, [1a:2], 3:1 mole ratio, two exothermic peaks were
observed on cooling, indicating some mixing and phase separation. Similar
results were observed for the mixtures when DC 8,11 PC was involved. The
major peaks relating to both sets of lipid mixture are compiled in
Table 2.

Table 2. Differential Scanning Calorimetric Data on Mixed
Lipid Systems

Lipid Ratio DA:A *	8,9 PC System Heating °C	Cooling °C	8,11 PC System Heating °C	Cooling °C
3:1	42.7, 40.4	35.7, 13.3	52.5, 50.5	44.5, 12.2, 9.2
2:1	36.2, 31.4	13.0	51.0	23.5
1:1	40.0, 31.4	23.0	50.5, 31.5	29.5
1:2	36.2, 31.4	18.1	31.5	24.8
1:3	31.4	17.8	31.5	21.8

* DA = Diacetylenic Lipid
  A = Acetylenic Lipid

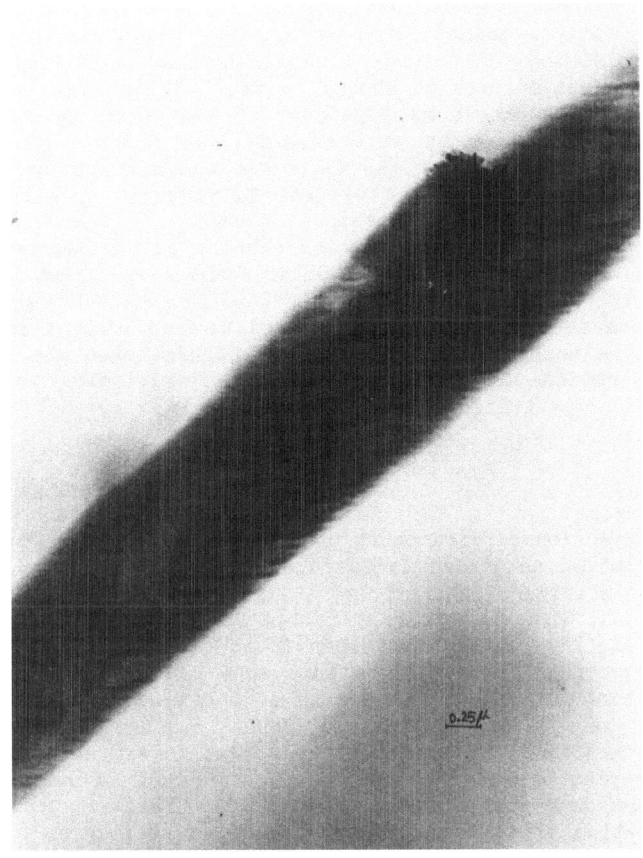

Figure 7. Cryo-Transmission Electron Micrograph of a Tubule
Microstructure from the Concentrated Aqueous Dispersion of DC 8,9 PC [1a] and DC 8 PC [2a] (9:1
molar ratio).

Table 3. Morphology of Microstructures in Concentrated
Aqueous Dispersions

Lipid Ratio DA:A	8,9 PC System	8,11 PC System
3:1	Small tubules, sheets & vesicles	Thick sheets & vesicles
2:1	Very small tubules & vesicles	Large sheets & vesicles
1:1	Very small tubules & vesicles	Sheets & vesicles
1:2	Vesicles	Vesicles
1:3	Vesicles	Vesicles

The microstructures obtained from the mixtures listed in Table 2 were examined by optical and electron microscopy. Diacetylenic PCs are known to form tubular microstructures when cooled slowly (approx. 1-2°C/min.) after heating the dispersion above the T_m.[12] It is also known that this phenomenon is concentration dependent.[20] For this reason dispersions obtained from the DSC pans were examined, as these high concentration samples had gone through the thermal cycle which initiates tubule formation. Table 3 illustrates the optical microscopic results obtained on these highly concentrated dispersions. Figure 7 is the cryo-transmission electron micrograph of a tubule which shows a patchy surface. Typically, a tubule has smooth surface with regular wrapping patterns.[12]

The above results clearly show that mixing of the acetylenic PC influences the morphology of the microstructures when the lipids are at high concentration. However, the vortexed mixed-lipid dispersions prepared at low concentration (2mg/mL) contained vesicles only.

SUMMARY

The interaction between short chain (6-8 carbon acyl chain) and long chain (synthetic, saturated and natural) phospholipids has been used to prepare stable unilamellar vesicles.[21] Upon mixing of short chain PC with long chain PC, formation of unilamellar vesicles has been observed and whose calorimetric behavior has been found similar to small unilamellar vesicle dispersions obtained from pure long chain PC. Diacetylenic PC mixtures with other lipids containing acyl chains similar or comparable with the 'm' segment of former lipid present a novel class of mixed lipid systems which have an impact on bilayer properties, such as phase behavior, polymerization and morphology. In the case of mixtures of other polymerizable and non-polymerizable lipids phase separation[22,23] and phase separation along with a decrease in polymerization efficiency has been reported.[24]

The present work provides a unique and an interesting system with multiple implications. The control over polymerization in bilayers may provide controlled release systems, efficient protein reincorporation in bilayers, etc. Further studies are underway to determine optimum lipid mixture ratios, concentration, and irradiation conditions required to produce stable microstructures for technological applications.

ACKNOWLEDGEMENTS

We wish to thank Ms. B. Herendeen for providing excellent technical assistance during the course of this work, Mr. R. Price for taking the electron micrographs, Mr. J. Georger for the film balance experiment and Drs. P. Schoen, E. Chang and J. M. Schnur for helpful discussions. This work was funded in part by Naval Research Laboratory Accelerated Research Initiative program and the Defence Advanced Research Projects Agency.

REFERENCES

1. For reviews on polymerized vesicles see: H. Bader, B. Hupfer & H. Ringsdorf, Advances in Polymer Science, **64**, 1 (1985); S. L. Regen, Polymer News, **10**, 68 (1984); H. Bader, H. Ringsdorf & B. Schmidt, Angew. Makromol. Chem., **123/124**, 457 (1984) and J. H. Fendler & P. Tundo, Acc. Chem. Res., **17**, 3 (1984).
2. S. L. Regen, A. Singh, G. Oehme & M. Singh, Biochem. Biophys. Res. Comm, **101**, 131 (1982); A. W. Dalziel, J. Georger, R. R. Price, A.

Singh & P. Yager in: S. C. Goheen, Ed., "Membrane Proteins", Bio-Rad Laboratories, Pub., 1986, p. 643.

3. S. L. Regen, B. Czech & A. Singh, J. Amer. Chem. Soc., **102**, 6638 (1980);

4. H. H. Hub, B. Hupfer, H. Koch & H. Ringsdorf, Angew. Chem., Int. Ed., **19**, 938 (1980).

5. D. S. Johnston, S. Sanghera, M. Pons & D. Chapman, Biochim. Biophys. Acta, 602, 57 (1980).

6. D. F. O'Brian, T. H. Whitesides & R. T. Klingbiel, J. Polym. Sci., Polym. Lett. Ed., 19, 95 (1981); E. Lopez, D. F. O'Brian & T. H. Whitesides, J. Amer. Chem. Soc., 104, 305 (1982).

7. S. L. Regen, A. Singh, G. Oehme & M. Singh, J. Amer. Chem. Soc., 104, 791 (1982)

8. A. Akimoto, K. Dorn, L. Gros & H. Ringsdorf, H. Schupp, Angew. Chem., Int. Ed. Engl., 20, 90 (1982).

9. L. Gros, H. Ringsdorf & H. Schupp, Angew. Chem., Int. Ed., **20**, 305 (1982).

10. K. Dorn, R. T. Klingbiel, D. P. Specht, P. N. Tyminski, H. Ringsdorf & D. F. O'Brian, J. Amer. Chem. Soc., **106**, 1627 (1984).

11. P. Tundo, D. J. Kippenberger, P. L. Klahn, N. E. Prieto, T. C. Jao & J. H. Fendler, J. Amer. Chem. Soc., **104**, 456 (1982).

12. P. Yager & P. E. Schoen, Mol. Cryst. Liq. Cryst., **106**, 371 (1984); P. Yager, P. E. Schoen, C. A. Davies, R. Price & A. Singh, Biophys. J., **48**, 899 (1985); J. M. Schnur, R. Price, P. Schoen, P. Yager, J. Calvert, J. Georger & A. Singh, Thin Solid Films, **152**, 181 (1987).

13. J. H. Georger, A. Singh, R. R. Price, J. M. Schnur, P. Yager & P. E. Schoen, J. Amer. Chem. Soc., **109**, 6169 (1987).

14. J. M. Schnur & A. Singh, Polym. Prepr., **26**, 186 (1985); A. Singh & J. M. Schnur, Polym. Prepr., **26**, 184 (1985); A. Singh, B. P. Singh, B. P. Gaber, R. Price, T. H. Burke, B. Herendeen, P. E. Schoen, J. M. Schnur & P. Yager, (1987) to appear in "Surfactants in Solution", K.L. Mittal, Ed.

15. A. Singh, R. Price, P. E. Schoen, P. Yager & J. M. Schnur, Polymer Prep., 27, 393 (1986).

16. A. Singh & J. M. Schnur, Synth. Commun., **16**, 847 (1986); C. M. Gupta, R. Radhakrishan & H. G. Khurana, Proc. Natl. Acad. Sci., U.S.A., **74**, 4315 (1977).

17. H. J. Cantow, Ed., Advances in Polymer Science, Volume 63, Springer-Verlag, Berlin, Heidelberg, 1984.

18. A. Singh & J. P. Sheridan, unpublished data.

19. P. E. Schoen & P. Yager, J. Polym. Sci., Polym. Phys. Ed., 23, 2203 (1985).

20. T. G. Burke, R. R. Price, J. P. Sheridan, A. S. Rudolph, A. W. Dalziel, A. Singh & P. E. Schoen, manuscript in preparation.

21. N. E. Gabriel & M. F. Roberts, Biochemistry, 25, 2812 (1986), N. E. Gabriel & M. F. Roberts, *ibid*, 23, 4011 (1984)

22. S. Marbrey & J. M. Sturtevant, Proc. Natl. Acad. Sci., USA., 73, 3862 (1976)

23. N. Seki, E. Tsuchida, K. Ukaji & T. Sekiya, Y. Nozawa, Polymer Bulletin, 13, 489 (1985).

24. H. Gaub, E. Sackmann, R. Bueschl & H. Ringsdorf, Biophys. J., **45**, 725 (1984).

GRAFT COPOLYMERS OF AMINO ACIDS ONTO NATURAL AND SYNTHETIC POLYMERS

William H. Daly and Soo Lee

Department of Chemistry
Louisiana State University
Baton Rouge, Louisiana 70803

By analogy with natural chitin-protein complexes, grafting of amino acids to natural polymers produces biodegradable biocomposites. The literature on grafting amino acid N-carboxyanhydrides (NCAs) to proteins, natural polymers and vinyl polymers is reviewed. Macroinitiators with primary amino substituents were synthesized by one of the following techniques: (a) cyanoethylation of cellulose followed by reduction to produce aminopropylcellulose [1], and (b) phthalimidation followed by hydrazinolysis to yield amino-methyl poly(arylene ether sulfone) [3]. Heterogeneous grafting of γ-benzyl-L-glutamate-N-carboxyanhydride (BLG-NCA) [8] to polymer [1] resulted in non-random distribution of amino acid residues; α-helical conformations were detected at low BLG-NCA/NH$_2$ ratios (<5 AA). Using molar ratios ranging from 1 to 100 of [8] relative to the amine concentration, grafting to polymer [3] was effected in anhydrous THF at room temperature under homogeneous conditions; high grafting efficiencies (>80%) were achieved. Polypeptides grafted to polymer [3] appeared to adopt the expected conformation for the chain length predicted by the BLG-NCA/NH$_2$ ratio. The benzyl ester functions on the BLG grafts are subject to direct modification with amine nucleophiles; studies with butylamine correlate reaction conditions with extent of ester vs. peptide cleavage. In the presence of 1-hydroxybenzo-triazole, aminolysis of the ester is favored and conversions to γ-amides up to 75% are achieved.

INTRODUCTION

One of the most ubiquitous natural polymers is chitin. Crustacean shells are very interesting composites of chitin, polypeptides or proteins, and an inorganic filler, calcium carbonate. Chitin has been found in the shells of over 150 mollusk species in amounts varying from 0.01 to 40% of the matrix dry weight.[1] Further, chitin is an important component of tendons and other stress bearing fibrous portions of marine animals, where the chitin molecules adopt a highly oriented structure.[2-4] The conformation and orientation of the matrix macromolecules were relatively poorly understood until the seminal X-ray and electron diffraction studies by Weiner,[5] who found that there is an association of chitin in its β-form (crystalline parallel chains) with proteins that adopt an antiparallel β-sheet conformation. The chitin polymer appears to be oriented approximately perpendicular to the protein-polypeptide chains; the crossed chain construction produces a mesh that contributes to the strength of the matrix. Transmission electron microscopy confirms that the ultrastructure of the matrix is a micro-mesh network of dense grains united by short, straight and thin organic connections.[6] The sheets of the matrix are composed of several different layers; the two surface layers are composed mainly of more soluble acidic constituents and the core comprises a thin layer of chitin sandwiched between two thicker layers of proteins (Figure 1).[7]

From a chemical point of view, there are two distinct structural units: (a) an acidic polypeptide fraction with a strong affinity for calcium ions called a mineralization matrix, and (b) a high molecular weight chitinoproteic complex called carrier protein, with no affinity for calcium, arranged in the form of sheets. The nature of the chitin-protein association is poorly understood, primarily because the form of the linkage between the two polymers has not been characterized completely. There are several potential sites in the polysaccharide polymer where covalent binding could occur, but binding to these sites has not been confirmed. Dissolution of native chitin composites is accompanied by degradation of both the protein and chitin components so efforts to ascertain the structure of the binding sites by solution techniques have failed.

Efforts directed toward development of model systems have provided useful insights. Hackmann has shown that covalently linked complexes form between N-acetylglucosamine and chitin when these materials are allowed to react with peptides containing aspartyl and histidyl residues,[8] but the structure of these complexes has not been determined. Brine and Austin showed that the predominant amino acids in residual chitin after

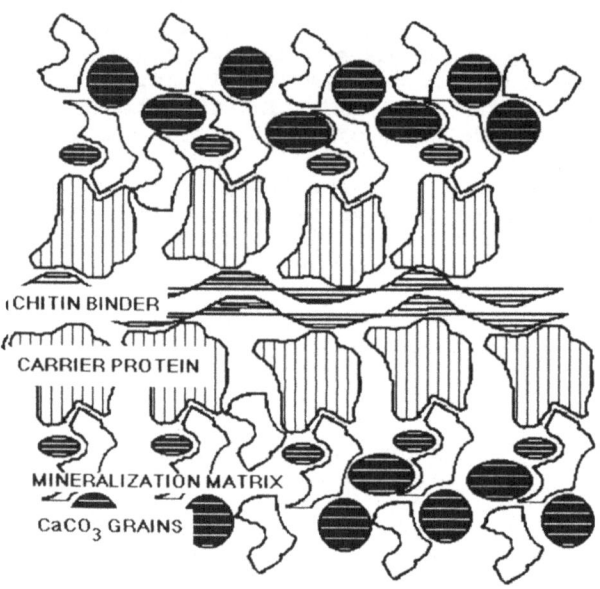

Figure 1. Crustacean Shell Structure.

partial alkaline hydrolysis were aspartic acid, serine and glycine, suggesting that these amino acids may be involved in the chitin-protein linkage.[9] In fact, these three amino acids comprise 35-50% of the amino acid residues in shell matrix. Formation of an glycosidic ester linkage between N-acetylglycosamine residues and β-carboxylic groups of aspartyl residue would appear the most likely structure of this linkage and indeed such structures have been proposed.[10] However, neither hydroxylamine nor lithium borohydride treatment of chitin protein complexes affected the strong interaction between the two polymers.[11] Since these reagents cleave ester linkages, some alternate type of bonding between chitin and proteins must be considered.

Recent results reported on the nature of the bond formation during sclerotization in insect cuticle are enlightening, but introduce further complexity to the protein chitin interactions.[12] Using CP-MAS ^{13}C and ^{15}N techniques, the relative concentrations of, and covalent interactions among catecholamine, protein and chitin in pupal cuticle of tobacco horn-worm, *Manduca secta*, were determined in situ. Proteins containing histidine and to a lesser extent, lysine residues couple via aromatic carbon-nitrogen bonds to catechol derivatives. Direct coupling of the protein to pupal chitin chains appears unlikely. Although the exact structure of the histidyl-catecholamine ring adduct is unknown, the NMR data are consistent with a product with the following structure:

The locus of the catecholamine-chitin carbon oxygen bond is drawn between the phenoxy carbon-3 and anhydroglucosamine carbon-4, but phenoxy carbon-4 as well as other anhydroglucosamine carbons could participate in the conjugate linkage.[12]

The formation of catechol adducts with chitin residues has received limited attention,[13] and although it is obviously important in under-standing the mechanism of natural chitinoprotein complexes, this route is not practical for the production of synthetic graft copolymers of amino acids onto polysaccharides as components for biocomposites. We believe that materials which will duplicate the strength and durability of chitin composites can be produced from more accessible cellulose derivatives by grafting techniques. Moreover, we are interested in utilizing the graft copolymers of amino acids onto natural and synthetic polymers as com-pletely biodegradable carriers for pharmacons and agricultural chemicals. Therefore, we have been applying more direct techniques to the synthesis of amino acid graft copolymers.

Genesis of Polypeptide Graft Copolymers

Multi-chain copolymers are defined as bundles of uniformly linear polymer chains attached to a polyfunctional core.[14] The branching should be introduced without concomitant crosslinking to assure the formation of soluble graft copolymers. Graft copolymers of amino acids should exhibit unique properties since both core and branch polymer chains can form rod-like, α-helical structures under certain conditions, and the overall conformation of the macromolecule is rigidly defined. Conditions can be selected to produce peptide grafts with narrow molecular weight distributions. Thus, a study of the hydrodynamic properties of poly-peptide graft copolymers should provide worthwhile data to confirm the theories of branched polymer dynamics.

In 1955, Katchalski, Sela and Gehatia first prepared several multi-chain poly(amino acids) by using polylysine or polyornithine as macro-initiator in the polymerization of N-carboxy-α-amino acid anhydrides (NCAs).[15] The macroinitiators were prepared by polymerization of the appropriate NCA to moderate DP (30-200). Graft polymerizations onto those polymers could be conducted in a 1:1 mixture of dioxane and diluted phosphate buffer (pH = 7), because NCAs are known to react with amines considerably faster than with water.[16,17] The structures of the grafts were confirmed by chromatographic separation of hydrolysates labeled at N-terminal sites with dinitrophenol. In each case, a sharp molecular weight distribution of multi-chain poly(amino acids) which contained grafts of up to an average degree of polymerization (DP) of 25 was ob-tained. Apparently the side chains were produced without encountering any termination during the grafting process. The viscosity of those multi-chain poly(amino acids) showed a peculiar non-linear concentration dependence, similar to the one found by Batzer for branched polyesters.[18] The unusual behavior was consistent with that expected for branch polymers with a high chain density.[19]

Several years later, Sela et al., reported that gelatin modified by attachment via its amino groups to short peptide chains of tyrosine, tryptophan, phenylalanine, and, to a less extent, cysteine, had consider-ably greater immunogenicity than unmodified gelatin.[20] Enhancement of immunogenicity due to an increase in rigidity of part of the active site in the molecule was proposed. Although polar amino acid residues did not generally enhance immunogenicity, enrichment of gelatin with both tyrosine and glutamic acid yielded a powerful antigen of very narrow specificity. To resolve the question concerning the contribution of gelatin itself towards the immunological properties of the new antigens, Sela et al. successfully used completely synthetic multi-chain poly(amino acids) as replacements for the gelatinous antigens.[21] They concluded that the overall shape of the molecules did not seem to be a critical factor and that the amino acid composition was the most important factor in determining immunogenicity.

To improve the graft yield and to avoid contamination by linear poly-(amino acids) formed as by-products in aqueous systems, a non-aqueous solvent system for peptides, anhydrous dimethyl sulfoxide, was employed for the preparation of multi-chain poly(amino acids) from polylysine and various NCAs by Tewksbury and Stahmann.[22,23] The multi-chain poly(amino acids) prepared under these conditions exhibited a single, broad molecular weight distribution, which is characteristic of the alkoxide initiated NCA polymerization used to prepare the macroinitiator.

In 1965, a number of multi-chain poly(amino acids) were also syn-thesized by reaction of NCAs with high molecular weight multifunctional

amines, such as polylysine (DP up to 700) or preformed multi-chain poly-
(amino acids).[24] The optimal conditions for removal of protecting benzyl
ester groups of multi-chain poly(amino acids) were also established,
i.e., HBr-treatment in glacial acetic acid was sufficient to remove
benzyl ester groups without cleaving peptide bonds. Yaron and Berger were
also pioneers in the study of the hydrodynamic, electrochemical, and
conformational properties of these synthetic protein models. Applying an
"equivalent ellipsoid" approach to interpretation of hydrodynamic
measurements, such as diffusion, partial specific volume, and dispersion,
reasonable values were calculated for the length of the resulting
polymers.[25,26] Electrochemical studies showed that the various ionizable
groups in the model polypeptides exhibited dissociation constants similar
to those observed for the corresponding groups in proteins. Helical
conformations were also detected by measuring optical rotations or
optical rotatory dispersions (ORD) when the DPs of the side chains were
long enough. The polyelectrolyte character of the models was apparent;
intrinsic viscosities of these polymers were strongly solvent dependent,
for example, that of multi-N^ϵ-poly(γ-benzyl-L-glutamyl)-poly(L-lysine)
was much larger in dichloroacetic acid than in N,N-dimethylacetamide.

More than a decade later, Sakamoto and Kuroyanagi studied the multi-
chain polymers produced by addition of N^ϵ-carbobenzyloxy-L-lysine NCA to
random poly(L-lysine-co-γ-methyl-L-glutamate) generated from selective
deblocking of the L-lysinylcarbobenzyloxy substituent with 36% HBr in
acetic acid at room temperature.[27] The branching intervals were controlled by the ratio γ-methyl-L-glutamate to N^ϵ-Cbz-lysine. The DPs of the
branch polymer chains were estimated by osmotic molecular weight and
amino acid analysis, and the α-helical conformational stability of the
copolymers was evaluated using ORD techniques. Multi-chain copoly(α-amino
acids) seemed to be more compactly shaped in a helix inducing solvent
than in a solvent favoring a random coil conformation, but the α-helical
conformation of multi-chain poly(α-amino acids) was shown to be less
stable than that of linear core poly(α-amino acids).

Polypeptide Grafting Onto Natural Polymers

A few methods are known for attaching amino acid units to the
hydroxyl group of polysaccharides, including the reaction of acid chlorides of amino acids with polyhydroxy polymers in a basic medium,[28-30] or
with aminated cellulose derivatives,[31] or amine derivatives,[32] or by
simple esterification of the polyhydroxy polymer with N-acetyl amino
acids.[33] Single amino acid substituents can not be considered grafts, at
best these derivatives could be used as macroinitiators.

The first attempts to produce a graft copolymer of poly(amino acids)
onto the natural polymers, such as cellulose, starch, and their derivatives, were carried out by Zilka and Avny in 1965.[33] Sodium methoxide
was known to be an initiator of NCA polymerization.[34,35] Therefore, they
proposed to use alkoxide derivatives of polysaccharides as macroinitiators for the graft copolymerization of NCA's of α-amino acids. All
known methods for production of alkoxide derivatives of natural polymers,
such as the reaction of polyhydroxy polymers with sodium metal in liquid
ammonia,[36] or exchange reactions between lower alkoxides and polyhydroxy
polymers,[37-39] were unsatisfactory for the subsequent graft copolymerization of NCAs, because any residual base would lead to homopolymerization. In addition, alkoxide derivatives of cellulose acetate[40] and
nitrocellulose[41] could not be obtained by these conventional methods due
to chemical degradation. Zilka et al.,[33] finally found that the reaction
of alkali metal naphthalenes [20] with polyhydroxy polymers in either

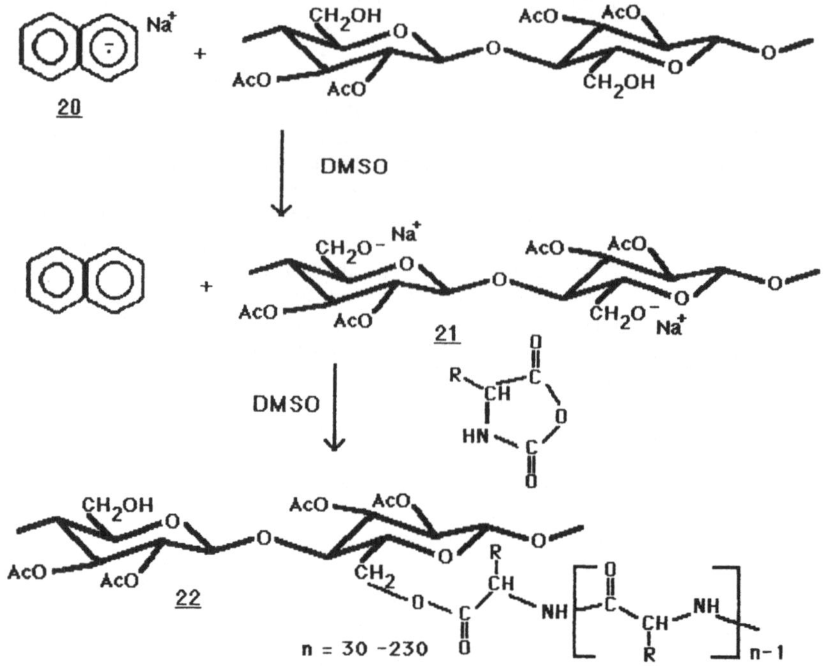

Scheme 1. Application of cellulosate macroinitiators.

DMSO or dioxane solutions, in analogy with the behavior of simple alcohols,[42] led to the formation of the desired polyalkoxides [21] (Scheme 1).

By using these macroinitiators, grafts of α-amino acids (phenyl-alanine, glycine, γ-benzyl-L-glutamate, sarcosine, and blocked cysteine) onto starch and cellulose acetate derivatives were obtained with high yield (>70%) in DMSO, dioxane, tetrahydrofuran, and DMF. Evaluation of the graft chain length in the products [22] revealed that less than 10% of the alkoxy groups were effective in initiating an NCA graft. Attempts to conduct the graft copolymerization of amino acids to a polyalkoxide of cellulose itself failed due to the heterogeneity of the system. There-fore, they used an amino derivative of cellulose xanthate, soluble in DMSO, DMSO-water and in 4% aqueous sodium hydroxide, as the macro-initiator. It is of interest to note that the graft copolymers obtained were not significantly contaminated with homopolypeptides even in 4% aqueous sodium hydroxide solution.

The possible mechanism for NCA initiation with polyalkoxy macro-initiators was also investigated by Zilka and Avny by studying low DP homogeneous graft copolymerization of NCA's of γ-benzyl-L-glutamate and ε-carbobenzyloxy-L-lysine on cellulose acetate alkoxide.[43,44] They found that the initiation reaction was a direct addition of the alkoxide to the C-5 carbonyl of the NCA, as evidenced by the formation of graft copolymer coupled by an ester link to the polysaccharide. This result must be considered contradictory evidence for the activated monomer mechanism suggested by Bamford et al.,[34] and Szwarc,[35] and supportive of the carbamate mechanism initially proposed by Idelson and Blout.[45] Although there are extensive discussions on NCA polymerization mechanisms in the literature several aspects of the propagation process remain unresolved.[46-49]

Recently, two papers describing graft copolymerization of γ-methyl-
or γ-benzyl-L-glutamate onto modified polysaccharides which contain
primary amino groups appeared. Kurita et al. reported the production of a
graft copolymer of γ-methyl-L-glutamate on a water-soluble 50% deacetylated chitin.[50] Relatively high grafting efficiency leading to the
formation of low DP (<6) side chains could be achieved in a homogeneous
mixed solvent medium like ethyl acetate/water. None of the resulting
copolymers were soluble in water, but they did swell in m-cresol. After
deblocking of the γ-methyl ester in 1M sodium carbonate at 70°C, the
poly(glutamic acid) derivatives were soluble in water and m-cresol.

High grafting efficiency (>85%) of amino acids onto cellulose was
achieved with aminoethyl- or aminopropylcellulose as macroinitiators for
NCA polymerization in a heterogeneous system (DMSO) at room temperature.[51] Using low D.S. (0.05) aminoethylcellulose, soluble grafts with
up to 18 γ-benzyl-L-glutamate residues could be obtained. The soluble
graft copolymers could be cast into films from dichloroacetic acid, trifluoroacetic acid, formic acid or LiCl-DMAC solutions. Since benzyl
esters are rather hydrophobic, the peptide grafts were modified with 2-
aminoethanol to produce the corresponding 2-hydroxyethyl-L-glutamine
(PHEG) grafts. The PHEG copolymers were twice as water absorbent, but
both types of graft copolymers exhibited excellent antithrombogenic
properties.

Polypeptide Grafting Onto Vinyl Polymers

Vinyl polymers with pendant primary amino groups have proven useful
for the variety of reactions.[52] If the primary amino group is aliphatic,
the polymerization of NCAs is initiated effectively by the nucleophilic
addition of amino group to the NCA and the resulting poly(α-amino acids)
carry the initiator fragment at the C-terminal. If polymers carrying
pendant amino groups are used as macroinitiators for the NCA polymerization, graft copolymers are formed in which the flexible vinyl hydrocarbon backbone constitutes the trunk and the poly(α-amino acids), which
assume α-helical conformations, are rathe rigid branches. Since the
trunk and the branches would not be expected to be compatible, the
resultant copolymers should form interesting phase separated domains.

One of the earliest reports of graft copolymers containing polypeptide side chains involved production of a macroinitiator by modification of poly(vinyl alcohol) [23] with 1,1-diethoxy-2-aminoethane [24].[53]
Low concentrations of the aminoacetalized poly(vinyl alcohol) [25] in
anhydrous ethyl acetate were used to initiate γ-methyl-D-glutamate as
shown on Scheme 2.

In the early 1980s, Imanishi described the preparation of a series of
vinyl backbone-peptide graft copolymers of phenylalanine and γ-benzyl-L-
glutamate with homo- or copoly(alkyl amines).[54] The hydrocarbon backbone
containing primary amino groups was synthesized by selectively blocking
one amine function on ethylene diamine [26] while converting the second
amine to an acrylamide [30] (Scheme 3). Polymerization and copolymerization of [30] with styrene, 2-vinylpyridine, acrylonitrile, methyl
methacrylate, and N-vinylpyrrolidone, followed by deblocking the polymers
[31] with HBr/HOAc or H_2/Pd, yielded polymers [32] with pendant primary
amine functions in a variety of environments.

The graft copolymerizations were carried out with various grafting
efficiencies (34.6-95.1%) in dichloromethane (DCM), chloroform, and DMF
at room temperature for 21 hrs. up to 210 hrs. The microstructure of the
graft copolymers was studied using transmission electron microscopy. A

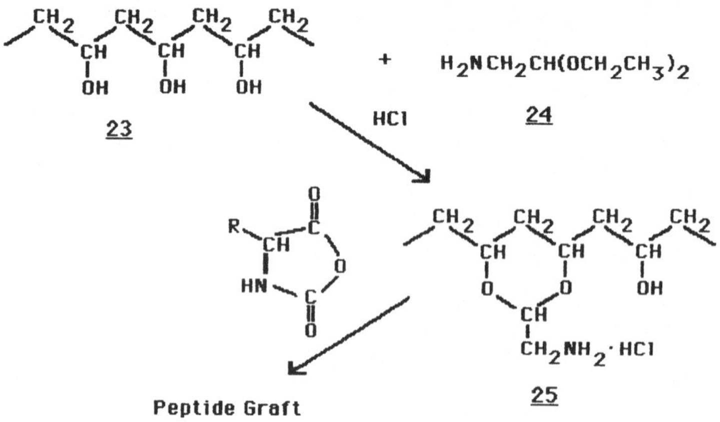

Scheme 2. Formation of aminoacetalized poly(vinyl alcohol).

micrograph of a film of copoly[(N-2-aminoethyl)acrylamide-styrene-g-[br]-
γ-benzyl-L-glutamate] cast from a tetrachloroethane and stained with
phosphotungstic acid showed the formation of crystalline, rod-like
domains made up of poly(γ-benzyl-L-glutamate) branches, placed in an
amorphous region made up of trunk polystyrene. Thus, the formation of
microdomains was confirmed.

Another approach to make homo- or copolymers which contain primary
amino functions was developed by Maeda and coworkers.[55] A lithium alkylamide catalyzed addition of mono N-alkyl-substituted ethylene diamines
[34] to 1,4-divinylbenzene [33] yielded a styrene derivative [35]
containing both tertiary and primary amino groups (Scheme 4).

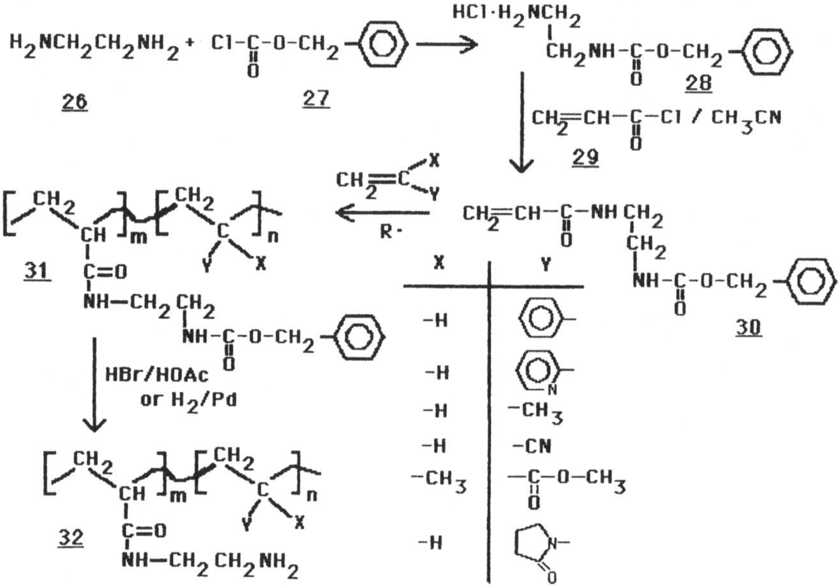

Scheme 3. Formation of polyacrylamides with amino
substituents.

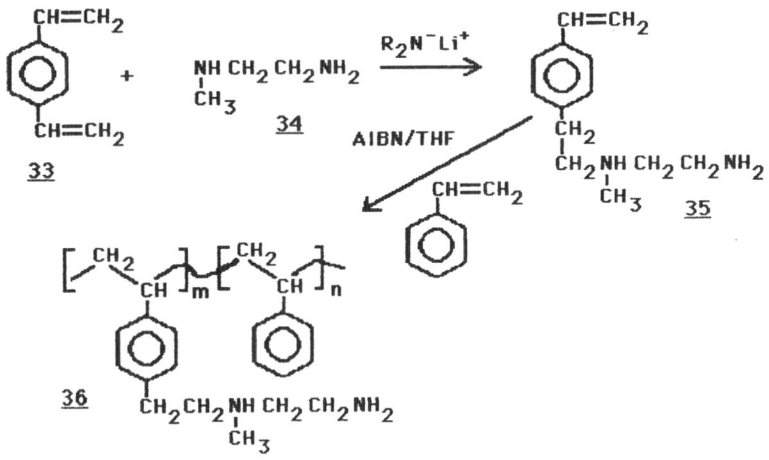

Scheme 4. Synthesis of ethylenediaminoethyl styrene.

By copolymerizing [35] with other vinyl monomers, such as styrene,[56,57] and butyl methacrylate,[56,58-60] copolymers [36] having varying amounts of reactive primary amino groups in the side chains were easily prepared. The tertiary amino group in the polymer substituent would be expected to initiate the NCA polymerization also. However, model studies using N,N-dimethylethylene diamine showed that the predominant initiation mode was induced by the primary amino group to produce poly-alanine with a 2-(dimethylamino)ethylamido end group.[61] Graft copolymers of poly(amino acids), poly(γ-benzyl-L-glutamate) and poly(γ-benzyl-L-aspartate) with desired peptide side chain DPs (5-17) were prepared in THF or THF-DCM at 30-35°C for 18 hrs. to 6 days by using [36] as a macro-initiator. This research group pioneered solution NMR characterization techniques for the grafted copolymers using trifluoroacetic acid (TFA)-CDCl$_3$ solvent mixtures.[57] The average number of amino acid residues in the poly(amino acid) grafts, determined by ^{1}H-NMR using the area ratio of protons on the styryl aromatic rings to that of α-CH (L-alanine) or benzylic CH$_2$ (γ-benzyl-L-glutamate, γ-benzyl-L-aspartate) substituents, was in fair agreement with the initial mole ratio of NCA to primary amino groups in [36]. Gel permeation chromatography showed that the products were contaminated by a very small amount of low molecular weight homo-poly(amino acid). This approach was employed to make permselective bio-membrane models from butyl methacrylate-[35] copolymer and NCAs.[58,59,60]

Recently, several other aminopolymers were synthesized for the NCA polymerization. Ichie and coworkers used copolymers of styrene-vinyl benzylamine and methyl methacrylate-vinyl benzylamine for NCA polymeriza-tion to study the kinetics of NCA polymerization with macroinitiators.[62] The polymerization was 1st-order with respect to monomer concentration and was much faster in nitrobenzene than in dioxane or THF. Kiba patented a new system for NCA polymerization with the different aminopolymers [38] produced according to Scheme 5.[63] He also claimed the ester exchange reaction of the resulting graft copolymer with ethylene cyanohydrin over p-toluene sulfonic acid.

Ogata et al. published several applications with graft copolymers of poly(γ-benzyl-L-glutamate) onto suspension polymerized crosslinked poly-styrene beads containing aminomethyl functions [39] (Scheme 6).[64-67] The benzyl ester group of the polypeptide side chain was converted either to benzyl amide by aminolysis or to free acid by hydrolysis and the effects

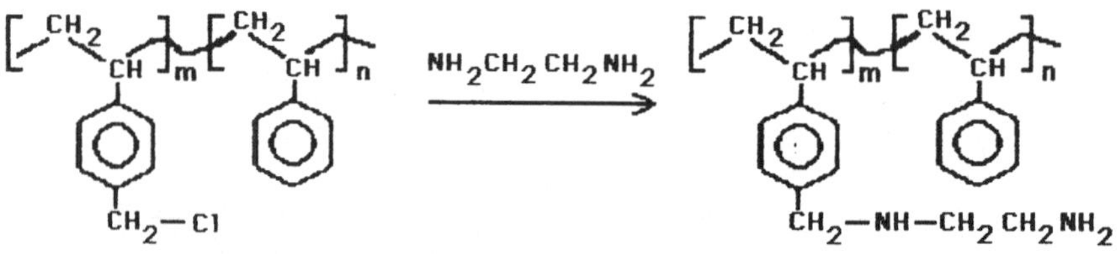

Scheme 5. Direct formation of poly(ethylenediaminomethyl-styrene).

of the polypeptide graft side chain functionality on the efficiency of optical resolution was evaluated.

Applications of Amino Acid Graft Copolymers

Limited reports concerning applications of the graft copolymers of amino acids onto natural and synthetic polymers have appeared. The reports focus on the following three possible applications: (1) adsorbents for chromatographic optical resolution of racemic mixtures, (2) permselective biomembranes, and (3) biomedical materials.

1. Applications for optical resolution of racemic mixture. Since conventional methods of resolution of racemic mixtures by fractional recrystallization of their corresponding diastermeric salts is often laborious, generates low yields, and does not always produce high optical purity, a direct chromatographical optical resolution method was desired. During the past decade, extensive research has been carried out in an effort to prepare novel chiral adsorbents based on silica gel for liquid

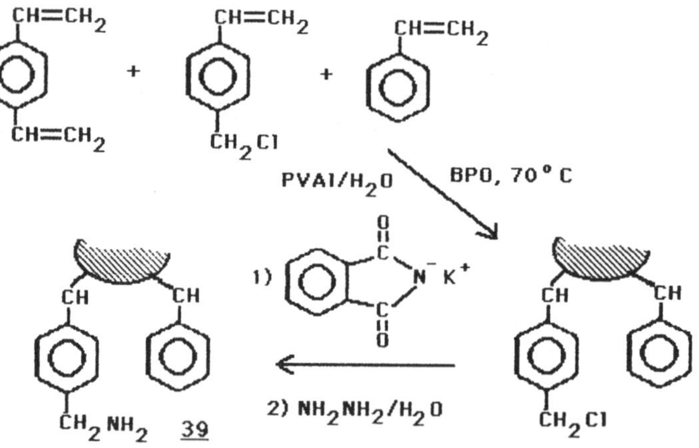

Scheme 6. Production of aminomethylated polystyrene beads.

chromatography.[68-75] Polymer-based adsorbents with highly ordered helical side chains, which amplify the chirality of poly(α-amino acids), should be very effective. A recognition interaction similar to that of natural enzymes between the poly(amino acid) helix and the various stereoisomers by hydrogen bond association may be anticipated.[67]

Kiba patented a chromatographical optical resolution method for a racemic mixture of D- and L-mandelic acid which employs high-pressure liquid chromatography using polystyrene-based adsorbents containing poly-(γ-methyl-L-glutamate) and poly[γ-(3-cyano)propyl-L-glutamate].[63] More recent publications describing applications of amino acid graft copolymers as adsorbents have been reported by Ogata and coworkers (64-67). They observed that polystyrene-based adsorbents incorporating several types of covalently immobilized poly(α-amino acids), such as poly(γ-benzyl-L-glutamate), poly(γ-N⁵-benzyl-L-glutamine), and poly-(glutamic acid), were useful for effecting the resolution of racemic mixtures like (R,S)-5-isopropylhydantoin,[64,66,67] and (D,L)-mandelic acid.[65] The DPs and functionality on the side chain of the incorporated poly(α-amino acids) were found to be the critical factors determining the extent of resolution. Reasonable resolution were accomplished on adsorbents with poly(amino acids), DP = 14 and 36; whereas, short grafts with a DP = 2 failed to effect resolution. Further, better optical resolution was obtained with a benzylamine modified adsorbent containing poly(N⁵-benzyl-L-glutamine) side chain than with adsorbents containing poly(γ-benzyl-L-glutamate) or poly(glutamic acid) side chain.

2. Applications as permselective biomembranes. Protein molecules may undergo reversible conformational changes to create a "hole" or a "channel" in the membrane for the specific substrate transported.[77] As an example of a synthetic membrane mimicking the function of biomembranes, i.e., specific, facilitated, active transport, Inoue and coworkers described the first case of pH-induced reversible conformational changes in the trans-membrane polypeptide domain of a synthetic membrane prepared from a copoly[(butyl methacrylate-g-[br]-(L-aspartic acid)].[78] The changes in conformation were confirmed using circular dichorism measurements. This synthetic graft copolymer was found to have microdomains of poly(amino acids) similar to biomembrane,[56] and was regarded as a trans-membrane for sodium cation,[69] and permselective membrane of sugars.[58] They also demonstrated regulation of solute permeability by a divalent cation, Ca++, in a polymer membrane of the graft copolymer of (L-glutamic acid) on a poly(butyl methacrylate) analog of [36].[59] Permeability of phenyl-1,2-ethanediol through this membrane was remarkably reduced in the presence of Ca++ and restored by addition of a competitive calcium binder, ethylenediaminetetraacetic acid.

3. Application in biomedical materials. In early 1980, Sakurai and his coworkers first showed the applicability of amino acid graft copolymers as biomedical membranes for a chromatographic cell separator.[79] Recently, Miyamoto et al. reported preliminary results on favorable blood compatibility of aminoethylcellulose graft copolymers of poly(γ-benzyl-L-glutamate) and poly(N⁵-2-hydroxyethyl-L-glutamine) with poly(amino acids) contents ranging from 7 to 60 mole%.[51] An in vivo method involving peripheral vein indwelling polyester sutures coated with these graft copolymers was employed. These graft copolymers were found to have excellent antithrombogenic properties and good absorbability; about 25% of the sample copolymers was absorbed within 4 weeks of implantation.

We are also interested in polymers with pendant reactive peptides as potential controlled release agents. Either the free amino function at the end of the peptide chains or the benzyl ester substituents on PBLG can be coupled with an appropriate pharmacon, which can be released in *vivo* by peptidases. Our attention was focused initially on cellulose derivatives in a effort to produce a completely biodegradable polymer delivery system; initial results on this problem appear promising. Unfortunately, the cellulose grafts are insoluble in most solvents, which makes characterization of the modified derivatives very difficult. Therefore, aminated poly(arylene ether) derivatives were employed as soluble macroinitiators in an effort to produce soluble graft copolymers, which could be cast into membranes. The soluble copolymers can be studied by numerous solution techniques, and some insight into the unique properties imparted by the peptide grafts can be gained.

Poly(γ-benzyl-L-glutamate), PBLG was selected as the representative peptide unit, because PBLG is not only a well characterized hydrophobic peptide known to adopt a several secondary structures, but also it can be converted readily into a number of derivatives ranging in properties from hydrophobic to hydrophilic. Hydrolysis of the benzyl ester should produce poly(glutamic acid) complexes capable of binding inorganic fillers; thus, strong biocomposites could be formed.

EXPERIMENTAL

Macroinitiators

Aminopropylcellulose [1] was prepared from cellulose by cyanoethylation, D.S.= 0.3, followed by reduction of the nitrile to [1], 1.6 meq/g NH$_2$, with a borane-THF complex (1.0 M in THF).[80] Direct phthalimido-methylation of poly(arylene ether sulfone) [5] was carried out at room temperature in a 50:50 v/v mixture of dichloromethane-trifluoroacetic acid using a trifluorosulfonic acid catalyst; by varying the ratio of N-hydroxymethylphthalimide to [5], the degree of functionalization (DF) was controlled to yield [6a-c], D.F. = 0.2, 0.5, or 1.0 respectively. Subsequent homogeneous hydrazinolysis of [6] in refluxing THF-ethanol yielded poly (2-aminomethyl-1,4-phenylene ether sulfone) [3a-c]. 0.447, 1.095, or 2.123 meq/g NH$_2$ (81). Poly(2-amino-1,4-phenylene ether sulfone) [2], D.F.= 0.3 (0.67 meq/g NH$_2$) was prepared by nitration of [5],[82] and reduction of the nitro substituents with SnCl$_2$ and concentrated HCl.[81] Treatment of BLG with phosgene in THF according to the procedure of Goodman[83] afforded N-carboxy-γ-benzyl-L-glutamic acid anhydride, BLG-NCA [8].

Graft Copolymerizations

Aminopropylcellulose [1], containing 1.6 meq/g NH$_2$, was slurried in 20 mL anhydrous THF and stirred at room temperature while a solution of BLG-NCA in 10 mL THF was added. Graft copolymerization was allowed to proceed at room temperature for 48 hours. After reducing the volume of mixture to a third under reduced pressure and pouring the slurry into ten-fold excess cold MeOH, the graft copolymers [9a-e], were recovered by filtration and dried at 25°C under vacuum for 24 hours. The results are summarized in Table 1.

The aminated poly(arylene ether sulfone) derivatives, [2] and [3], were dissolved in anhydrous THF before adding the BLG-NCA solution. The copolymerizations remained homogeneous except in the cases when the BLG-NCA/NH$_2$ ratios were greater than 15. The copolymers were isolated as described above; the results are reported in Tables 2 and 3.

Table 1. Graft copolymers of γ-benzyl-L-glutamate on aminopropylcellulose, [1], D. S. = 0.3

Structure	(a) grams	NCA grams	NCA/APC (m/m)	%Grafting Efficiency	DP (b)	Conformation
9a	1.076	0.424(c)	0.94	89.0	0.8	α-Helix
9b	0.687	0.813	2.81	80.2	2.3	α-Helix
9c	0.504	0.995	4.67	76.7	3.6	α-Helix
9d	0.303	1.197	9.38	87.6	8.2	β-sheet + α-Helix
9e	0.169	1.331	18.7	70.5	13.2	α-Helix + β-sheet

(a). Aminopropylcellulose, 1.6 meq/g of NH$_2$.
(b). Average D.P. of grafts based upon weight gain.
(c). Reaction conditions: total reactant conc., 1.5 g/25 mL
of THF, R.T., 48 hrs.

Modification of Graft Copolymers

Graft copolymer [**14a**] was converted to the corresponding poly[(amino-methyl arylene ether sulfone)-g-[br]-(N^5-butyl-γ-L-glutamine)] [**15a**] by stirring a solution on the copolymer (0.1 meq benzyl ester/2 mL solvent) in 12.5 V/V% DMSO-THF with the designated amine at 55°C; the results are summarized in Table 4. The extent of aminolysis and peptide cleavage was estimated by ^{1}H NMR (DMSO-d$_6$) using the resonances at 5.04 ppm (benzylic CH$_2$ of PBLG), 1.64 ppm (CH$_3$ of polysulfone backbone) and 0.79 ppm (CH$_3$ of butyl group).

Table 2. Graft copolymers of γ-benzyl-L-glutamate with poly-
(aminoarylene ether sulfone), [2].

Structure	(a) grams	NCA grams	NCA/NH$_2$ (m/m)	%Grafting Efficiency	DP values (b)	(c)	Conformation
10a	0.53(d)	0.47(d)	5	10.0	0.3	0.5	Random + β-Sheet
10b	0.36	0.64	10	30.0	3.4	3.0	β-Sheet
10c	0.22	0.78	20	25.0	6.2	5.0	β-Sheet
10d	0.10	0.90	50	26.0	13.6	13.0	α-Helix

(a). Polymer was poly(aminoarylene ether sulfone), 0.67 meq/g
of NH$_2$, substrate for samples [10a-d].
(b). Average D.P. of grafts based upon weight gain.
(c). Average D.P. of grafts based upon ^{1}H NMR.
(d). Reaction conditions: total reactant conc., 1.00 g/30 mL
THF, R.T., 48 hrs.

Table 3. Graft copolymers of γ-benzyl-L-glutamate with poly-(aminomethylphenyl arylene ether sulfones), [3a-c].

Structure	(a) grams	NCA grams	(b)	%Grafting Efficiency	DP values (d)	(e)	(c) (cps)	Conformation
12a(f)	0.642	0.358	1	90.0	0.8	0.9		Random
12b	0.375	0.625	3	93.3	2.5	2.8		Random
12c	0.204	0.796	7	100.0	6.6	7.0		Random
12d	0.152	0.848	10	90.0	8.1	9.0		β-Sheet
12e	0.082	0.918	20	82.0	16.3	16.4		β-Sheet + α-Helix
13a(g)	0.739	0.261	3	83.3	2.9	2.5	1.84	Random
13b	0.630	0.370	5	90.0	4.7	4.5	1.89	Random + β-Sheet
13c	0.460	0.540	10	95.0	9.8	9.5	1.79	β-Sheet + α-Helix
13d	0.362	0.638	15	90.7	13.4	13.6	1.79	β-Sheet + α-Helix
13e	0.254	0.746	25	96.0	23.6	24.0	1.93	α-Helix
13f	0.145	0.855	50	88.0	48.3	44.0	2.27	α-Helix
13g	0.078	0.922	100	85.0	95.5	85.0	2.26	α-Helix
14a(h)	9.00	10.38	4	97.5	3.6	3.9		Random + β-Sheet
14b	1.5	5.92	13.7	98.5	12.8	13.5		β-Sheet + α-Helix

(a). Poly(aminomethylene arylene ether sulfone), [3c], 2.123 meq/g NH$_2$ for [12a-e]; [3a], 0.447 meq/g NH$_2$ for [13a-g]; [3b], 1.095 meq/g NH$_2$ for [14a-b].
(b). Molar ratio of NCA:AMPS.
(c). 2.5% in pyridine at 25°C, Wells-Brookfield Viscometer (Spindle, CP-40; angle 0.8°, volume 0.5 mL; shear rate 450 sec^{-1}.
(d). Average D.P. of grafts based upon weight gain.
(e). Average D.P. of grafts based upon ^{1}H NMR.
(f). Reaction conditions: total reactant conc., 1.00 g/25mL of THF, R.T., 24 hrs.
(g). Reaction conditions: total reactant conc., 1.00 g/30mL of THF, R.T., 48 hrs.
(h). Reaction conditions: total reactant conc., 7.00 g/100mL of THF, R.T., 48 hrs.

RESULTS AND DISCUSSION

Cellulose Graft Copolymers

Grafting of BLG-NCA to aminopropylcellulose [1] could be accomplished at room temperature in the dried THF (Scheme 7). The cellulose derivative did not appear swollen in THF but there were enough active amino sites accessible on the surface to allow the reaction to proceed without difficulty. The graft copolymers were not soluble in most solvents, but did swell in THF, DMSO, and pyridine. Infrared spectra were very useful in confirming the extent of grafting and for identifying the secondary structure of the peptide units grafted. Several publications document the

Table 4. Homogeneous aminolysis of poly[(aminomethylarylene
ether sulfone)-g-[br]-(γ-benzyl-L-glutamate)], [14a],
with n-butylamine.(a)

n-Butylamine gram (meq)		Reaction Time, hrs.	Average Branch Composition			Cleavage (b) %
			Benzyl(c)	Butyl(d)	Total	
0.000		0	3.9	0.0	3.9	0.0
0.293	(4.0)	24	3.2	0.6	3.8	1.6
0.586	(8.0)		1.9	1.8	3.7	5.1
1.170	(16.0)		1.7	2.2	3.9	0.0
1.755	(24.0)		1.5	2.0	3.5	10.3
2.925	(40.0)		0.4	3.2	3.6	7.7
0.586	(8.0)	5	3.6	0.3	3.9	0.0
		12	2.2	1.5	3.7	5.1
		48	1.5	1.9	3.4	12.8
		72	1.1	2.1	3.2	17.9
		96	1.0	2.1	3.1	20.5
		120	0.9	2.2	3.1	20.5
		144	0.9	2.1	3.0	23.1
		204	0.4	2.0	2.4	38.5
0.64	(8.8)(e)	6	1.4	2.5	3.9	0.0
		11	1.1	2.8	3.9	0.0
		24	0.9	2.9	3.8	2.6
		48	0.8	3.0	3.8	2.6
		72	0.7	3.1	3.8	2.6
		96	0.5	3.3	3.8	2.6

(a). Poly[(aminomethylarylene ether sulfone)-g-[br]-(γ-Benzyl-
L-glutamate)], [14a], D.F.=0.5, Ave. DP=3.9, 0.2 g (0.44
meq) in 8mL of DMSO/THF = (12.5v/v%; Temp. = 55°C.
(b). % Amino acids lost.
(c). Average number of γ-Benzyl-L-glutamate residues per graft
based upon ^{1}H NMR.
(d). Average number of N^5-n-butyl-L-glutamate residues per
graft based upon ^{1}H NMR.
(e). 1.2 eq. 1-hydroxybenzotriazole/eq. peptide unit added.

critical chain lengths for β-sheet (4-10 amino acids) or α-helix (>11
amino acids) formation and identify the IR bands in the amide region
associated with a given conformation.[84-88] The aminopropylcellulose
grafts exhibited strong peaks at 1655 and 1550 cm^{-1} for amide I and amide
II bands, respectively, suggesting an α-helical conformation even though
the theoretical DP of the grafts was calculated to be less than 5.
Apparently the actual percentage of amino functional groups, which are
effective initiators is much lower than that determined by titration, and
a few grafts with DPs >15 are formed. The appearance of β-sheet structures at high BLG-NCA/APC ratios suggests that the rate of initiation is
much slower than that of propagation due to the heterogeneous system, but
incorporation of a few grafts enhances the accessibility of the amine
sites. Thus, long chain grafts are produced initially followed by short
chains initiated by the amine groups unveiled by the graft induced
swelling of the cellulose matrix. Both the insolubility and the obvious
variation in graft structure forced us to seek a more tractable system to
utilize in characterization of peptide graft copolymers.

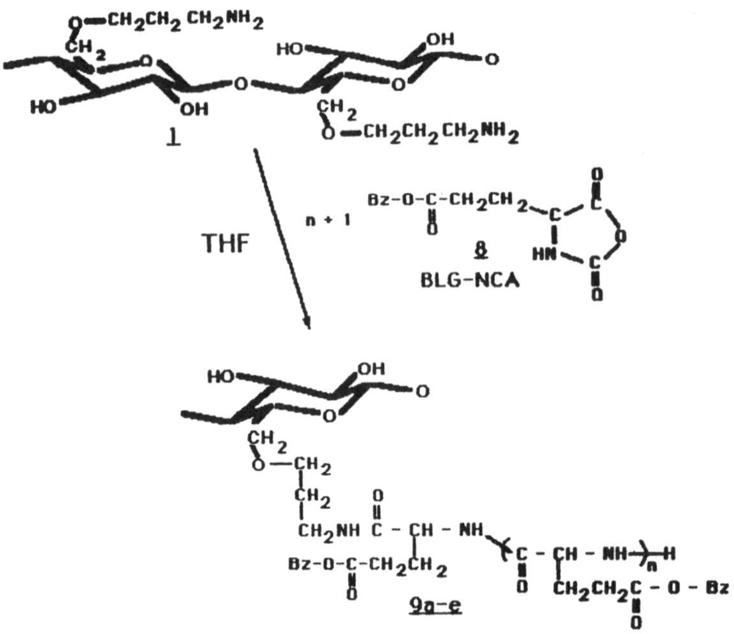

O—CH$_2$CH$_2$ CH$_2$NH$_2$
CH$_2$
HO   OH   O
HO   OH
1

THF

n + 1

Bz-O-C-CH$_2$CH$_2$
8
BLG-NCA

HO   OH   O
CH$_2$
O—CH$_2$
CH$_2$
CH$_2$NH C - CH - NH
Bz-O-C-CH$_2$CH$_2$ C - CH - NH-$\rangle_n$ H
CH$_2$CH$_2$C - O - Bz
9a-e

Scheme 7. Reaction of BLG-NCA with aminopropylcellulose.

Poly(arylene ether) Graft Copolymers

Soluble, well characterized polymers with primary amine substituents, [2,3], were used to test the accessibility theory. Poly(2-amino-1,4-phenylene ether sulfone) [2], prepared by reduction of the corresponding nitro derivative, dissolved readily in THF and CHCl$_3$; intrinsic viscosity measurements indicated that little change in molecular weight·occurred during the reduction. However, we observed that very low NCA grafting efficiencies were obtained with [2] as the macroinitiator (Table 2). The nucleophilicity of these aromatic polyamines is not high enough to initiate the polymerization of NCAs effectively. Further, in contrast to the results obtained with aminopropylcellulose, a termination reaction limited the length of the peptide grafts. Even in the presence of a fifty-fold excess of BLG-NCA, the average DP of the grafts was only 13.

The more interesting soluble macroinitiator for polymerization of BLG-NCA was [3], which has a primary aliphatic amino function. The phthalimidomethylation of poly(arylene ether sulfone), [5], with N-hydroxylmethylphalimide in dichloromethane-trifluoroacetic acid could be controlled to any desired degree of substitution, although some reduction in the molecular weight of the substituted polymers was detected by viscosity measurements. The aminomethyl substituents were released by hydrazinolysis of the phthalimide substituents in mixture of THF and ethanol. The aminomethylated polymers with low amine contents (DF <1) are soluble in CHCl$_3$, dioxane, THF, DMSO, and pyridine. Using [3c], DF = 1.0, graft copolymers [12a-e] were synthesized (Table 3). The average DP of the grafts appeared to be correlated directly with the BLG-NCA: amine feed ratio. The conformations of the BLG grafts were assigned from the IR spectra of films. The graft copolymers [12a-e] were soluble in hot pyridine and 5 v/v% TFA in CHCl$_3$. However, attempts to confirm the DPs of BLG grafted to the poly(arylene ether sulfone) backbone by comparison of the integrations of ^{1}H NMR peaks at 5.04 ppm (benzylic H's of BLG) and 1.70 ppm (methyl H's of back bone polymer) were thwarted on these densely

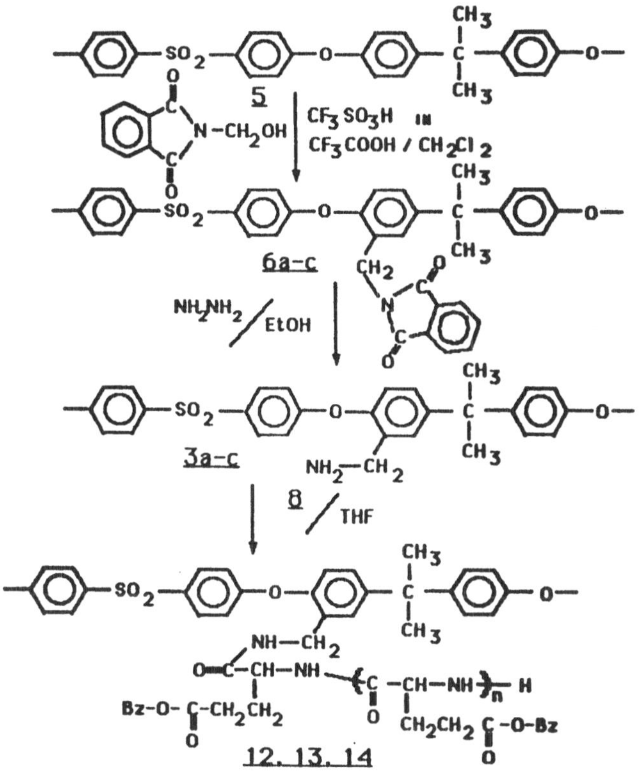

Scheme 8. Preparation and modification of poly(aminomethylarylene ether sulfone)

grafted copolymers due to the relatively high contents of PBLG units
relative to the backbone.

With polymer [3c], DF = 0.2, loading on the backbone was reduced and
a better balance was achieved between graft and backbone properties.
(Table 3). These copolymers, [13a-e], were soluble in pyridine and DMSO;
copolymers with a low DP (<15 PBLG units), were also soluble in CHCl₃.
The graft copolymerizations were carried out with greater than 90%
efficiency and the structures of the peptides were consistent with the
average DPs calculated from the feed ratios. The secondary conformation
of the PBLG units was identified using IR and NMR spectroscopy. A dis-
ordered structure, which has an amine I band at 1660 cm^{-1} and amide II
at 1535 cm^{-1}, was prominent for copolymers with 2.5 or 4 PBLG units
grafted exhibited amide I band at 1700 and 1630 cm^{-1}, and amide II band
at 1530 cm^{-1}, characteristic of the antiparallel β-structure. Infrared
spectra of copolymers with more than 15 amino acids in the PBLG units
showed strong bands at 1655 cm^{-1} and 1550 cm^{-1}, characteristic of the α-
helical conformation of BLG units.

Solution Properties of the Graft Copolymers

Since the infrared studies of films revealed the presence of helical
grafts in the solid state, we elected to study the structure of the
copolymers in solution by NMR. Studies with oligopeptides in dilute solution reveal resolvable amide (NH) and α-methine (α-CH) resonances with

267

differing chemical shifts for the random and α-helical conformations.[89] Since the backbone polymer would hold the grafts in close proximity, similar high dilution measurements would not be possible. On the other hand some indication of the intermolecular bonding should be evident. The spectra of [13c] in a 5 w/v% deuterochloroform solution was essentially featureless. Addition of trifluoroacetic acid was required to sharpen the α-CH and interestingly, the benzylic CH₂ resonances. Up to 3 v/v% TFA could be added to the CDCl₃ solution without disrupting the α-helical conformation, (α-CH = 3.94 ppm). Transformation of the α-helical conformation to a random coil structure could be effected by increasing the amount of trifluoroacetic acid in the chloroform-d solution.[90] At 10 v/v% TFA the chemical shift of the α-methine reached 4.6 ppm and further additions of TFA failed to produce any change, indicating that the grafts were in the random coil conformation. The conformations, however, were not changed when the concentrations of the grafted copolymers in 3 v/v% TFA-CDCl₃ were varied within the ranges of 0.3–11 w/v%.

Determination of the average DP for the peptide grafts involves quantitation of the backbone and peptide resonances. These measurements were made in 10 v/v% TFA/CDCl₃ because the most accurate comparisons were obtained with the peptide in a random coil conformation. A typical spectrum is shown in Figure 2. The resonances associated with the poly-(arylene ether sulfone) backbone are reasonably well resolved with the exception of an overlap in the aromatic region with the aromatic protons attached to the benzyl ester and the amide protons of the peptide backbone. The average DP was calculated from the ratio of the ratio of the benzyl CH₂ protons to the geminal CH₃ protons in the backbone polymer.

The viscosities of the graft copolymers were evaluated under various shear conditions to ascertain if the grafts promoted aggregation at low shear. As is often the case with graft copolymers, the viscosities observed at high shear rates for the copolymers did not vary much from those of the backbone (Table 3). Both the starting backbone and the graft copolymers exhibited some shear thinning at high shear rates. The recovery of the low shear viscosity was instantaneous when the shear was reduced on the backbone polymer in the stirred system. In contrast, copolymer [13e] required 3–8 minutes to recover the initial low shear viscosity. Thus, there is some indication of aggregation, but the effect is not pronounced.

Amidation of PLBG Grafts

Utilization of the graft copolymers as controlled delivery systems depends upon facile modification of the PBLG grafts. Aminolysis of the benzyl ester on PBLG homo- and copolymers with ammonia and various amines leads to the formation of γ-amides.[91] In fact, Scheraga has used 3-amino-propanol and 4-aminobutanol extensively to prepare water soluble polypeptides.[92] However, when we attempted this transformation with graft copolymer [14a], the derivative precipitated rapidly from either THF or DMSO-THF solutions, indicating that crosslinking via transesterification occurred. As the reaction proceeded, the sample redissolved in DMSO-THF, but precipitated when we added water for dialysis. Anticipating that the hydroxyethylamine was not sufficiently hydrophilic to pull the backbone polymer into aqueous solution, we allowed [14a] to react with tris-(hydroxymethyl)aminomethane in DMSO; conversions to the corresponding amide of greater than 50% produced an adduct which would swell in water but homogeneous aqueous solutions could not be obtained until substitution >95% was achieved. Clearly the backbone polymer plays an important role in the solution properties of the graft copolymers.

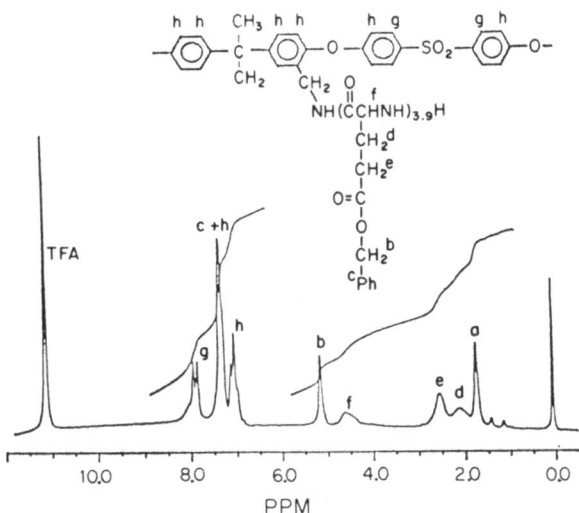

Figure 2. A typical proton NMR spectrum of [14a] (10 w/v%) in
10 v/v% TFA-CDCl3 at 297°K.

The rate of aminolysis of [14a] was studied under hetero- and homogeneous conditions using butylamine as a model nucleophile (Scheme 9).
Although the term aminolysis is applied primarily to cleavage of the γ-
benzyl ester, a side reaction which can become significant is cleavage of
the peptide chain by transamidation. By working with copolymers with
short chain grafts, we were able to monitor both processes by NMR.
Aminolysis of the benzyl ester lead to the disappearance of the benzylic
CH₂ resonances (5.04 ppm) and the appearance of butyl CH₃ at 0.79 ppm
(Figure 3). The ratio of peptide to backbone polymer could be monitored
by comparing resonances at 1.64 ppm with the geminal CH₃ of the backbone.

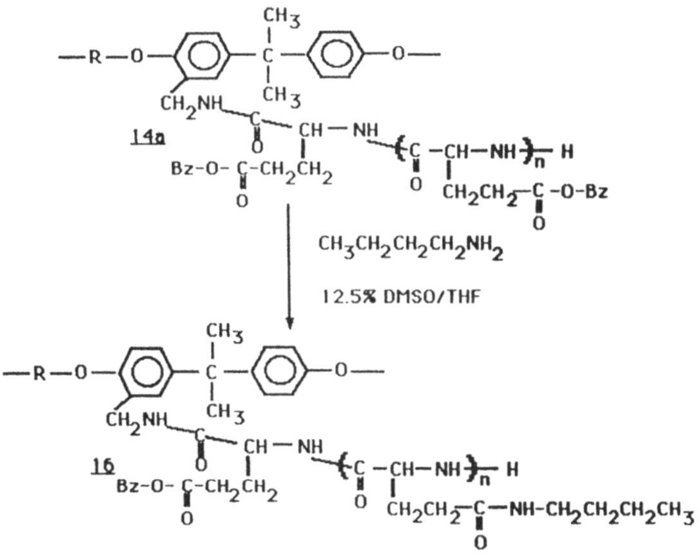

Scheme 9. Aminolysis of PBLG grafts.

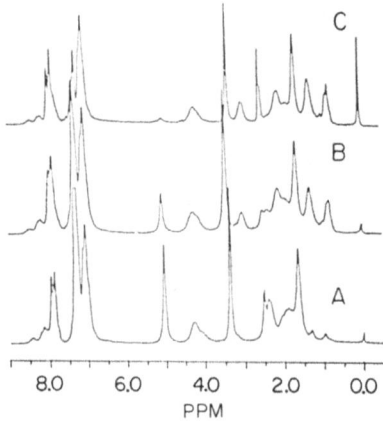

Figure 3. Proton NMR spectra (in DMSO-d6) of partially amidated graft copolymers from [14a]. (A, 3.9 BLG units; B, 1.9 BLG + 1.8 BuLG units; C, 0.4 BLG + 2.0 BuLG units; where BuLG = N5-n-butyl-L-glutamine).

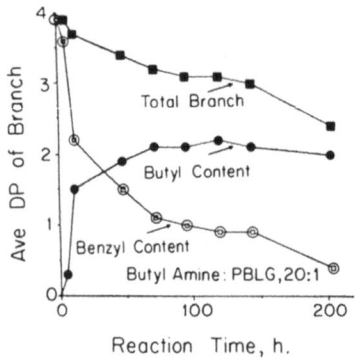

Figure 4. Influence of reaction times on the aminolysis of [14a] with n-butylamine in 12.5 v/v% DMSO-THF at 55°C.

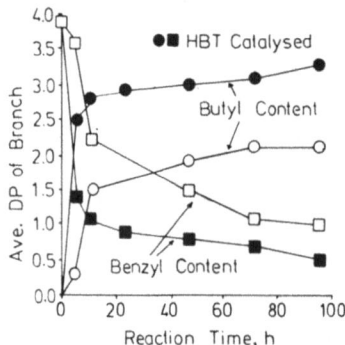

Figure 5. Influence of 1-hydroxybenzotriazole on the amino-lysis of [14a] with n-butylamine in 12.5 v/v% DMSO-THF at 55°C.

When the aminolysis of [14a] was conducted in TFA, the product precipitated when approximately 40% of the benzyl ester had reacted. Conversion of the benzyl ester to amide reached 50% within 24 hrs. and did not change significantly thereafter. However, the extent of peptide chain cleavage continued to increase from a value 7.7% to 17.9% over a total reaction time of 144 hrs. When the product precipitated, the access to the benzyl ester was impeded and subsequent activity was focused on the peptide bonds. Addition of 12.5% DMSO to the THF produced a solvent mixture which dissolved by reactants and products in all conversion ranges. Thus, it was possible to study the aminolysis of [14a] under homogeneous conditions in this solvent mixture.

The influence of reactant ratios and reaction times was studied in the 12.5 v/v% DMSO-THF solvent mixture (Table 4). Note that the extent of peptide cleavage can be minimized by using very large excesses, i.e. >50:1, of the amine. In fact if a hundred fold excess is used, an 82% conversion of the benzyl ester to amide can be achieved in 24 hrs. at 55°C. However, if a twenty fold excess of amine is used and the reaction is allowed to run for several days, significant loss of peptide units are observed (Figure 4). Only 56% of the benzyl ester initially present is converted to amide.

The aminolysis of the γ-benzyl ester can be catalyzed by 1-hydroxybenzotriazole [15].[93] When 1.2 eq. of [15] was added to a solution of [14a] with a twenty fold excess of butyl amine, 64%, 72% and 75% conversion of the benzyl ester to amide was obtained in 6, 11, and 24 hrs., respectively (Figure 5). Cleavage of the peptide bonds was minimized under these conditions. The average DP of the peptide branches in [14a] is four, but only three of the amino acid residues are reacting rapidly. It appears that the amino acid bound directly to the backbone polymer is subject to more steric hindrance and may be more difficult to transform.

CONCLUSIONS

A soluble macroinitiator, poly(aminomethylarylene ether sulfone) was effective in initiating the polymerization of the NCA of γ-benzyl-L-glutamate to produce soluble graft copolymers. The average DP of the peptide grafts could be predicted from the BLG-NCA/amine ratio. Infrared and NMR spectroscopies can be used to determine the conformations of the PBLG grafts. The secondary conformations depend primarily on the length of PBLG chain; little influence of the backbone polymer on the peptide orientation could be detected. The γ-benzyl ester could be modified by aminolysis, particularly in the presence of 1-hydroxybenzotriazole.

Aminopropylcellulose also served as a macroinitiator for NCA polymerization with high grafting efficiency. However, conformational data showed that the chain length of the peptide grafts was not a simple function of the BLG-NCA/amine ratio, and the graft copolymers remain insoluble.

REFERENCES

1. M. Poulicek, M. F. Voss-Foucart & Ch. Jeuniaux in: "*Chitin in Nature and Technology*", R. Muzzarelli, Ch. Jeuniaux, & G.W.Gooday, Eds., Plenum Publ. Corp., New York, 1986; pp. 7-13.
2. C. Ramakrishnan & N. Prasad, Biochem. Biophys. Acta, **261**, 123 (1972).
3. H. Bittiger, E. Husemann, & A. Kuppel, J. Polym. Sci., Part C, **28**, 45 (1969).

4. N. E. Dweltz, J. R. Colvin, & A. G. McInnes, Can. J. Chem., **46**, 1513 (1968).
5. S. Weiner, Amer. Zool., **24**, 945 (1984).
6. G. Goffinet, Ch. Gregoire & M. F. Voss-Foucart, Arch. Internat. Physiol. Biochem., **85**, 849 (1977).
7. H. Nakanara, G. Bevelander & M. Kakei, Venus, **39**, 205 (1982).
8. R. H. Hackman, Austr. J. Biol. Sci, **8**, 83 (1955); **13**, 568 (1960).
9. C. J. Brine & P. R. Austin, Comp. Biochem. Physiol., **70B**, 173 (1981).
10. A. Gottschalk, W.H. Murphy, & E.R.B. Graham, Nature, **194**, 1051 (1962).
11. M. M. Atwood & H. Zola, Comp. Biochem. Physiol., **20**, 993 (1967).
12. J. Schaefer, K. J. Kramer, J. R. Garbow, G. S. Jacob, E. O. Stejskal, T. L. Hopkins & R. D. Speirs, Science, **235**, 1200 (1987).
13. T. Kato, S. Ito, & K. Fujita, Biochem. Biophys. Acta, **881**, 415 (1986).
14. J. R. Schaefgen & P. J. Flory, J. Amer. Chem. Soc., **70**, 2709 (1984).
15. M. Sela, E. Katchalski & M. Gehatia, J. Amer. Chem. Soc., **78**, 746 (1955).
16. F. Wessely, K. Riedl & M. Gehatia, Monatsh, **81**, 861 (1950).
17. R. R. Becker & M. A. Stahmann, J. Biol. Chem., **204**, 737 (1953).
18. H. Batzer, Makromol. Chem., **12**, 145 (1954).
19. G. S. Grest, K. Kremer & T. A. Witten, Macromolecules, **20**, 1376 (1987).
20. R. Arnon & M. Sela, Biochem. J., **75**, 91, (1960),; **77**, 394 (1960).
21. M. Sela, S. Fuchs, & R. Arnon, Biochem. J., **85**, 223 (1962).
22. D. A. Tewksbury & M. A. Stahmann, Arch. Biochem. Biophys., **105**, 527 (1964).
23. J. W. Stewart & M. A. Stahmann in: "*Polyamino Acids, Polypeptides and Proteins*", M. A. Stahmann, Ed., Univ. of Wisconsin, Madison, Wisconsin, 1962; p. 102.
24. A. Yaron, & A. Berger, Biochem. Biophys. Acta, **107**, 307 (1965).
25. W. Moffitt & J. T. Yang, Proc. Natl. Acad. Sci. U.S.A., **42**, 596 (1956).
26. P. Urnes & P. Doty, Advan. Protein Chem., **16**, 401 (1961).
27. M. Sakamoto & Y. Kuroyanagi, J. Polym. Sci., Polym. Chem. Ed., **16**, 1107 (1978).
28. Lin-Yan, V. A. Derevitskaya & Z. A. Rogovin, Vysokomol. Soed., **1**, 157 (1959).
29. Z. A. Rogovin, V. A. Derevitskaya, S. Tun, C. Wei-Gan & L. S. Galbraikh, J. Polym. Sci., **53**, 117 (1961).
30. Z. A. Rogovin, J. Polym. Sci., **48**, 443 (1960).
31. P. Karrer & W. Wehrili, Helv. Chim. Acta., **9**, 591 (1926).
32. T. S. Gardner, J. Polym. Sci., **1**, 121 (1946).
33. Y. Avny & A. Zilka, Israel J. Chem., **3**, 207 (1965/66).
34. C. H. Bamford. E. Elliot & W. E. Hanby, in: "*Synthetic Polypeptides*", Academic Press., New York, 1956; p. 62.
35. M. Szwarc, Adv. Polym. Sci., **4**, 1 (1965).
36. I. E. Muskat, J. Amer. Chem. Soc., **56**, 2449 (1934).
37. V. A. Derevitskaya. M. Prokof'eva & Z. A. Rogovin, Zh. Obshch. Khim., **28**, 1368 (1958); Chem. Abst., **52**, 17698i.
38. C. A. Harris & C. B. Purves, Paper Trade J., **110**, 29 (1940); Chem. Abst. **34**, 25873.
39. R. F. Schwenker, Jr., T. Kinoshita, K. Barlingand & E. Pacsu, J. Polym. Sci., **51**, 185 (1961).
40. L. F. Audrieth & J. Kleinberg, in: "*Nonaqueous Solvents*", Wiley & Sons, New York, 1953, p. 111.
41. E. Ott, H. M. Spurin & M. W. Graffin, in "*Cellulose*", Vol. II, 2nd Ed., Interscience publ., New York, 1954, p. 751.
42. D. E. Paul, D. Lipkin & S. I. Weiseman, J. Amer. Chem. Soc., **78**, 116 (1956).
43. Y. Avny & A. Zilka, Europ. Polym. J., **2**, 367 (1966).

44. Y. Avny & A. Zilka, Europ. Polym. J., **2**, 355 (1966).
45. M. Idelson & E. R. Blout, J. Am. Chem. Soc., **79**, 3948 (1957).
46. M. Goodman & E. Peggion, Pure & Appl. Chem., **53**, 699 (1981).
47. Y. Imanishi, Pure & Appl. Chem., **53**, 715 (1981).
48. H. Sekiguchi, Pure & Appl. Chem., **53**, 1689 (1981).
49. H. J. Harwood, Polym. Preprints, **25** (1), 212 (1984).
50. K. Kurita, M. Kanari & Y. Koyama, Polym. Bull., **14**, 511 (1985).
51. T. Miyamoto, S.-I. Takahashi, S.-I. Tsuji, H. Ito & H. Inagaki, J. Appl. Polym. Sci., **31**, 2303 (1986).
52. D. J. Dawson, R. D. Gless & R. E. Wingard, Jr., J. Amer. Chem. Soc., **98**, 5996 (1976).
53. Y. Yamashita, Polym. Preprints, **16** (1), 429 (1975).
54. Y. Imanishi, T. Kimura & T. Higashimura, Polymer, **22**, 1407 (1981).
55. M. Maeda, Y. Nitadori & T. Tsuruta, Makromol. Chem., **181**, 2251 (1980).
56. M. Maeda & S. Inoue, Makromol. Chem., Rapid. Comm., **2**, 537 (1981).
57. M. Kimura, T. Egashira, T. Nishimura, M. Maeda & S. Inoue, Makromol. Chem., **183**, 1393 (1982).
58. D.-W. Chung, S. Higuchi, M. Maeda & S. Inoue, J. Amer. Chem. Soc., **108**, 5823 (1986).
59. M. Maeda, M. Aoyama & S. Inoue, Makromol. Chem., **187**, 2137 (1986).
60. S. Higuchi, T. Mozawa, M. Maeda & S. Inoue, Macromolecules, **19**, 2263 (1986).
61. S. Inoue & Y. Kawano, Makromol. Chem., **180**, 1405 (1979).
62. M. Takaki, R. Asami, M. Ichigawa & T. Ichie, Kobunshi Ronbunshi, **40**, 703 (1983); Chem. Abst., **100**, 156970k.
63. H. Kiba, Jpn. Kokai Tokyo Koho, JP 62,38238, 19 Feb., 1987; Chem. Abst., **106**, 158442n.
64. H. Kiniwa, Y. Doi, T. Nishikaji & N. Ogata, Nippon Kagaku Kaishi, 3, 460 (1987); Chem. Abst., **106**, 206954e.
65. H. Kiniwa, T. Nishikaji & N. Ogata, J. Polym. Sci., Polym. Chem., **25**, 2689 (1987).
66. H. Kiniwa, T. Nishikaji & N. Ogata, Makromol. Chem., **188**, 1841; **188**, 1851 (1987).
67. H. Kiniwa, T. Nishikaji & N. Ogata, J. Polym. Sci., Polym. Chem., **25**, 2953 (1987).
68. M. P. Scheider & H. Bippi, J. Amer. Chem. Soc., **102**, 7363 (1980).
69. Y. Okamoto, S. Honda, I. Okamoto, H. Yuki, S. Murata, R. Noyori & H. Takaya, J. Amer. Chem. Soc., **103**, 6971 (1981).
70. W. H. Pirkle, J. M. Finn, J. L. Schneider & B. C. Hamper, J. Amer. Chem. Soc., **103**, 3964 (1981).
71. S. Allenmark, B. Bomgren & H. Boren, J. Chromatography, **264**, 63 (1983).
72. N. Oi & H. Kitahara, J. Chromatography, **265**, 117 (1983).
73. Y. Okamoto, M. Kawashima, K. Yamamoto & K. Hatada, Chem. Lett., 5, 739 (1984).
74. Y. Okamoto, M. Kawashima & K. Hatada, J. Amer. Chem. Soc., **106**, 5357 (1984).
75. W. H. Pirkle, C. J. Welch, G. S. Mahler, A. I. Meyer, L. M. Fuentes & M. Boes, J. Org. Chem., **49**, 2504 (1984).
76. Y. Okamoto, M. Kawashima, R. Abratani, K. Hatada, T. Nishiyama & M. Masuda, Chem. Lett., 7, 1237 (1986).
77. W. R. Penrose, R. Zand & D. L. Oxender, J. Biol. Chem., **245**, 1432 (1970).
78. M. Maeda, M. Kimura, Y. Hareyama & S. Inoue, J. Amer. Chem. Soc., **106**, 251 (1984).
79. K. Kataoka, M. Maeda, T. Nishimura, Y. Nitadori, T. Tsuruta, T. Akaike & Y. Sakurai, J. Biomed. Mater. Res., **14**, 817 (1980).
80. W. H. Daly & A. Munir, J. Polym. Sci. Chem. Ed., **22**, 975 (1984).
81. W. H. Daly, Soo Lee, & C. Rungaroonthaikul in: "*Chemical Reactions on*

Polymers", J. Benham and J. Kinstle, Eds., ACS Symposium Series, 394, Washington, D.C., 1988; Chapter 1.

82. J. V. Crivello, J. Org. Chem., **46**, 3056 (1981).
83. W. D. Fuller, M. S. Verlander & M. Goodman, Biopolymers, **15**, 1869 (1976).
84. J. S. Balcerski, E. S. Pysh, G. M. Bonora & C. Toniolo, J. Amer. Chem. Soc., **98**, 3470 (1976).
85. M. Palumbo, S. D. Rim, G. M. Bonora & C. Toniolo, Makromol. Chem., **177**, 1477 (1976).
86. C. Toniolo & M. Palumbo, Biopolymers, **16**, 219 (1977).
87. R. Katakai, J. C. S. Perkins Trans. I, 905 (1976).
88. T. Ozaki, A. Shoji & M. Furukawa, Makromol. Chem., **183**, 781 (1982).
89. A. Riveiro, R.F. Saltman & M. Goodman, Biopolymers, **19**, 1771 (1980).
90. J. A. Ferretti & B. W. Ninhan, Macromolecules, **3**, 30 (1970).
91. H. Block, "*Poly(γ-benzyl-L-glutamate) and Other Glutamic Acid Containing Polymers*", Gordon and Breach, New York, 1983; p. 56.
92. A. Kidera, M. Mochizuki, R. Hasegawa, T. Hayashi, H. Sato, A. Nakajima, R. A. Fredrickson, S. P. Powers, S. Lee & H. A. Sheraga; Macromolecules, **16**, 162 (1983) and references mentioned therein.
93. Y. Kobayashi, F. Cardinaux, B. O. Zweifel & H. A. Scheraga, Macromolecules, **10**, 1271 (1977).

RADIATION AND PHOTOCHEMICAL METHODS FOR SYNTHESIZING NOVEL BIOACTIVE POLYMERS FOR MEDICAL APPLICATIONS

P. Dworjanyn and J. L. Garnett

School of Chemistry
The University of South Wales
Kensington, N.S.W. Australia 2033

The use of ionizing radiation and ultraviolet to synthesize polymers possessing novel structures is becoming
increasingly important in a wide variety of fields. The concept is particularly useful in grafting reactions where specific groups can be incorporated into polymers in a one-step
process for the subsequent attachment of biologically active
molecules, such as enzymes, etc. In all of this work, the
ability to lower the exposure of the polymer system to radiation during the grafting reaction is valuable for both the
ionizing radiation and the photochemical systems. The development of additives for this purpose has been extensive over
the past ten years. Thus, inorganic acids, salts and polyfunctional monomers in additive amounts (1%) can enhance UV
and radiation grafting of monomers to backbone polymers. In
this paper, the effect of specific organic compounds as additives for increasing the grafting yields is discussed and
compared with the enhancement properties of earlier additives. Styrene in methanol has been used as the representative monomer with the polyolefins and cellulose as the typical backbone polymers in the presence of ionizing radiation
and ultraviolet light. The mechanism of the additive effect
and its possible use in the synthesis of polymers capable of
immobilizing bioactive materials is discussed.

INTRODUCTION

The ability to incorporate functional groups into polymers to permit
the attachment of molecules of biological significance is of value in a
wide variety of medical applications, e.g. slow drug release, enzyme
immobilization etc.[1-3] Techniques involving ionizing radiation and photochemical procedures are becoming increasingly important as initiators for
these processes, both grafting[4-7] and direct irradiation[6] being employed
to achieve the required polymer properties. In these radiation processes,
methods for reducing the total dose absorbed by the substrate are continuously being investigated especially for ionizing radiation work where
excess exposure may result in appreciable degradation of components in
the system.

275

In the present paper, the use of novel additives for reducing the dose required to achieve a particular percentage graft in both ionizing radiation and UV systems will be discussed. In particular, the value of specific organic compounds as additives for this work will be reported for the first time. Previously inorganic acids[6] and certain inorganic salts[8] were found to enhance both radiation and UV grafting of monomers to backbone polymers. Inclusion of polyfunctional monomers (PFMs) in additive amounts in these monomer solutions resulted in synergistic effects in grafting.[9] The ramifications of all of these additive effects will be considered in the preparation of graft copolymers, especially for the synthesis of novel bioactive polymers for medical application.

EXPERIMENTAL

The following modifications of previously reported grafting methods were used.[6] For the gamma irradiation work, all grafting experiments were performed in pyrex tubes (15 x 2.5 cm) with styrene/solvent solutions (20 mL) at 20°C. The trunk polymer films (4 x 2.5 cm) were fully immersed in the monomer solutions and the pyrex tubes stoppered for irradiation, which was performed immediately after preparation in a cobalt-60 source. The pyrex tubes were uniformly positioned on a circular rack around the source such as that the polymer films were perpendicular to the plane of the radiation. At the completion of the grafting, the films were immediately removed from solution, washed in an appropriate solvent to remove trapped homopolymer and extracted in a soxhlet apparatus for 72 hours. If acid had been used as additive, the films were washed with methanol/dioxane (1:1) prior to soxhlet treatment. With the polyolefin films at high graft of polystyrene (>50%), the films were soaked in chloroform at 50°C for a further 3 hours after soxhlet extraction to ensure complete removal of homopolymer. The films were dried in air, then at 45°C to constant weight.

For the UV studies, sample solutions (monomer/solvent, 20mL) were prepared in pyrex tubes, as before with the gamma irradiation system, and the tubes positioned on a motor driven ventilated circulating drum at a distance of 24 cm, unless otherwise stated, from the UV source (90W, high pressure Hg type 93110E E_2, Philips). The polymer films were so positioned that, during irradiation, the surfaces of the films were perpendicular to the incident radiation. After irradiation, films were treated as for the gamma work.

RESULTS AND DISCUSSION

When styrene in methanol is photografted to polyethylene film, inclusion of acid leads to a significant enhancement in graft at almost all monomer concentrations studied (Table 1). The increase in yield is particularly evident with the monomer solution corresponding to the Trommsdorff peak (35%). If mineral acid is replaced by a lithium salt such as the perchlorate, a similar enhancement in copolymerization yield is observed, however, the pattern of the variation in grafting increase with monomer concentration is different from that of the acid. The replacement of UV with ionizing radiation from a cobalt-60 source as initiator for the same grafting reaction leads to analogous grafting enhancement with both acid and lithium perchlorate additives, the increase in yield being significant at the lower monomer concentrations.

276

Table 1. Ultraviolet and radiation grafting of styrene in methanol to polyethylene using acid and lithium perchlorate as additives.

Styrene in methanol (% v/v)	Graft (%)					
	UV (a)			Radiation (b)		
	N.A.	H+ (0.05 m)	Li+ (0.1 m)	N.A.	H+ (0.05 m)	Li+ (0.1 m)
15	6	5	9	34	42	28
20	8	14	16	60	77	68
25	10	16	28	78	140	122
30	17	25	31	142	160	102
35	20	35	24	139	116	91
40	19	24	17	119	92	80

(a) For UV work, low density polyethylene film (0.12 mm) was irradiated for 10 hrs. at 24 cm from a 90 w lamp using benzoin ethyl ether (1 % w/v) as sensitizer at 20°C with sulfuric acid.

(b) For ionizing radiation work, irradiation in air at a dose rate of 3.3×10^4 rad/hr to a total dose of 1.8×10^5 rad at 20°C.

When cellulose replaced polyethylene as backbone polymer, similar acid and lithium perchlorate additive effects are observed for the grafting of styrene in methanol under both UV and ionizing radiation conditions (Table 2). Cellulose is less reactive than polyethylene in these copolymerization reactions, thus higher UV and radiation doses are required with cellulose to achieve yields comparable to those observed with polyethylene. The fact that both cellulose and polyethylene exhibit these additive effects, as do other backbone polymers,[1,6] indicates that the phenomenon is of general application in these grafting processes.

In early studies of the role of acid in these reactions,[6] the enhancement effect was attributed to increased hydrogen atom yields leading to the creation of more grafting sites. The more recent discovery of the lithium salt effect and more extensive work on the mechanism of the reaction, especially UV grafting, has indicated that both acid and salt effects in UV and ionizing radiation grafting systems can be explained by the following model, using cellulose as representative polymer system.

In any grafting system at one time, there is an equilibrium concentration of monomer absorbed within the grafting region of the backbone polymer. This grafting region may be continually changing as grafting proceeds. Thus, in grafting styrene to cellulose, during the initial part of the reaction, the grafting region will be initially cellulosic in nature; however, as the reaction proceeds, the grafting region becomes more styrenated. The degree to which monomer is absorbed by the grafting

Table 2. Ultraviolet and radiation grafting of styrene in methanol to cellulose using acid and lithium perchlorate as additives.

Styrene in methanol (% v/v)	Graft (%)					
	UV (a)			Radiation (b)		
	N.A.	H+	LiClO₄	N.A.	H+	LiClO₄
15	–	–	–	32	34	54
20	11	23	38	66	120	155
25	–	–	–	106	153	159
30	25	20	41	112	95	96
35	–	–	–	110	60	80
40	32	18	38	82	52	72

(a) For UV work, cellulose (Whatman No. 41 filter paper) irradiated for 15 hrs. at 24 cm from 90 W lamp at 20°C with benzoin ethyl ether (1% w/v) sensitizer and sulfuric acid (0.1 m), lithium perchlorate (0.2 m).

(b) For ionizing radiation work, irradiation in air at a dose rate of 3.3×10^4 rad/hr to a total dose of 5.0×10^5 rad at 20°C.

region will therefore depend on the chemical structure of the region at the specific time of grafting. Experimental information currently available indicates that increased partitioning of monomer occurs in the graft region when ionic salts are dissolved in the bulk grafting solution. Thus, higher concentrations of monomer are available for grafting at a particular backbone polymer site. Partitioning depends on the polarities of monomer, substrate, and solvent, and also on the concentration of ionic solute. Metal salts such as LiClO₄ are more effective than acids in enhancing photografting due to the overall monomer partitioning effect. It is thus the effect of these ionic solutes on partitioning which is predominantly responsible for the observed increase in photografting yields in the presence of these additives. Because of the complexity of the effect, it is obvious that processes based on changes in physical parameters of the backbone polymer, especially with substrates such as cellulose, will also contribute to the overall mechanism of the salt additive effect, but these contributions will be of minor significance compared with the partitioning process.

Support for the above model is provided by the data in Table 3 where an organic additive, urea, is shown to enhance the photografting of styrene and methanol to polypropylene significantly. This is the first report of the use of an organic additive for this purpose. Interestingly, in preliminary experiments, thiourea does not exhibit the same enhancement properties as urea in these reactions, presumably due to strong complex between the monomer and the additive, the resulting complex being sterically limited in the diffusion process. The other important result in Table 3 is that a flow additive (FC-430, a fluorinated alkyl ester) which is frequently used in UV curable surface coatings also enhances the

Table 3. Effect of urea and flow additive (FC-430) on UV grafting of styrene in methanol to polypropylene.

Styrene (% v/v)	Graft (%) (a)		
	N.A.	Urea	Urea + FC-430 (b)
20	0	0	0
30	0	30	23
40	0	46	53
50	0	19	16
60	0	13	19
70	0	11	10

(a) Irradiation 8hrs. at 24 cm from 90 W lamp using benzoin ethyl ether (1% w/v) as sensitizer with polypropylene film (0.06 mm). No graft formed without a sensitizer.

(b) Fluorinated alkyl ester from 3M company.

grafting at two monomer concentrations. This observation suggests that during UV curing of monomer mixtures containing FC-430, concurrent grafting will be enhanced, thus improving the properties of the finished film.

Finally when polyfunctional monomers such as divinylbenzene (DVB) are used in additive amounts (1% v/v) in the acid grafting solutions, synergistic effects in grafting yield are observed, both acid and DVB enhancing grafting by different mechanistic pathways (Table 4). Thus with polyfunctional monomers, such as DVB, in additive amounts, branching of the grafted polystyrene can occur when one end of the DVB, anchored during grafting, is bonded to the growing chain. The other end is saturated and free to initiate new chain growth. Grafting is thus enhanced mainly through the branching of the grafted polystyrene chain.

Overall, in terms of the use of the current range of additives in grafting work, especially for biological applications, the present work is important since there is now a wider range of additives posing different physical properties which can be successfully used in a preparation context. In this respect each of the additives acts in a complementary fashion. Thus acid cannot be used with acid sensitive backbone polymers and lithium salts have limited solubilities in the grafting solutions. In such systems, the discovery of urea as a new additive for enhancing grafting can be of significant benefit.

ACKNOWLEDGMENT

The authors thank the Australian Institute of Nuclear Science and Engineering and the Australian Research Grants Committee for the support of this research.

Table 4. Synergistic effect of acid with polyfunctional monomers in the radiation grafting of styrene to polyethylene. (a)

Styrene in methanol (% v/v)	Graft (%)			
	N.A.	H$_2$SO$_4$ (0.2 m)	DVB (1% v/v)	DVB + H$_2$SO$_4$
20	14	19	15	27
30	37	51	41	58
40	76	81	74	119
50	109	134	136	188
60	89	119	121	156
70	89	73	–	112

(a) Irradiated to 2.4×10^5 rad at dose of 4.1×10^4 rad/hr. with divinylbenzene (DVB). Film as in Table 1.

REFERENCES

1. C. H. Ang, J. L. Garnett, R. Levot & M. A. Long, J. Macromol. Sci.-Chem., **A17**, 87 (1982).
2. I. Kaetsu, Radiat. Phys. Chem., **25**, 517 (1985).
3. A. S. Hoffman & B. D. Ratner, Radiat. Phys. Chem., **14**, 831 (1979).
4. V. Stannett, "*Graft Polymerization of Ligocellulose Fibers*", D. N.-S. Hon, Ed., Am. Chem. Soc. Symp. Ser. 187, Am. Chem. Soc., Washington, DC, 1982, p. 3.
5. A. Hebeish and J. T. Guthrie, "*The Chemistry and Technology of Cellulosic Copolymers*", Springer-Verlag, Berlin, 1980.
6. J. L. Garnett, Radiat. Phys. Chem., **14**, 79 (1979).
7. J. C. Arthur, Jr., "*Graft Polymerization of Lignocellulose Fibers*", D. N.-S. Hon, Ed., Am. Chem. Soc. Symp, Ser. 187, Am. Chem. Soc., Washington, DC, 1982, p. 21.
8. J. L. Garnett, S. V. Jankiewicz, M. A. Long & D. F. Sangster, J. Polymer Sci., Polym. Lett., 23, 563, (1985).
9. C. H. Ang, J. L. Garnett, R. Levot & M. A. Long, J. Polym. Sci., Polym. Lett., **21**, 257 (1983).

SURFACE TREATMENT OF PMMA WITH POLYVINYLPYRROLIDONE AND A TITANIUM COMPOUND AND ITS EFFECT ON BLOOD COMPATIBILITY

Debra A. Wrobleski,[a] David L. Cash,[a] Norman Elliott,[a] Ram Kossowsky,[c] Jerry E. London,[b] Bruce E. Lehnert,[b] & David V. Duchane[a]

(a) Material and Technology Division and
(b) Life Sciences Division
     Los Alamos National Laboratory
     Los Alamos, NM 87545
(c) Penn State University
     State College, PA 16801

The surfaces of poly(methyl methacrylate) (PMMA) have been modified through a chemical infusion process by treatment of the sample with a solution containing varying amounts of titanium (IV) isopropoxide and poly(vinylpyrrolidone) (PVP). The resulting sample is modified in the outermost 150–325 micron region while the underlying polymeric material is unchanged. The chemical infusion process, a solvent based surface modification technique, is described in detail along with a study correlating treatment conditions with penetration depth. The treated samples were characterized by scanning electron microscopy, optical microscopy, and neutron activation analysis. These samples were evaluated for blood compatibility using two biological assays: (1) an adherence assay in which the adherence of human polymorphonuclear leukocytes to the samples was determined, and (2) a dynamic hemolysis assay using rat blood erythrocytes to determine the hemolytic activity of the samples. Based on the results of these assays, the PMMA samples treated with PVP alone resulted in an improvement in reactivity with the blood cells in a manner comparable to Tecoflex[R], a commercially available polymer with relatively benign characteristics.

INTRODUCTION

Polymeric materials are used in a wide range of medical applications, because of their unique physical properties such as strength, elasticity, and pliability. A potential application could include small diameter vascular implants if one of the major problems of polymeric biomaterials in contact with blood, thrombus formation,[1] could be overcome. Although the underlying processes are not completely understood, an initial step in the thrombogenic sequence is the adsorption of plasma proteins to the surface of a material followed by adhesion of platelets and/or leukocytes.[2,3] The extent of thrombosis, in turn, is related to the

281

surface properties of the polymer exposed to blood. The properties recognized as contributing to thrombosis include surface charge and polarity, surface energy, hydrophilicity, chemical composition, and surface roughness.[4] Due to the detrimental consequences of one or more of these surface properties, even the best commercially available polymers continue to show limited blood compatibility.[5]

Approaches to modify the surfaces of polymers by heparinization[6] (coating the surface with the polysaccharide heparin) or biolization[7] (coating with a denatured natural polymer like albumin) have shown promise, although the question of long term stability has limited the use of such preparations in prostheses.[8] Our approach to surface modification uses a technique originally intended to smooth polymer surfaces, the chemical infusion process.[9,10] This technique can introduce normally insoluble materials into the outermost layer of a polymeric material, thereby, altering the surface without changing its bulk physical properties. Using this process, we decided to impregnate a polymeric surface with biocompatible materials in our attempt to improve its blood compatibility.

Poly(vinylpyrrolidone) (PVP) and titanium dioxide were selected as target materials for incorporation in the polymer's surface in that it could potentially provide a non-thrombogenic surface. PVP was chosen in our experiments because of its intrinsic blood compatibility. The synthesis of PVP was developed in Germany during the late nineteen thirties. It was used extensively as a blood plasma substitute or blood volume expander during World War II by the German army and is responsible for saving thousands of lives.[11,12] In fact, a follow-up study of people who had received transfusions of PVP solution showed no permanent kidney or liver damage.[13] Moreover, this polymer has been used as a retardant vehicle in the administration of antibiotics and other drugs (e.g., PVP causes penicillin to be retained in the blood stream longer) thereby reducing the frequency of injections necessary.[11] Therefore, because of its benign nature, PVP showed promise as a material for further investigation.

Titanium dioxide was considered as a potential material for incorporation into the polymer's surface because of the unusually low bioreactivity and non-toxic nature of titanium in soft tissue which is attributed to the high thermodynamic stability of the protective surface oxide.[14-17] Moreover, in a study of the dielectric properties of various cardiovascular implant materials, strong correlations were found between materials that demonstrate antithrombogenicity and their dielectric constants.[18] Exposure of these material surfaces to blood proteins produced pronounced electrokinetic and dielectric charge. This bioelectric charge transfer was believed to be crucial in determining thrombosis. It has also been proposed that intrinsic electroconduction and semiconduction might be involved in the biocompatibility of materials.[19] Therefore, titanium dioxide with its high thermodynamic stability, low reactivity, and high dielectric constant of the order of 110 may provide a stable, low thrombogenic surface on polymer surfaces.

One of the characteristics of the infusion technique is that the materials entrapped in the surface may slowly diffuse out of the infused layer if they are volatile or highly mobile. One way to change permanently the surface is to employ polymeric infusant materials that may become chain entangled with the host polymer or to use soluble infusant compounds that can be chemically transformed into an insoluble material that is unable to diffuse into the surrounding solution. We have explored both of these methods by examining the infusion of poly(vinylpyrrolidone) (PVP) and titanium (IV) isopropoxide (which readily converts into titanium dioxide) into a poly(methyl methacrylate) (PMMA) substrate. Our initial results, in terms of how such modifications of the PMMA affect blood cell interactions, are presented here.

EXPERIMENTAL

1. Chemical Infusion

A. Materials and Methods. PMMA: Plexiglas VM[R] was purchased from Rohm & Haas (Philadelphia, PA) and injection molded into a disk shape, 26 mm in diameter and 3.2 mm thick. The diameter was machined back to 22.2 mm and cleaned in a soap solution followed by several rinses with deionized water. The samples were air dried prior to use. Titanium (IV) isopropoxide and poly(vinylpyrrolidone), (PVP, molecular weight 10,000) were purchased from Aldrich Chemical, Co. The former was used as received while PVP was dried at 80°C for 24 hours in vacuo prior to solution preparation. Baker reagent grade isopropyl alcohol (IPA) and acetone were dried over Drierite[R], distilled, and handled under argon. All solutions containing titanium were prepared under an atmosphere of anhydrous argon.

B. Procedure. Two solutions are required for the chemical infusion process. The diluent solution was prepared by addition of titanium (IV) isopropoxide to a 35% solution PVP (w/w) in IPA. The amount of titanium (IV) isopropoxide was varied from 0 to 50% by weight. The starting solution was prepared by adding 35% acetone by weight to the diluent solution. The infusion system (pictured in Figure 1) is initially charged with this starting solution. The apparatus consists of two glass tubes connected by silicone tubing. In order to ensure complete mixing, the solution in one tube is mechanically stirred or statically stirred by addition of 2 mm glass beads to the mixing tube while the other tube holds the samples. The PMMA sample disks are mounted in a series of ring-like retainers. The rings are fabricated from Kovar (29% Ni, 17% Co, 54% Fe), linked together with nylon mono-filament line, and suspended in the solution from a rubber septum. One peristaltic pump circulates the solution in the infusion chamber while a second pump adds the diluent solution in small increments. In this manner, the solution in the apparatus gradually becomes richer in diluent. The total volume of 325 mL for the system requires about 7 hours dilution time at a rate of 2 mL/min for complete replacement of the starting solution with the diluent. The final solution contains greater than 95% diluent. Upon removal from the final solution, the samples were rinsed with IPA or deionized water for samples with or without titanium in the diluent solution, respectively. With this approach, samples were prepared from diluent solutions containing PVP with concentrations of 0, 10, 20, 40, and 50% titanium (IV) isopropoxide.

C. Sample Characterization. The treated samples were examined by optical microscopy, scanning electron microscopy, and neutron activation analysis (NAA). Samples were cross-sectioned and cut to an appropriate size for analysis by means of a cut-off wheel equipped with a diamond wafering blade. Cross-sections of the samples were examined by optical microscopy and with a Nikon Profile Projector, H-14B, to determine the depth of infusion. Samples for scanning electron microscopy were cross-sectioned, mounted in epoxy, and polished. The prepared samples were analyzed with a Hitachi Model S-520LB scanning electron microscope. Digital integration of the Ti X-ray signal from a lithium drifted, silicon detector was performed. Each image was integrated approximately 6-8 hours. Samples for NAA were cut in a rectangular shape (approx. 15 x 7 mm). The analytical results were calibrated against NBS coal calibration standard #1632A with a certified value of 1750 ppm for titanium

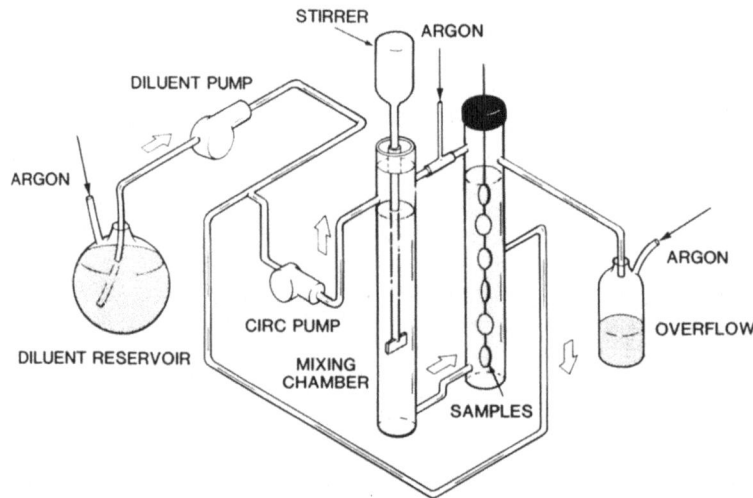

Figure 1. Schematic of the chemical infusion apparatus used
for infusion of moisture sensitive additives such
as titanium (IV) isopropoxide.

and NBS fly ash calibration standard #1633A with a value of 0.8% for
titanium.

2. Biological Assays

A. Testing Chamber. The blood testing chamber shown in Figure 2 consists of eight cylindrical wells machined into a Teflon[R] block. Flat
disks (22.2 mm X 3.2 mm) of the material of interest are placed in the
bottom of the Teflon[R] ports, then an inner sleeve of Tecoflex[R], a commercially available biocompatible polyurethane, is placed in the port to
secure the disk and contain the test cell suspensions. The cylindrical
sleeves were prepared by injection molding Tecoflex[R] EG 60D purchased
from Thermedics, Inc., Woburn, MA. The screw cap can be tightened with a
torque wrench to a torque of 7 inch-ounces in order to provide a uniform
pressure on the test disks so that distortion of the samples and leakage
are minimized or prevented, respectively. Aliquots of suspensions of
blood cellular constituents may be added to the chamber to assay interactions of the blood components with the test samples.

B. Leukocyte Adherence Assay. Human polymorphonuclear neutrophils
(PMN) were isolated from whole blood using Neutrophil Isolation Medium,
(Los Alamos Diagnostics, Los Alamos, NM) according to procedures provided
by the supplier. The isolated cells were washed in divalent cation-free
phosphate buffered saline (PBS, pH = 7.3) and contaminating erythrocytes
were lysed by hypotonic shock. Thereafter, the PMN were adjusted to a
concentration of 3.6×10^5/mL in 0.5% bovine serum albumin (Sigma Chem.
Co., St. Louis. MO) in minimum essential medium buffered with 3-(N-mor-
pholino)propane sulfonic acid (pH = 7.3). Routinely, greater than 90% of
the cells were PMN and the viabilities of the cells ascertained by trypan
blue exclusion exceeded 95%. The cell adherence assay procedure was a
modified version of that previously described by Lehnert and Ferin.[20] One
mL of the PMN suspension was placed in the test chamber, Figure 2, with
the polymer disk being tested mounted in the bottom of a well. The sample
disks were secured in place as described above. The test chamber was pre-
warmed to 37°C in a water bath (Hotpack Shaker) before the cells were

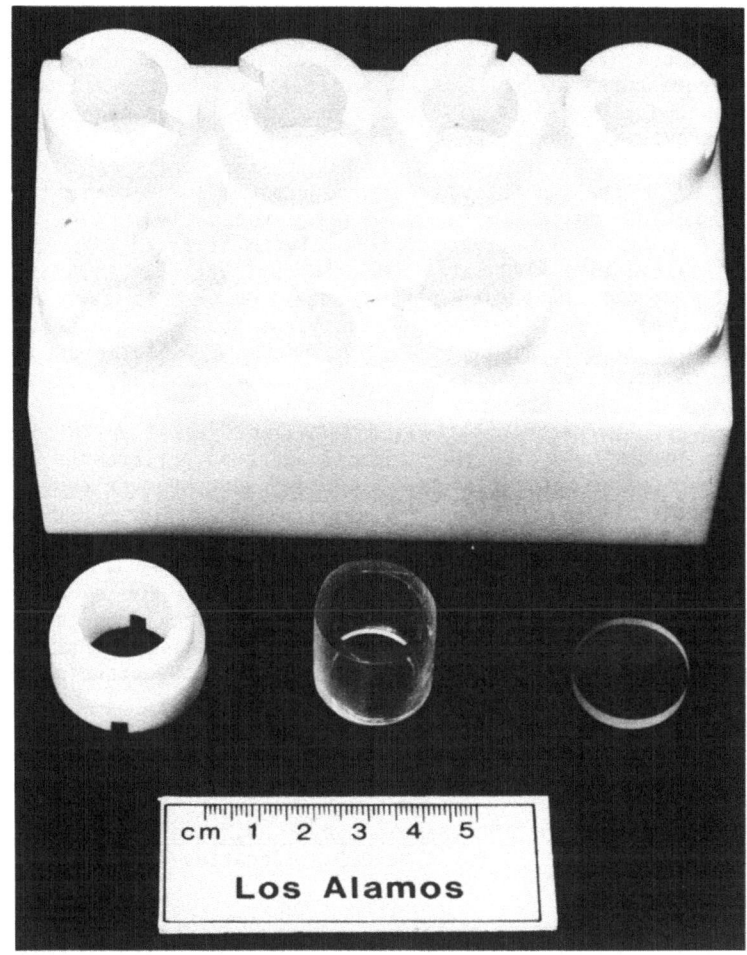

Figure 2. The Teflon[R] blood testing chamber with eight cylindrical sample wells. From left to right, a threaded cap, Tecoflex[R] sleeve, and a sample disk are shown in front.

added. Following the addition of the cells, the chamber was maintained in the water bath for 30 min. After the 30 min period, the chambers were oscillated for 50 sec. at 1.8 Hz. The culture fluids containing nonadherent cells were aspirated with a pipette from the test chambers and placed in test tubes on ice. Adherent cells were calculated from the total number of cells initially added to each well minus the nonadherent cell numbers following the oscillation phase of the assay.

C. Hemolysis Assay. The hemolysis of erythrocytes was quantitated spectrophotometrically using a modification of the hemolysis assay described by Harington and colleagues[21] and red blood cells obtained from adult, male, specific-pathogen-free Fischer-344 rats. Rat whole blood was collected from pentobarbital sodium-anesthetized animals by cardiac puncture and subsequently placed in glass tubes containing the anti-coagulant ethylenediamine tetraacetic acid. The blood cells were washed three times with PBS and the buffer layer was removed following each centrifugation cycle (5-7 min at 400g). The washed erythrocytes were then resuspended to a nominal 1% initial concentration. Routinely, 1 mL aliquots of these daily erythrocyte suspensions were mixed with 4 mL of distilled water and the absorbance (Beckman Model DUR, Fullerton, CA) of the lysed preparations was measured at 530 nm. All original suspension volumes were further adjusted with PBS to give a standardized 0.3 absorbance units reading, as previously described.[21,22]

One mL of the red blood cell suspensions was placed in a chamber well, Figure 2, containing a given sample disk. For each sample disk type, 4-8 disks were analyzed for hemolytic activity. The test samples were maintained in a 37°C water bath and oscillated at 1.2 Hz for 60 min. After the 60 min incubation period, the fluids from each chamber well were aspirated, transferred to polypropylene tubes, and centrifuged for 5 min at 400 g in order to remove intact erythrocytes. The absorbencies of the supernatants were determined at 530 nm, as previously indicated. PBS only was used as a reference blank. Positive control for 100% hemolysis consisted of supernatants retrieved from water-lysed erythrocyte pellets that were centrifuged from the original adjusted erythrocyte suspensions. Other controls consisted of 1 mL aliquots of erythrocyte suspensions that were incubated in glass tubes with particulate silica (Min-U-SilR) at a mass concentration of 2.5 mg/mL. These samples were also incubated in the water bath at 37°C for 60 min while being oscillated in the same manner as the test chamber containing the disks. Controls for spontaneous hemolysis due to normal cell fragility (negative control) consisted of supernatants from red blood cell suspensions that were maintained in polypropylene tubes and processed in the same manner as the other samples.

The percent hemolysis in the various sample preparations was calculated from the following relationship, where O.D. is the optical density:

$$\% \text{ Hemolysis} = \frac{100 \, [\text{Sample O.D.} - \text{Negative Control O.D.}]}{\text{Positive O.D.} - \text{Negative Control O.D.}}$$

RESULTS AND DISCUSSION

The chemical infusion process was first developed to smooth the surfaces of PMMA rod for use as mandrels for physical vapor deposition of thin metal foils. This technique requires selection of an appropriate solvent for the polymer to act as the solvent component. A second solvent is chosen as a poor solvent for the polymer and will be referred to as the non-solvent component. The non-solvent component must be miscible with the solvent and any additives must be initially soluble in the solvent/non-solvent mixture. This starting solution causes the polymer matrix to swell and, thereby, facilitates the diffusion of the insoluble additives into the treated sector. As the infusion process proceeds, the initial solution is gradually replaced with the non-solvent mixture until the solution consists of greater than 95% diluent. During this latter phase of the process, the solvent diffuses out of the polymer, which results in the restoration of the polymer's surface rigidity. At the end of the process, the polymer samples are removed from the bath, rinsed with the non-solvent to remove additives adsorbed on the surface, and allowed to dry.

The proper combination of solvent, non-solvent, and polymeric additive must be selected, in order to smooth a polymer's surface. The first solvent system that gave a smooth surface was a solution containing poly-(ethylene glycol) (PEG), water, and acetone. In addition to smoothing the surface, it was noted that the additives (PEG and water) were incorporated in the sample. This was observed as the weight gain of the sample,

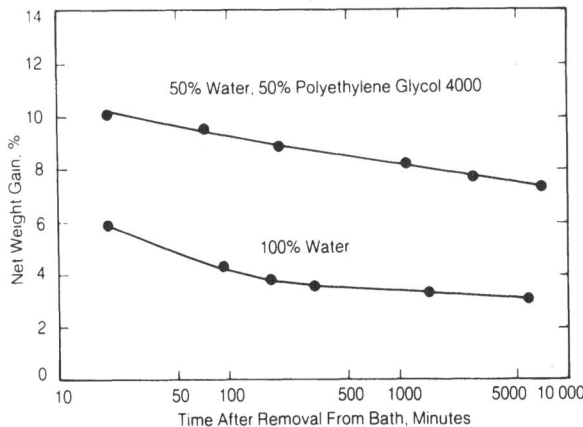

Figure 3. Plot of net weight gain (%) in 1/4" PMMA rod versus
time elapsed after removal from the final treatment
solution. Data is indicated for an infusion experiment in which PMMA is treated with a diluent solution containing 50%/50% water/poly(ethylene glycol)
(above) and 100% water (below).

Figure 3. During the first day after removal from the bath, a weight loss
was observed, which most likely was due to evaporation of the volatile
components such as the acetone and water used in the treatment bath. As
indicated in Figure 3, the sample treated with water alone had an overall
weight gain lower than the sample also containing PEG. These observations
demonstrate how polymeric additives or non-volatile materials can be
incorporated in the infused sector. We decided to use this technique in
our attempts to improve the biocompatibility of PMMA surfaces.

In order to demonstrate how uniformly the infusion process modified
the polymer samples, we examined the relationship of the rate of dilution
on the penetration depth of the infusant in the infused sector. The results for a series of infusion experiments with PVP alone are shown in
Table 1. The concentration of the starting solution and diluent solution
for all of these samples, as indicated in the experimental section, were
identical. The only parameter varied was the rate at which the diluent
solution was added to the system. Overall, these studies revealed that
the penetration depth is inversely proportional to the dilution rate.
Thus, the infusion depth can be controlled by regulating the rate of
dilution. Moreover, the infused region is uniformly treated as seen in
the constant value for the percentage weight gain in the infused region.

Table 1. Variation of penetration depth of PVP with dilution
parameters.

Dilution time (min)	Penetration depth (micron)	% Penetration	Total % weight gain	% Weight gain in infused region
530	324	13.7	2.0	14.6
400	288	11.7	1.7	14.6
250	145	5.8	0.82	14.2

The uniform treatment of the infused sector indicates that the process is diffusion controlled and reproducible sample preparations may be expected from the process.

The modification of surfaces required choosing infusion solvents and additives likely to improve their blood compatibility. Poly(vinylpyrrolidone) and titanium dioxide were selected for incorporation in the polymer surface because of the reasons cited previously. Since titanium dioxide is insoluble in all common solvents, a soluble titanium alkoxide compound, titanium (IV) isopropoxide, was chosen as the additive. By preparing solutions with anhydrous solvents, we were able to exploit the hydrolysis reaction indicated in Equation 1 to convert the soluble titanium alkoxide compound into the insoluble titanium dioxide. Because this hydrolysis reaction is very favorable, the infusion apparatus must be rigorously kept free from moisture. Upon infusion of a PMMA sample with a solution containing titanium, the sample becomes opaque. Three samples infused with PVP alone and with PVP and concentrations of 5 and 50% titanium alkoxide in the diluent solution are shown in Figure 4. The opaque nature of these samples can be attributed to the titanium alkoxide being converted into titanium dioxide. By looking at the cross-section of an infused sample, the infused sector can be easily seen; the sample in Figure 5 clearly shows that only the outermost layer is modified during the chemical infusion process.

$$Ti(OR)_4 + 2H_2O \longrightarrow TiO_2 + 4ROH \qquad \text{(Equation 1)}$$

$$\text{Where } R = CH(CH_3)_2$$

The surfaces of the samples containing PVP, both with and without titanium, are much smoother than those without PVP. Deletion of PVP leads to a rough, uneven surface unsuitable for blood interaction studies. We examined cross-sections of samples treated with titanium solutions with and without PVP by scanning electron microscopy. In order to further verify that the titanium was incorporated in the infused sector and to

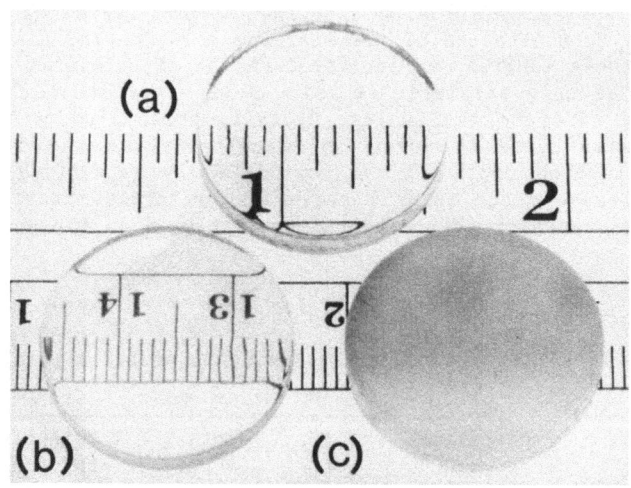

Figure 4. Three PMMA disks after treatment by the chemical infusion process with 35% PVP and (a) 0, (b) 5, and (c) 50% titanium (IV) isopropoxide in the diluent solution.

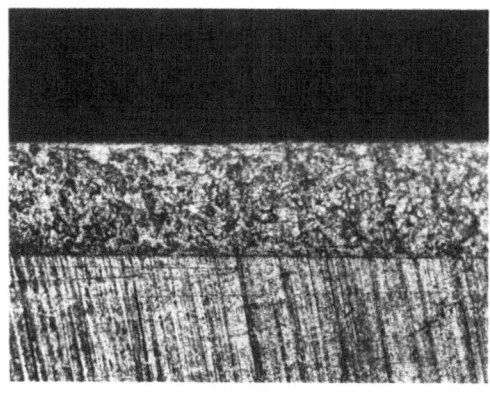

500 µm

Figure 5. Cross section of a PMMA disk treated with a diluent
solution containing 40% titanium (IV) isopropoxide
and 21% PVP at 100x magnification. The top of the
sample is the boundary between the top (dark) and
middle layers. The middle layer corresponds to the
infused sector of 280 µm while the bottom layer is
the untreated polymer. Note the sharp interface
between the infused region and the untreated PMMA
region.

characterize its distribution in the sample, the sample preparations were
examined using energy dispersive X-ray analysis. The results of this
study are shown in Figure 6. The titanium X-ray image, Figure 6b, of the
same area of the sample as the scanning electron micrographs, indicates
that the gray colored regions in the SEM, Figure 6a, correspond to domains of high titanium concentration, whereas the dark regions correspond
to domains of lower titanium concentration. A comparison of the SEM of a
sample treated with titanium along with PVP and without PVP is shown in
Figure 7. There is a significant decrease in particle size between the
sample without PVP and the sample containing PVP. The largest particles
are about 60 µm for the sample without PVP while the largest particle is
about 30 µm with PVP. In addition, the range of particle sizes is greater
without PVP while more uniform particle size is evident with PVP. The PVP
appears to distribute the titanium more uniformly, although a gradient is
observed across the infused sector with smaller particles near the inside
edge and with larger particles in the center of the infused region. This
could be due to PVP aiding in dispersing the water in the polymer, therefore, resulting in a smaller amount of titanium alkoxide being hydrolyzed
to TiO_2 in a given area. Part of the PVP improvement in dispersion is
most likely due to coordination of the pyrrolidone, amide group of PVP to
titanium facilitating formation of smaller particles. This is evident in
the bright, orange color observed in solutions containing PVP and titanium (IV) isopropoxide (colorless) in IPA. Coordination compounds of
Ti^{4+} are often brightly colored.[23] The complexation property of PVP for
pharmaceuticals and toxic chemicals has been recognized in its ability to
complex iodine, thus reducing its oral toxicity while maintaining its
germicidal properties.[11] Most importantly, the overall surface of the
sample is smoother with the PVP additive.

All of the titanium containing samples were subjected to neutron
activation analysis to quantitatively determine the amounts of titanium
incorporated in the infused layers. Samples were prepared as previously

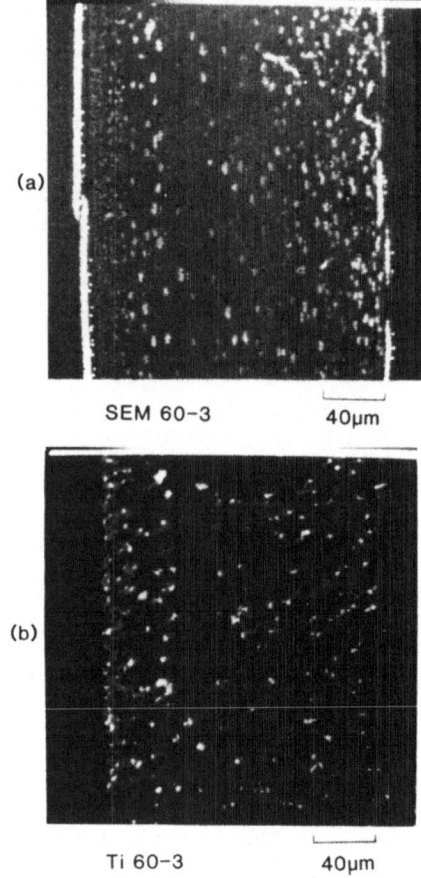

SEM 60-3   40µm

Ti 60-3   40µm

Figure 6. (a) SEM and (b) titanium X-ray image (map) of the
same area of a sample containing PVP and 4.1%
titanium in the infused region. Note the correlation of the gray image (brighter regions) in the
SEM with regions of high titanium concentration in
the Ti X-ray image photo. The solid white lines in
the SEM are artifacts due to cracks in the untreated PMMA sample (left side), separation of the top
of the sample from the mounting epoxy (right side)
and intensity scale (top) and contain no titanium.

described and the percentages of the infused region for each sample were
determined. The results are given in parts per million or µgm of titanium
per gm of sample. Using the percent of the sample which is infused and
the concentration of titanium in the sample, the percent titanium in the
infused sector was estimated. This information is compiled in Table 2
along with the concentration of titanium in the diluent solution. By
plotting the titanium concentration in the diluent solution versus the
concentration of titanium in the infused sector, a linear relationship
with a slope of 0.38 is evident, Figure 8. Accordingly, ~38% of the titanium and diluent solution was incorporated in the infused sector, or
38% of the infused layer and the surface is modified in the process.
Figure 9 illustrates this notion graphically by representing the infusant
modified portion of the infused region with a shaded circle while the
unmodified polymeric domains are represented by open circles. Thus, the
process alters a significant portion of the surface of the polymer. The

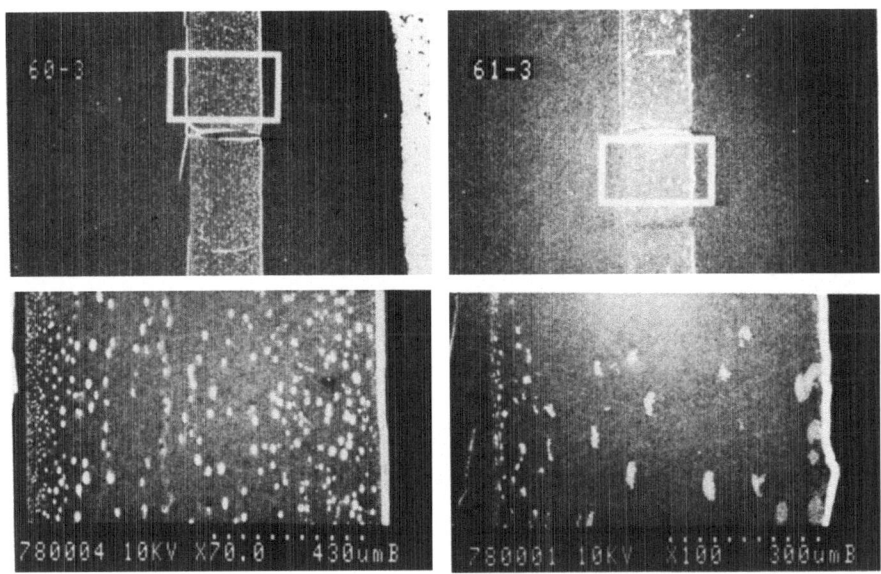

4.2% Ti with PVP   2.1% Ti without PVP

Figure 7. The scanning electron micrographs of two samples
are shown with the mounting epoxy on the right of
the photo, the infused sector in the center, and
the untreated PMMA on the left. The top half of
each photo shows low magnification of the sample
while the region in the white box is shown under
higher magnification in the bottom half of each
photo. The white lines on the right and left side
of each photo correspond to artifacts due to separation of the epoxy from the surface of the
sample and cracks in the PMMA, respectively. The
enhanced dispersion and improved uniformity of size
of the titanium particles in the infused region is
clearly seen when comparing a sample containing PVP
with 4.2% titanium (left) in the infused region
with PMMA samples containing no PVP with 2.1%
titanium (right).

Table 2. Titanium concentration in diluent solution and in
the infused region.

Diluent solution (weight %)		Percent of sample infused	[Ti] in sample (ppm)	[Ti] in infused region (weight %)
[Ti(OPr)$_4$]	[Ti]			
5	0.8	23	250	0.11
10	1.7	19	950	0.51
20	3.4	20	2370	1.2
40	6.7	16	4270	2.6
50	8.4	17	5010	2.9

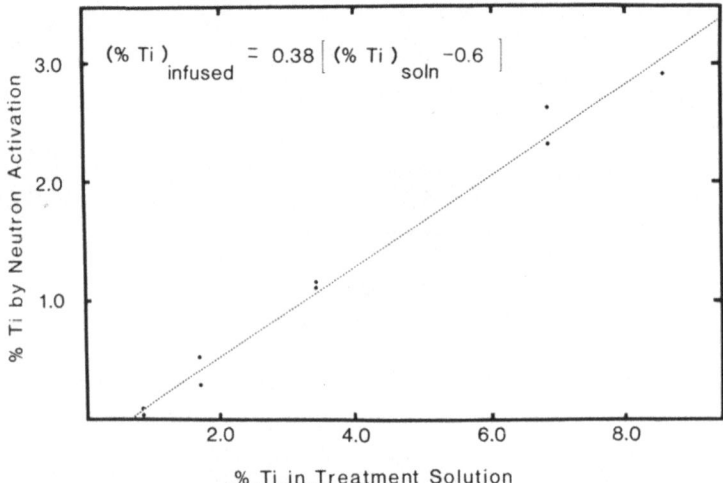

$$(\% \text{ Ti})_{\text{infused}} = 0.38 \left[(\% \text{ Ti})_{\text{soln}} -0.6 \right]$$

.%. Ti.in. Treatment. Solution

Figure 8. Plot of [Ti] in diluent solution versus the [Ti] in
the infused region. The non-zero x-intercept re-
flects a systematic degradation of titanium alkoxide by adsorbed water in the apparatus.

results of the biological assays are an indication of how this infusion
process actually modifies the surface of the polymer.

Infusion of the PMMA samples with titanium (Ti) did not appear to
significantly alter the adherence of human polymorphonuclear leukocytes
(PMN) in a directional manner consistent with changing Ti concentration
in the infused region. Greater than 70% of the PMN adhered to all the Ti
treated disks and to the parent PMMA substrate, Figure 10. Similarly,
~70% or more of the PMN also adhered to the Teflon[R] and the polystyrene
disks, and to the commercially available polystyrene culture plates pretreated by the manufacturer with electrostatic charge. On the other hand,
surface smoothing and infusion of the PMMA substrate with poly(vinylpyrrolidone) substantially reduced the adherence of the PMN. Essentially

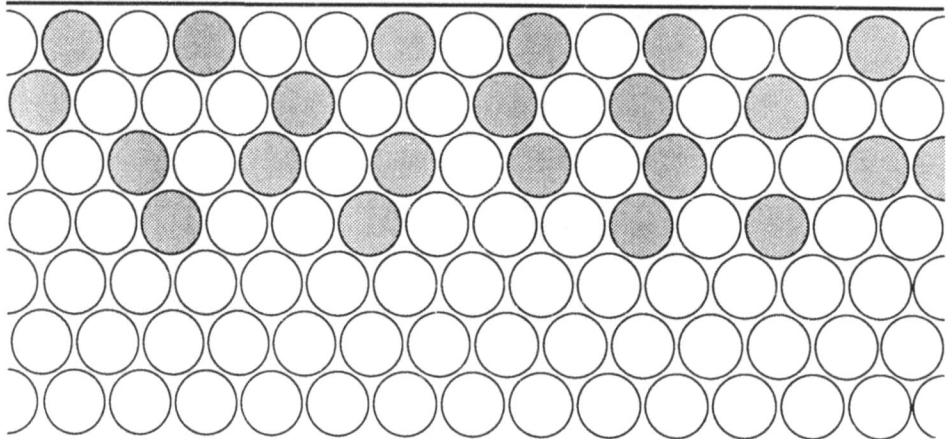

Figure 9. Schematic representation of the infused sector of a
polymer in which the infusant-modified region is
represented by a shaded circle and the pure polymeric region by an open circle.

292

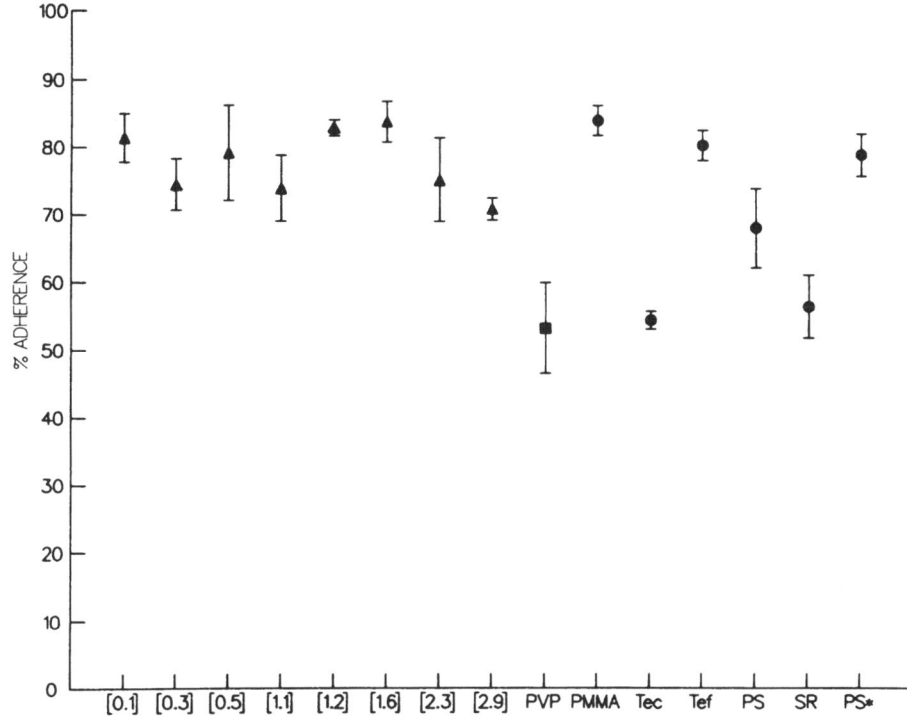

Figure 10. Percentages of human polymorphonuclear leukocytes that adhered to the various substrate preparations. △, titanium infused PMMA substrates; , titanium concentration in the infused region; PVP, poly(vinylpyrrolidone) infused PMMA substrate; PMMA, poly(methyl methacrylate) substrate; Tec, Tecoflex[R]; Tef, Teflon[R]; PS, Polystyrene; SR, Dow Corning Medical Grade silicone rubber; PS*, Falcon[R] polystyrene tissue culture plates. Each of the above values represent the mean ± S.E.M. of 4-8 samples of each type of substrate.

identical to the Tecoflex[R] and silicone rubber substrates, only ~50% of the PMN adhered to the PVP-treated disks.

Infusion of the PMMA substrate with varying concentrations of Ti did not result in any consistent increases or decreases in the hemolytic activities of the disks as a function of Ti concentration in the infused region, Figure 11. All substrates tested lysed ~2-6% of the rat erythrocytes with the outstanding exception of polystyrene, which caused ~9% of the red blood cells to lyse. Thus, these preliminary biological studies suggest that the incorporation of PVP into a polymer's surface by the infusion process may favorably increase the polymer's compatibility with blood.

SUMMARY

The chemical infusion process can modify a significant fraction (~38%) of the treated region and the surface of PMMA as indicated in the cell adherence assay. This was elucidated by the detection of titanium in

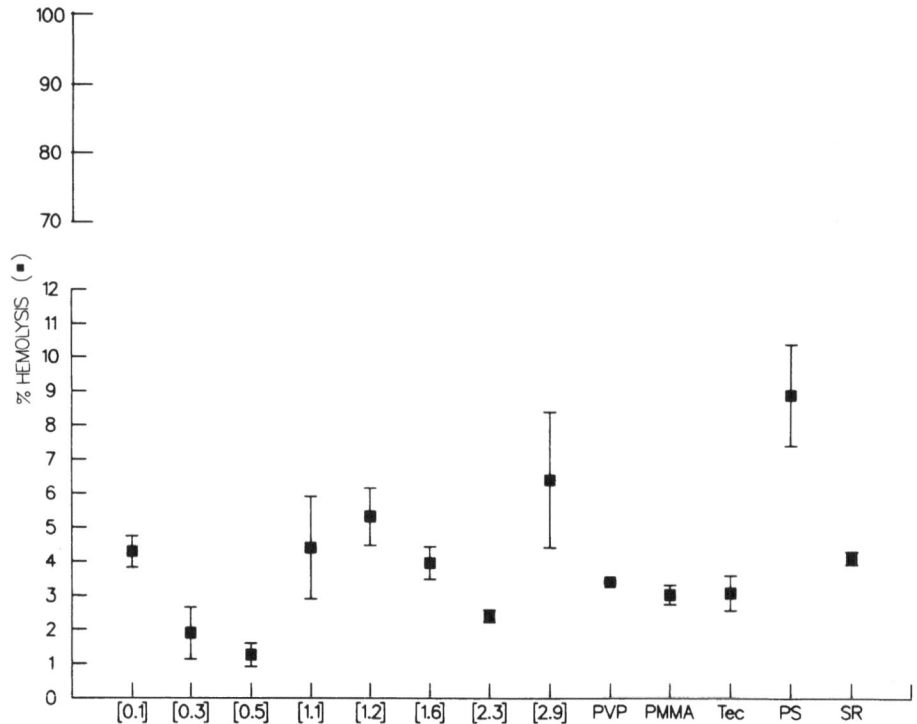

Figure 11. Percent hemolysis following incubations of rat erythrocytes with the various substrates. , titanium concentration in infused region of PMMA; PVP, poly(vinylpyrrolidone) infused PMMA substrate; PMMA, poly(methyl methacrylate) substrate; Tec, Tecoflex[R]; PS, Polystyrene; SR, Dow Corning Medical Grade silicone rubber; PS*, Falcon[R] polystyrene tissue culture plates; H₂O, water hemolyzed erythrocytes; Si, silica treated erythrocytes. Each of the above values represent the mean ± S.E.M. of 4-8 samples of each type of substrate or preparation.

the surface of the polymer by neutron activation analysis and its distribution in the infused region by scanning electron microscopy. All the tested materials indicated that the infusion process does not significantly change the surfaces with regard to rupture of cell membranes. Most importantly, the PVP-treated samples showed a substantial improvement in bioreactivity as seen in the reduction of the adherence of PMNs to the samples. Therefore, these preliminary biological tests suggest that, through the addition of PVP to the polymer's surface by the infusion process, the blood compatibility of PMMA may be substantially increased.

ACKNOWLEDGMENT

We would like to thank Keith Abel of Los Alamos National Laboratory for the neutron activation analysis of the titanium infused samples. This work was performed under the auspices of the U. S. Department of Energy.

REFERENCES

1. L. Vroman, A. L. Adams, M. Klings, G. C. Fischer, P. C. Munoz & R. P. Solensky, Ann. N. Y. Acad. Sci., **283**, 65 (1977).
2. *Guidlines for Blood-Material Interactions*, U. S. Department of Health and Human Services, N.H.L.B.I., N.I.H., 1985, No. 85-2185/September.
3. M. Szycher in: *Biocompatible Polymers, Metals, and Composites*, M. Szycher, Ed., Technomic Publishing Co. Inc., Lancaster, PA, 1983, Chapter 1, p. 1.
4. A. S. Hoffman in: *Biomaterials: Interfacial Phenomena and Applications*, S. L. Cooper & N. A. Peppas, Eds., ACS Adv. Chem. Ser. No. 199, 1982, Chapter 1, p. 3.
5. A. S. Hoffman in: *Polymeric Materials and Artificial Organs*, C. G. Gebelein, Ed., ACS Symp. No. 256, Amer. Chem. Soc., Washington, D.C., 1984, p. 13.
6. M. F. A. Goosen & M. V. Sefton in: *Biomaterials: Interfacial Phenomena and Applications*, S. L. Cooper & N. A. Peppas, Eds., ACS Adv. Chem. Ser. No. 199, 1982, Chapter 11, p. 147.
7. H. E. Kambic, S. Murabayashi & Y. Nose in: *Biocompatible Polymers, Metals, and Composites*, M. Szycher, Ed., Technomic Publishing Co. Inc., Lancaster, PA, 1983, Chapter 8, p. 179.
8. C. G. Gebelein & D. Murphy, Polym. Mater. Sci. Eng., 53, 415 (1985).
9. D. V. Duchane, J. Vac. Sci. Tech., **18**, 1183 (1981).
10. D. V. Duchane, U. S. Patent No. 4,376,751 (1983).
11. J. L. Azorlosa & A. J. Martinelli in: *Water-Soluble Resins*, R. L. Davidson & M. Sittig, Eds., Van Nostrand Reinhold Co., New York, 1968, Chapter 7, p. 131.
12. Encycl. Polymer Science & Tech., Vol. **14**, John Wiley & Sons, New York, 1971, p. 239.
13. L. W. Burnette, Proc. Sci. Sect. T. G. S., **38**, 1 (1962).
14. P. G. Laing, A. B. Ferguson & E. S. Hodge, J. Biomed. Mat. Res., **1**, 135 (1967).
15. P. J. Aragon & S. F. Hulbert, J. Biomed. Mat. Res., **6**, 155 (1972).
16. J. Black, *Biological Performance of Materials. Fundamentals of Biocompatibility*, Dekker, New York, 1981.
17. D. F. Williams, *Biocompatibility of Implant Materials*, CRC Press, Boca Raton, FA, 1981.
18. H. L. Milligan, W. T. Cleminshaw & K. W. Edmark, J. Biomed. Mat. Res., **7**, 445 (1973).
19. S. D. Bruck, Ann. N. Y. Acad. Sci., **1976**, 332.
20. B. E. Lehnert & J. Ferin, J. Reticuloendothel. Soc., 33, 293 (1983).
21. J. S. Harington, K. Miller & G. Macnab, Environ. Res., **4**, 95 (1971).
22. R. P. Nolan, A. M. Langer & J. S. Harington, Environ. Res., 26, 503 (1981).
23. F. A. Cotton & G. Wilkinson, *Advanced Inorganic Chemistry*, John Wiley & Sons, New York, 1980, Chapter 21, p. 694.

UROKINASE:AT-III:PGE₁:METHYL DOPA COMPLEX IMMOBILIZED ALBUMIN-BLENDED

UROKINASE:AT-III:PGE$_1$:METHYL DOPA COMPLEX IMMOBILIZED ALBUMIN-BLENDED

CHITOSAN MEMBRANES - ANTITHROMBOTIC AND PERMEABILITY PROPERTIES

Thomas Chandy and Chandra P. Sharma*

Division of Biosurface Technology
Sree Chitra Tirunal Institute for
Medical Sciences and Technology
Poojapura, Trivandrum 695012, India

The search for a nonthrombogenic membrane having high permselectivity for hemodialysis applications continues to be a field of extensive investigation. A series of membranes was prepared by air drying the thin layers of albumin:chitosan [a (1→4)-2-amino-2-deoxy-β-D-glucan] blends in various proportions. The albumin blended chitosan membranes showed high permeability properties for low molecular weight compounds. Complexes having fibrinolytic, anticoagulant and antiplatelet activities were prepared by repeated modification of urokinase with antithrombin-III, and methyl dopa:PGE$_1$. A nonthrombogenic albumin:chitosan blended membrane was derived by immobilizing this bioactive complex on them, via the carbodiimide functional moiety. This novel membrane demonstrated good permeability properties for small molecules and showed a dramatic reduction in platelet attachment. Such membranes that have drug complexes immobilized on them may have wider applications in the hemodialysis of patients with hypertension, as well as providing improved permeability and blood compatibility. Carbodiimide crosslinked membranes have shown improved mechanical properties with the least interference with their permeability. Other proteins, such as gelatin and collagen, were similarly blended with chitosan to make membranes which also demonstrated improved permeability characteristics, when compared with those of the standard cellulose membranes.

INTRODUCTION

Recent developments in the design of artificial kidney systems have made possible repetitive hemodialysis and the sustaining of life of chronic kidney failure patients. The most important part of the artificial kidney is the semipermeable membrane itself, where commercially available regenerated cellulose and cuprophan have been used since the time of the development of the artificial kidney until the present. Because the primary action of the cellulose membrane is that of a sieve,

---

* To whom inquiries should be sent.

there is little selectivity in the separation of two closely related molecules except when their size is approximately that of the size of the pore.[1] Hence, novel membranes need to be developed for better control of transport, ease of formability and inherent blood compatibility.

Hirano, et al, prepared a series of membranes from chitin and its derivatives which showed improved dialysis properties.[2,3] They observed that the permeability properties of N-acetyl chitosan membranes were similar to those of Amicon Diaflomembrane UM10 (Amicon Ltd., England).[3] The most serious problem in using these artificial membranes is the surface induced thrombosis, where heparinization of blood is needed to prevent clotting, and people who are susceptible to internal hemorrhaging can be dialyzed only at great risk. Hence, the most challenging problem still existing with all membranes now in use is their compatibility with the blood.

Recently, complexes having wider applications in therapeutics have been described by Maksimenko and Torchilin.[4] They prepared a wide range of water soluble urokinase derivatives of a wide action spectrum, (urokinase:sodium nitroprusside, urokinase:heparin:sodium nitroprusside, etc.) having both fibrinolytic, hypotensive and anticoagulant effects simultaneously. We also prepared a complex by repeated modification of urokinase with antithrombin III:methyl dopa:prostaglandin E_1, which showed fibrinolytic, anticoagulant and antiplatelet effects simultaneously, in addition to the normal antihypertensive action of methyl dopa.[5] Recent studies have indicated that protein blended chitosan membranes have superior permeability properties.[6]

Here we report an attempt to immobilize an urokinase:antithrombin III:PGE_1:methyl dopa conjugate on albumin blended chitosan membranes and the evaluation of their antithrombotic and permeability properties. Further studies have also been undertaken to improve the mechanical properties of the albumin blended chitosan membranes through optimum cross-linking with carbodiimide. A novel approach of producing other protein blends of chitosan, as non-thrombogenic membranes, for improved permeability had been demonstrated and compared to that of the standard cellulose membranes.

MATERIALS AND METHODS

Materials

Chitosan (a $(1 \rightarrow 4)$-2-amino-2-deoxy-β-D-glucan), which is one of the most abundant polysaccharides in nature, albumin (human, Fraction V, 96-99% pure), urokinase (~100,000 Iu/vial and MW = 54,000), antithrombin-III (heparin cofactor, Factor Xa inhibitor), collagen (from calf skin, acid soluble, type III), 1-ethyl-3,3'-dimethylaminopropyl-carbodiimide and PGE_1 were obtained from Sigma, USA. Sembrina (methyl dopa, antihypertensive drug) was obtained from Boehringer-Knoll Ltd.; gelatin powder was obtained from S. D. Fine Chemicals, India. All other chemicals used were of the analytical grade.

Preparation of Membranes

Chitosan was dissolved in 2% acetic acid and was mixed thoroughly in the presence of 2% albumin by varying their ratios at room temperature. The various mixtures were spread over a clean plate and dried at 50°C to form uniform thin films. The membranes were removed from the plate by soaking in 0.5M NaOH solution at room temperature, washed with water, then finally with ethanol and kept under vacuum at 4°C until use. A membrane having chitosan:albumin in the ratio of 7:3 was chosen for further immobilization, complexation and crosslinking studies. Similarly, other protein blended chitosan membranes were prepared by mixing either of the proteins (gelatin or collagen) in a ratio of 7:3 chitosan:protein and were spread over glass plates to give the thin membranes.

Immobilization of Urokinase Complex

The urokinase:antithrombin-III:PGE$_1$:methyl dopa complex was prepared as reported earlier.[5] Briefly, 200 µg antithrombin-III and 20,000 units of urokinase were dissolved in 2.0 mL of 0.1M phosphate buffer, pH = 7.4, and the mixture was incubated, with stirring, in the presence of 0.1% glutaraldehyde for 5 hrs at 4°C. The excess glutaraldehyde was removed by dialysis and further modification of the urokinase:antithrombin-III complex was performed by the preliminary activation of their carboxyl groups with carbodiimide.[4] For this purpose, 300 mg of 1-ethyl-3,3'-dimethylaminopropyl-carbodiimide was added at 4°C to a solution containing 2 mL of 200 ug PGE$_1$ and 100 mg methyl dopa in a phosphate buffer (pH = 7.4) and then incubated for 16 hrs at 4°C. The complex was dialyzed and concentrated using ultrafiltration at 4°C.

The carboxyl groups of the albumin blended chitosan membranes were activated with carbodiimide.[4] The membranes were dipped in a solution containing 1% carbodiimide, in 0.05M phosphate buffer (pH = 8.3) for 30 min. at 4°C, and the excess diimide was washed from the membrane with buffer solution. The complex was dissolved in phosphate buffer (pH = 8.3) and added to the previously equilibrated, activated albumin blended chitosan membranes, and kept 5 hrs. at 4°C for coupling. At the end of this process, the unbound complex was washed off with buffer. These membranes were used for platelet adhesion studies and permeability evaluation. A few albumin:chitosan membranes were also exposed to carbodiimide for various time intervals to evaluate the effect of crosslinking on their permeability properties.

Platelet Adhesion Studies With Washed Platelets

Calf blood platelets were isolated by differential centrifugation, within 2 hrs. after collection, from citrated blood as described elsewhere,[7] and washed with tyrode solution (0.055M D-glucose, 0.138M NaCl, 0.012M NaCO$_3$, 0.0018M CaCl$_2$, 0.0049M MgCl$_2$, 0.0027M KCl, 0.00036M NaH$_2$PO$_4$; pH = 7.4) for the adhesion studies.[7,8] Briefly, 10 mL of blood was collected and added to 1.0 mL of 3.8% sodium citrate and centrifuged at 700 x g for 10 minutes. The supernatant liquid, having platelet rich plasma (PRP), was centrifuged at 1000 x g for 10 minutes and the white blood cell button was removed. The PRP was again centrifuged at 2000 x g for 10 minutes to get the platelet button which was washed three times with tyrode solution and suspended in the same solution. The concentration of platelets was determined by staining them using trypan blue (one volume of 1% trypan blue to 9 volumes of platelet suspension), and counting the unstained viable cells with a hemocytometer. The platelet suspensions (approx. 1.0 x 10^8 platelets/mL) were exposed to various chitosan membranes for 15 min. at room temperature (about 30°C). The surfaces were then rinsed with 0.1M phosphate buffer (pH = 7.4). Next, the platelets were fixed with 2.5% glutaraldehyde and stained with Coomassie blue G. The number of platelets adhering to the substrates were counted using an optical microscope.

Permeability Test for the Membranes

A dialysis cell was used for determining the permeability properties of various compounds, as a function of time, at room temperature. The membrane was clamped between the two compartments using multiple supporting and sealing devices. One compartment was filled with distilled water and the other with a mixture of solutes containing urea (100 mg%, MW = 60), creatinine (10 mg%, MW = 113), uric acid (10 mg%, MW = 168) and glucose (100 mg%, MW = 180). The permeability of solutes through the membrane was analyzed spectrophotometrically at intervals of 1,2,4,6 and 16 hrs. employing a diacetyl monoxime reagent for urea,[9] alkaline picric acid for creatinine,[10], the o-toluidine method for glucose,[11] and the Folin-Wu modified method for uric acid.[10] The permeability percentages were then calculated.[3] The same membrane was used for all the times studied, by changing the solutions in the upper and lower compartments. The leaching of the immobilized complex from the membrane was also checked by analyzing the solutions for the absorption at 280 nm.

The mechanical properties of the membranes were determined by the ASTM standard method protocol using a Chatillon universal test stand model UTSE-2.[12] The membranes were cut in the form of standard dumbbell shaped specimens, having as the length between the grips of 2.55 cm, a width of 0.5 cm and employing a cross head speed of 1 inch/min. The tensile stress and the tensile strength (percentage of elongation) were calculated.

RESULTS AND DISCUSSION

Table 1 depicts the permeability percentage of urea through various albumin blended chitosan membranes as a function of crosslinking time, using carbodiimide, during a 6 hour dialysis period. Urea diffused through all the membranes to the extent of 60 to 78%. However, further modification employing carbodiimide did not modify the permeability rates for the treatments up to 4 hrs., but did cause a slight reduction for the 16 hr. treated cases. An increase in albumin content caused a slight decline in urea permeability, in the untreated cases, although the carbodiimide treated membranes did not show this change. The permeability percentages of uric acid through these membranes is shown in Table 2. Here we see that the uric acid permeation was greater with the albumin blended membranes, although carbodiimide treatment did not show significant changes.

Table 1. The permeability (%) of urea through various albumin blended chitosan membranes (6 hour dialysis).

Membranes	Ratio	Crosslinking time with carbodiimide			
		0 hrs.	1 hr.	4 hrs.	16 hrs.
Chitosan only	10:0	78.82	72.72	72.03	65.77
Chitosan:Albumin	9:1	61.83	61.24	64.82	60.40
Chitosan:Albumin	8:2	67.03	71.77	72.03	59.73
Chitosan:Albumin	7:3	69.02	74.64	70.14	63.08
Chitosan:Albumin	6:4	67.22	70.81	72.03	58.38
Chitosan:Albumin	5:5	62.08	72.72	73.93	59.73

Table 2. The permeability (%) of uric acid through various
albumin blended chitosan membranes (6 hour dialysis).

Membranes	Ratio	Crosslinking time with carbodiimide			
		0 hrs.	1 hr.	4 hrs.	16 hrs.
Chitosan only	10:0	39.48	40.83	43.65	41.59
Chitosan:Albumin	9:1	37.06	42.49	36.55	40.76
Chitosan:Albumin	8:2	44.25	46.66	40.10	41.36
Chitosan:Albumin	7:3	53.67	47.49	49.74	42.49
Chitosan:Albumin	6:4	48.10	47.08	47.20	40.79
Chitosan:Albumin	5:5	43.03	45.83	48.22	39.09

It appears that the permeability of uric acid is greater in the
albumin blended cases compared with the bare chitosan membranes. For this
reason, further studies were performed with chitosan:albumin blends in
the ratio of 7:3, where the maximum permeability rates for these small
molecules was observed. It was observed earlier that albumin blended
membranes have permeability properties similar to those of other protein
blended membranes for the small molecules, although the water content is
less here than with the gelatin blends or the bare chitosan membranes.[6]
It is possible that many factors govern the permeability of the solutes
through the membranes, such as the amount of solute dissolved in the
bound water.

The results of the platelet adhesion to the urokinase complex
modified albumin blended chitosan membranes is shown in Table 3. The
number of adhering platelets seen on the urokinase derivative immobilized
surface has been dramatically reduced when compared with the albumin
blended membrane. The permeability of various molecules through the
albumin blended chitosan and the urokinase derivative immobilized membranes, as a function of time, is demonstrated in Figures 1 and 2,
respectively. It is evident from these studies that the urokinase complex
modified membranes had similar permeability properties to those of the

Table 3. Platelet Adhesion to Various Modified Chitosan
Membranes.

Surfaces	Mean Platelets[a] ± S.D.
Bare Chitosan (CM)	27.5 ± 3.2
Albumin Blended Chitosan Membrane (ACM)	17.5 ± 3.2
Complex Immobilized ACM	7.7 ± 3.5

(a) Platelet suspension exposed to various substrates. The
values are expressed as the average of the number of
platelets adhered to the surface per mm² ± the standard
deviation. At least 25 observations were made on duplicate experiments.

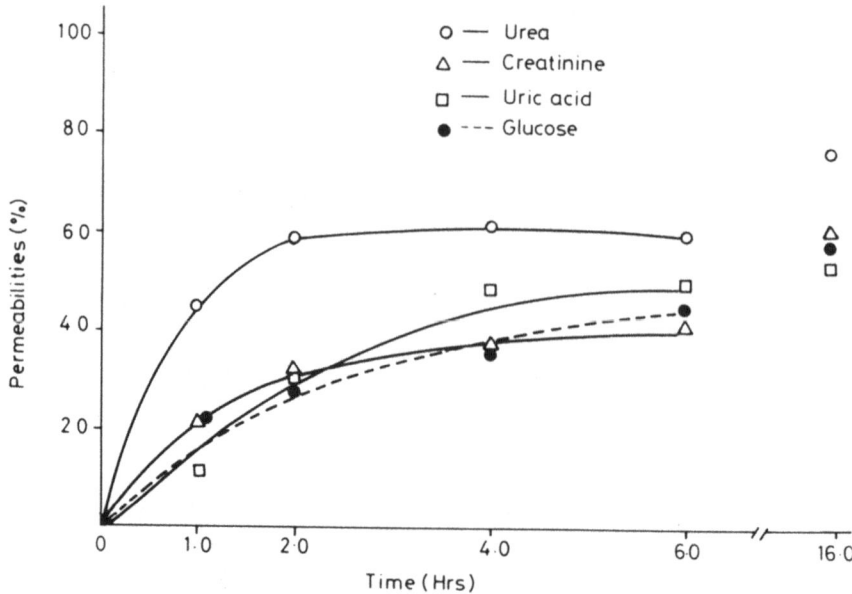

Figure 1. Permeability of various compounds through albumin
blended chitosan membrane as a fumction of time
(from a mixture of compounds).

albumin blended membranes for small molecules. Moreover, the permeability
of urea was greater in the urokinase derivative immobilized case,
although a slight reduction in the uric acid permeation had been
observed. The leakage of the urokinase complex from the substrate is also
negligible, as shown in Figure 3.

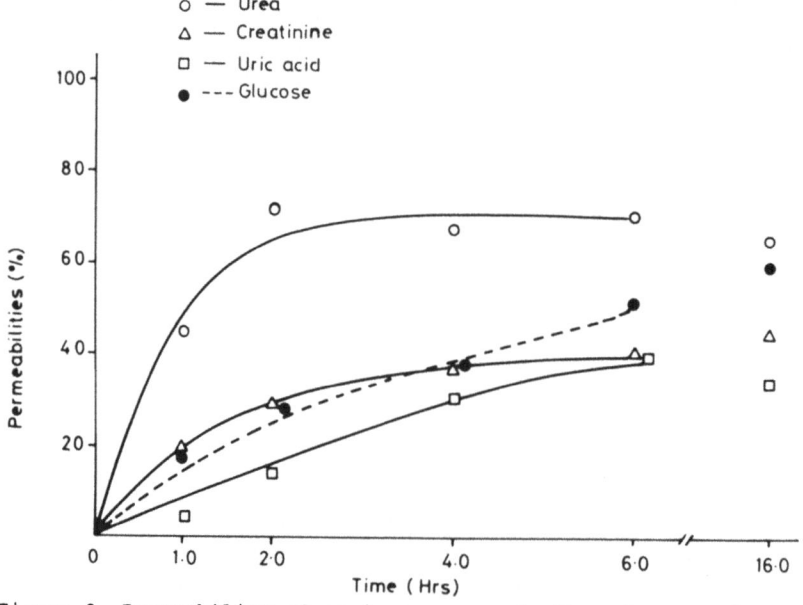

Figure 2. Permeability of various compounds through a complex
immobilized albumin blended chitosan membrane as a
function of time (from a mixture of compounds).

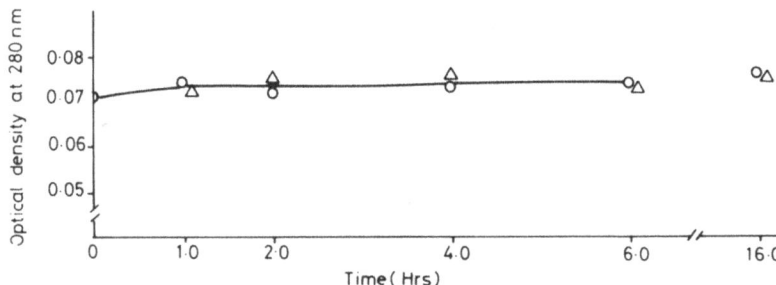

Figure 3. Leakage of the immobilized complex with time,
during dialysis, from the complex immobilized albumin blended chitosan membrane, to the permeant
solution.

The permeability of various molecules, like urea, creatinine and uric
acid though the albumin blended chitosan membranes, as a function of
time, is depicted in Figures 4, 5 and 6, respectively. It appears that
the permeability of all these molecules through the albumin blended membranes was greater when compared with the bare chitosan membrane.
However, the changes were not significant with an increase in the albumin
content. The mechanical properties of these blended membranes were also
evaluated as represented in Table 4. It appears that an increased amount
of albumin in the blend caused a reduction in tensile stress and strain.
In order to improve the strength of the membrane, chemical crosslinking
was tried by exposing the membranes for various time intervals to cabro-
diimide. It appears that the mechanical properties of the membranes were
increased by crosslinking and that an optimum time of 16 hrs. may be

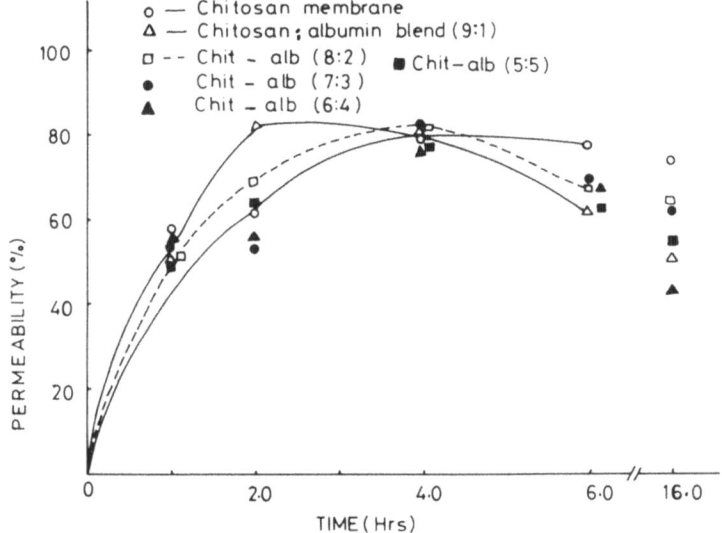

Figure 4. Permeability of urea through various ratios of the
albumin blended chitosan membranes (from a mixture
of urea, uric acid and creatinine).

303

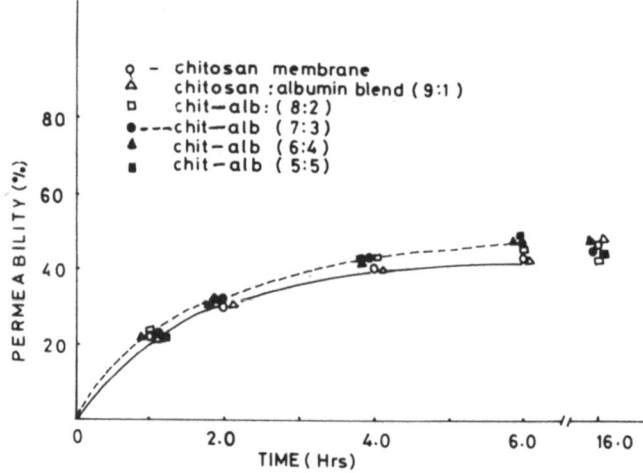

Figure 5. Permeability of creatinine through various ratios
of the albumin blended chitosan membranes (from a
mixture of urea, uric acid and creatinine).

sufficient for the improved mechanical properties without adversely
affecting the permeability.

The permeability of various molecules through the albumin blended
chitosan membranes, as a function of time after 6 hrs. carbodiimide
crosslinking, is shown in Figures 7, 8 and 9, respectively. These results
suggest that the permeability was not significantly affected with 4 hrs.
crosslinking. However, prolonged crosslinking for 16 hrs. had slightly
reduced the permeability of the solutes through these membranes, as shown
in Figures 10, 11 and 12, in comparison with uncrosslinked membranes.

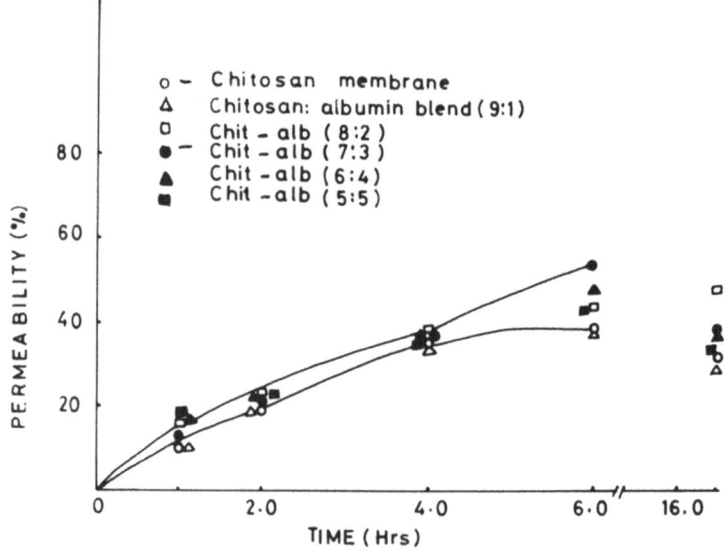

Figure 6. Permeability of uric acid through various ratios of
albumin blended chitosan membranes (from a mixture
of urea, uric acid and creatinine).

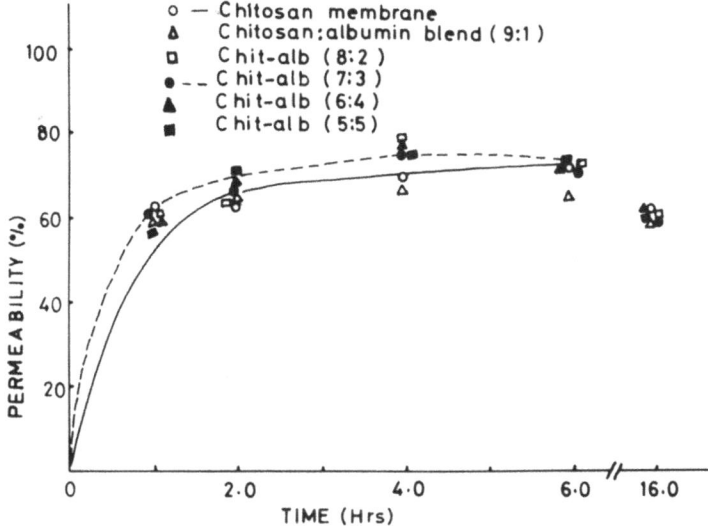

Figure 7. Permeability of urea through various ratios of albumin blended chitosan membranes crosslinked for 4 hours with EDC (from a mixture of urea, uric acid and creatinine).

Table 4. Mechanical Properties of Various Chitosan Membranes.

Membranes	Ratio	Tensile Stress (Kg/cm²) n = 5	Tensile Strain (% elong.) n = 5
Chitosan only	10:0	176.9 ± 9.6	18.8 ± 3.8
Chitosan:Albumin	9:1	164.5 ± 4.7	10.3 ± 0.2
Chitosan:Albumin	8:2	154.7 ± 5.2	18.1 ± 4.7
Chitosan:Albumin	7:3	139.2 ± 13.0	16.8 ± 5.1
Chitosan:Albumin	6:4	92.9 ± 1.9	5.7 ± 1.1
Chitosan:Albumin	5:5	87.7 ± 2.9	5.4 ± 0.7
Chitosan:Albumin Crosslinked 4 hrs.	7:3	247.7 ± 3.9	20.9 ± 0.3
Chitosan:Albumin Crosslinked 16 hrs.	7:3	298.2 ± 11.1	18.0 ± 0.8
Chitosan:Gelatin Crosslinked 16 hrs.	7:3	252.2 ± 21.9	23.99 ± 0.7
Standard Cellulose Membrane		575.6 ± 39.5	35.5 ± 4.5

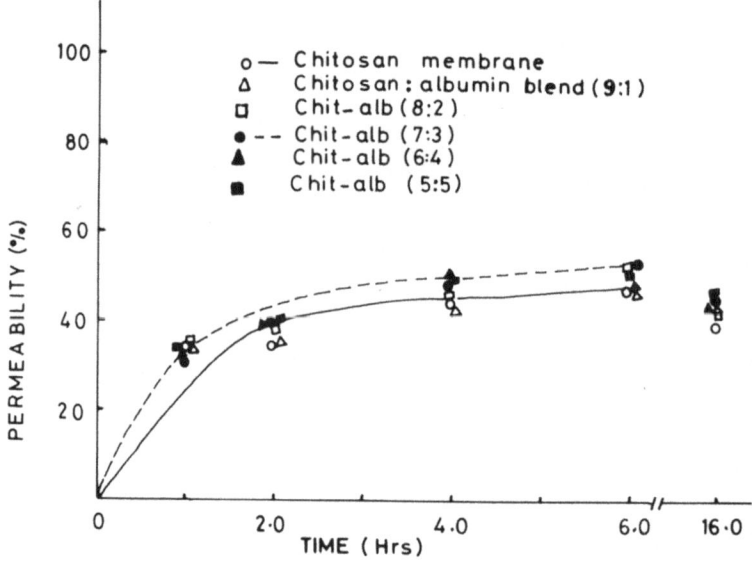

Figure 8. Permeability of creatinine through various ratios of albumin blended chitosan membranes crosslinked for 4 hours with EDC (from a mixture of urea, uric acid and creatinine).

However, it appears from Table 4 that the 16 hrs. crosslinking had signi-ficantly improved the dry strength of the membranes. Hence, the membranes having a chitosan:albumin ratio of 7:3 and crosslinked with carbodiimide for 16 hrs. were chosen for further studies.

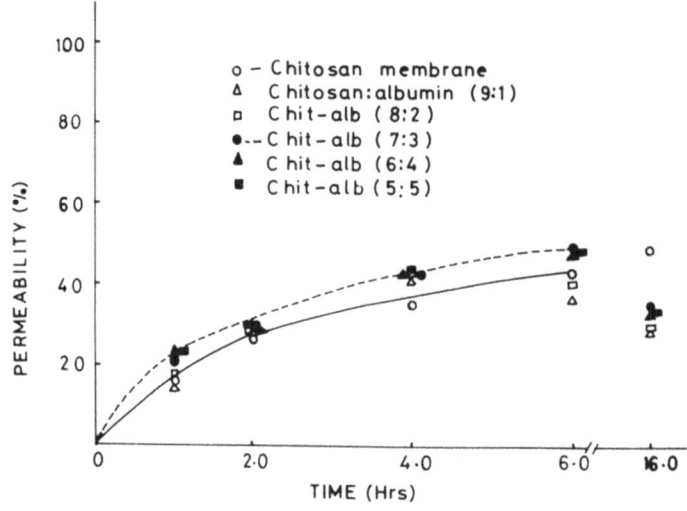

Figure 9. Permeability of uric acid through various ratios of albumin blended chitosan membranes crosslinked 4 hours with EDC (from a mixture of urea, uric acid and creatinine).

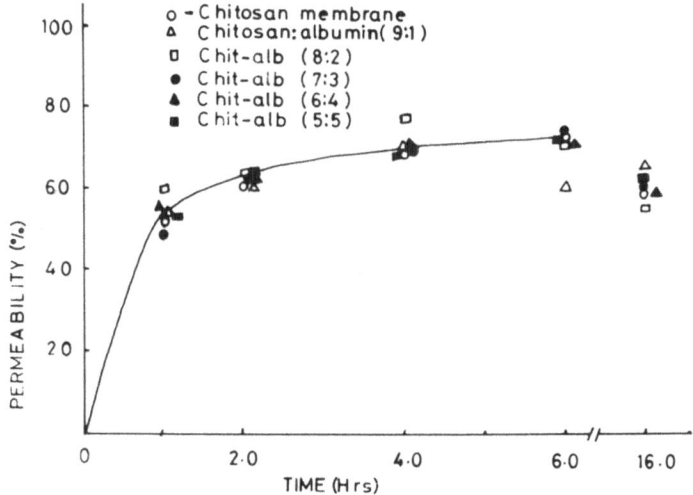

Figure 10. Permeability of urea through various ratios of albumin blended chitosan membranes crosslinked 16 hours with EDC (from a mixture of urea, uric acid and creatinine).

The use of other proteins, such as gelatin, collagen, etc., to prepare chitosan blended membranes was tried in a 7:3 ratio (chitosan: protein) and the results were compared to the standard cellulose membranes. The permeability, as a function of time, of various molecules, such as urea, creatinine, uric acid, glucose and albumin, through such membranes is shown in Figures 13, 14, 15, 16 and 17, respectively. It appears that the protein blended membranes exhibited improved permeability properties with respect to small molecules compared to the standard cellulose membrane or bare chitosan. These protein blended membranes

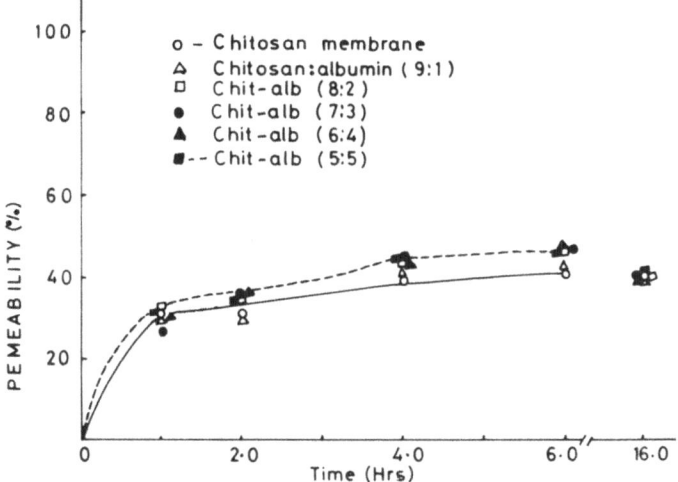

Figure 11. Permeability of creatinine through various ratios of albumin blended chitosan membranes crosslinked 16 hours with EDC (from a mixture of urea, uric acid and creatinine).

307

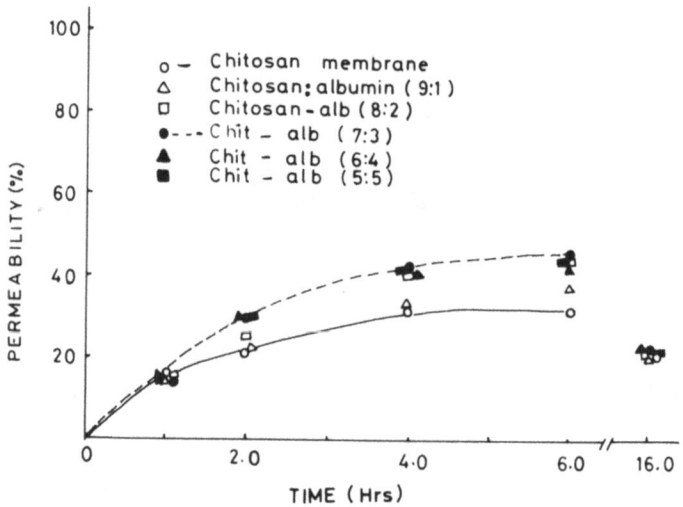

Figure 12. Permeability of uric acid through various ratios
of albumin blended chitosan membranes crosslinked
16 hours with EDC (from a mixture of urea, uric
acid and creatinine).

also inhibited the passage of large molecules such as albumin (MW =
69,000), although a slight increase had been observed with the gelatin
blended membranes compared to the standard membrane.

Albumin and gelatin are being widely used for modifying the polymeric
substrates to improve their blood compatibility because of their passive
nature in attaching the platelets.[13,14] Collagen has been tried as a
membrane and demostrated superior permeability of solutes.[15] Thus it
appears that the protein blended membranes may be superior with respect
to compatibility and permeability.

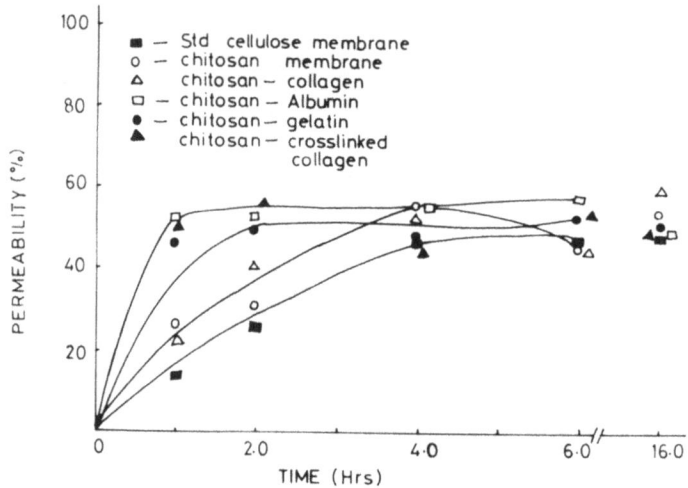

Figure 13. Permeability of urea through various chitosan
membranes as a function of time (from a mixture of
urea, uric acid and creatinine).

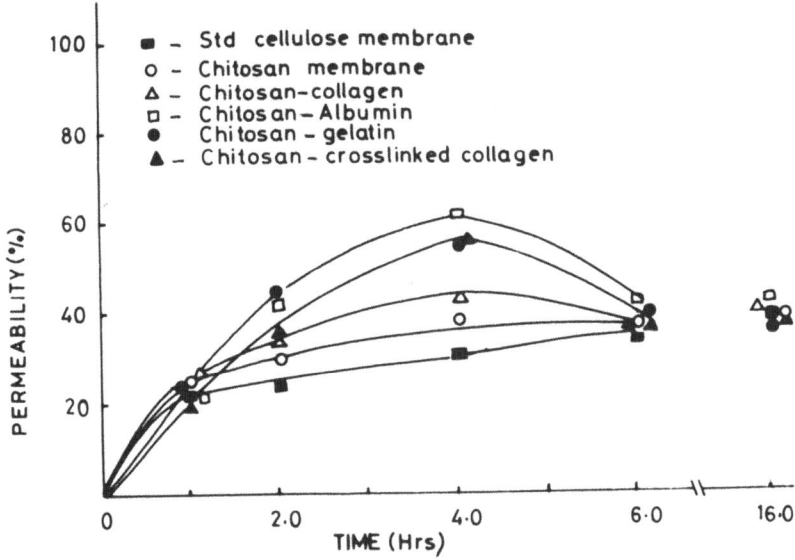

Figure 14. Permeability of creatinine through various
chitosan membranes as a function of time (from a
mixture of urea, uric acid and creatinine).

In conclusion, the present studies suggest that protein blended
chitosan membranes have superior permeability properties for the smaller
molecules compared to the standard cellulose membranes. It also seems
that membranes having drug complexes immobilized on them may have wider
applications in the hemodialysis of patients with hypertension, as well
as offering improved permeability and blood compatibility. This may also
be useful for patients who are liable to internal hemorrhaging on

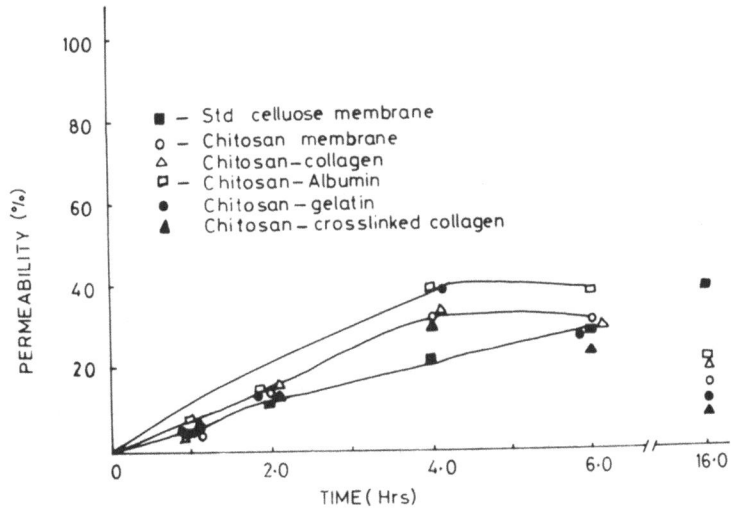

Figure 15. Permeability of uric acid through various chitosan
membranes as a function of time (from a mixture of
urea, uric acid and creatinine).

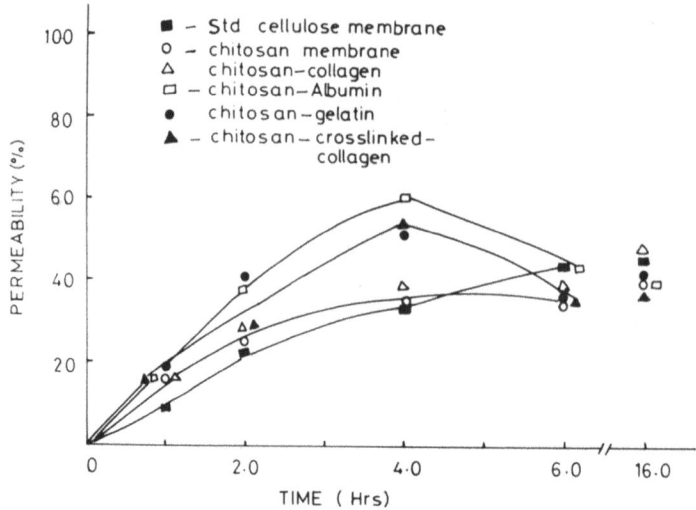

Figure 16. Permeability of glucose through various chitosan
membranes as a function of time (from a mixture of
glucose, albumin, urea, uric acid and creatinine).

heparinization, resulting in a reduction or the absence in the use of
heparin during dialysis. Finally, complexes having multiple actions, such
as the urokinase:antithrombin III:PGE₁:methyl dopa, may be used to
improve the blood compatibility of existing membranes.

ACKNOWLEDGEMENTS

We appreciate the help from Dr. A. V. Lal for providing calf blood.
This work was funded by DST, India.

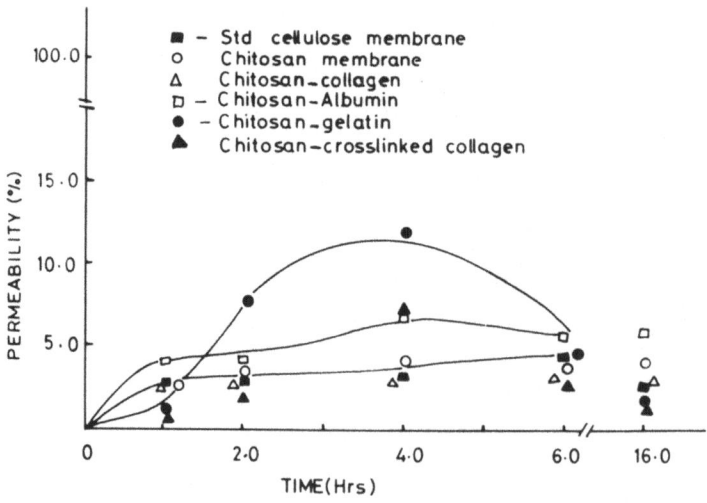

Figure 17. Permeability of albumin through various chitosan
membranes as a function of time (from a mixture of
glucose, albumin, urea, uric acid and creatinine).

310

REFERENCES

1. S. M. Hudson & L. A. Cuculo, J. Macromol. Sci., Revs. Macromol. Sci., **C18**, 1 (1980).
2. S. Hirano, Agric. Biol. Chem., **42**, 1939 (1978).
3. S. Hirano, K. Tobetto, M. Hasegawa & N. Matsuda, J. Biomed. Mater. Res., **14**, 477 (1980).
4. A. V. Maksimenko & V. P. Torchilin, Throm. Res., **38**, 277(1985).
5. C. P. Sharma & T. Chandy, J. Biomed. Mater. Res., submitted.
6. C. P. Sharma & T. Chandy, Trans. Soc. Biomaterials, **10**, 31 (1987).
7. T. Chandy & C. P. Sharma, Throm. Res., **41**, 9 (1986).
8. E. S. Lee & S. W. Kim, Trans. Am. Soc. Artificial Organs, **XXV**, 124 (1979).
9. G. B. Latting, Am J. Clin. Path., **41**, 565 (1964).
10. P. B. Hawk, "Physiological Chemistry", 14th Ed., B. L. Oser. Ed., McGraw Hill, New York ,1965.
11. J. D. Bauer, P. G. Ackermann & G. Toro, "Clinical Laboratory Methods", 8th Ed., C. V. Mosby Co., St. Louis, 1974, p. 384.
12. ASTM-D 638-80, "Annual Book of ASTM Standards", **35**, 250 (1982).
13. M. A. Packham, G. Evans, M. P. Glynn & I. F. Mustard, J. Lab. Clin. Med., **73**, 686 (1969).
14. H. Kambic, G. Picha, R. Kiraly, I. Koshino & Y. Nose, Trans. Am. Soc. Artificial Organs, **XXII**, 664 (1976).
15. T. Kon, G. L. Mrava, D. Webber & Y. Nose, J. Biomed. Mater.Res., **4**, 13 (1970).

CONTROL OF SKIN WOUND CONTRACTION RATE BY CRITICALLY INSOLUBLE COLLAGEN

MATRICES

I. V. Yannas, E. Lee and M. Dionne Bentz

Fibers and Polymers Laboratories
Massachusetts Institute of Technology
Cambridge, MA 02139

Several porous graft copolymers of collagen and chondroitin 6-sulfate were prepared and contacted with freshly excised subcutaneous muscle tissue in a standard guinea pig wound healing model. The degradation rate in collagenase of the copolymers was varied over a wide range by controlling the conditions of crosslinking in glutaraldehyde during polymer preparation. The average pore diameter was maintained at a constant level in the series. The kinetics of skin wound contraction were studied up to about 200 days following grafting with members of the series. We conclude that wound contraction is delayed significantly provided that the highly porous copolymers remain largely insoluble (undegraded) for a critical period following contact with tissue. The data are consistent with a requirement for an insolubility period of minimal duration. Although the absolute length of the critical period was not determined it was independently estimated at 10-15 days.

INTRODUCTION

When a polymeric material is first contacted with living tissue following a surgical procedure, the local biochemical environment is most probably characteristic of a local inflammatory response.[1] Irrespective of how reactive the exogenous polymeric material may be towards the tissues with which it is in contact, an inflammatory response of significant magnitude is virtually guaranteed following the trauma of the surgical procedure which is normally required for implantation of the material at the desired organ site. One of the earliest events following skin trauma is the synthesis of collagenase.[2] To enhance understanding of the mechanism by which certain graft copolymers of collagen and a glycosaminoglycan (GAG) induce partial regeneration of skin[3,4] when contacted with full-thickness skin wounds, it is, therefore, necessary to study the interaction between these collagen-based copolymers and collagenase.[5]

Certain bacterial collagenases have been available commercially for several years whereas mammalian collagenases are not readily available. The mechanism of collagenolysis in these two classes of enzymes is different.[6] In previous work we have, however, shown the presence of an empirical correlation between the rate of degradation of various cross-linked collagens by bacterial collagenase *in vitro* and the rate at which these collagens are degraded *in vivo* following surgical implantation.[7] Accordingly, we have used the *in vitro* reaction in our present study as a simple empirical probe to answer the question: Is there a critical period of insolubility (resistance to catastrophic degradation) for polymers which delay wound contraction? The *in vitro* assay provided a convenient empirical metric for resistance to degradation of a large number of collagen based polymers and its use thereby afforded an answer to the question posed above.

An early version of the *in vitro* collagenase degradation assay was based on measurement of stress relaxation of a strip of test polymer immersed in a standardized collagenase bath.[1,8] Previously, Tobolsky[9] had used such a device to study the chemical stress relaxation of natural rubber in the presence of ozone. In spite of its immediate utility as a screening probe in our early research[1,5] this experimental arrangement was eventually replaced by a more reproducible assay. The latter is an adaptation of a colorimetric procedure originally developed by Mandl and coworkers.[10]

Previously we have hypothesized that matrices which possess biological activity degrade at a rate which is comparable to the rate of synthesis of new tissue following trauma.[11,12] We have argued that an excessively rapid degradation rate converts the graft to a liquid-like state earlier than required by the physicochemical criteria for an effective wound cover; on the other hand, a particularly slow degradation rate is associated with an enzymatically intractable cover which is walled off by fibrotic tissue and is eventually separated physically.[11,12] In this study we tested the hypothesis that the degradation rate of a biologically active wound cover must not exceed a maximum level.

Our results showed that polymers which degraded very rapidly in collagenase were not biologically active, i.e., they did not delay contraction of full-thickness skin wounds. Only polymers which possessed a minimal resistance to degradation were capable of delaying wound contraction. Our finding supports the hypothesis that collagen matrices are biologically active provided that they persist as insoluble matrices over a minimal period. This hypothesis has implications not only in efforts to control other wound healing processes but probably also in efforts to understand developmental processes in biology as well.

MATERIALS AND METHODS

Collagen-*graft*-chondroitin 6-sulfate polymers were prepared as described in detail elsewhere.[5,13] Porous sheets were prepared by freeze drying and were exposed to 105°C under vacuum, a procedure which insolubilizes the CG ionic complex, probably by amide condensation reactions between carboxylic groups on GAG and ε-amino groups of lysyl residues of collagen.[13,15] The porous CG sheet was knife-coated with a 0.25-mm thick layer of poly(dimethyl siloxane) prepolymer fluid (Silastic Medical A, Dow Corning, Midland, MI) which was subsequently cured to an elastomer by immersion in 0.05M aqueous acetic acid. This was followed by immersion into a bath of aqueous glutaraldehyde (reagent grade, Aldrich, Milwaukee, WI) in 0.05M aqueous acetic acid. Exposure to glutaraldehyde induces collagen chains to undergo covalent crosslinking, presumably by attack on ε-amino groups of lysyl residues and formation of quaternary pyridinium residues.[16]

Increase of the residence time in the glutaraldehyde bath from 0 to 24 h yielded polymers varying widely in their crosslink density, as reflected in values of the average molecular weight between crosslinks, M_c, which ranged from *ca.* 40,000 to *ca.* 12,000, respectively. Following rinsing in deionized water over 24 h the glutaraldehyde concentration in the rinse water was found to be considerably less than 5 ppm using the reagent 4-amino-3-hydrazino-5-mercapto-1,2,4-triazole (Purpald, Aldrich, Milwaukee, MI).[17]

The average pore diameter d was determined by first embedding the porous membrane in methyl methacrylate, sectioning to a thickness of 5 μm, mounting on a glass slide and staining with 1% toluidine blue. Slides were 5 examined under a light microscope using an image analyzer and results obtained agreed with data from a previously described method[18] based on viewing in the scanning electron microscope. The average pore diameter of the copolymer series studied averaged 450 ± 60 μm.

The degradation rate in collagenase was determined by first incubating the finely comminuted polymer for 5 h at 37°C in a stirred 0.08% w/v solution of bacterial collagenase from *Clostridium histolyticum* (GIBCO, Grand Island, NY) in a buffer, pH = 7.4.[10,19] Following filtration to separate out undigested substrate particles aliquots were treated by addition of a colored solution of ninhydrin and hydrindantin at pH = 5.5. The resulting colored solution was incubated in a boiling water bath at 20 min and 50% w/w propanol/water was then added. The solution was allowed to stand at room temperature for 15 min and the transmittance at 500 nm was recorded. Values of the degradation rate, R, thereby obtained were expressed as enzyme units which were calibrated using a 0.002M aqueous solution of L-leucine.[19] One enzyme unit liberates amino acids from collagen which are equivalent in ninhydrin color to 1.0 μM L-leucine in 5 h at pH = 7.4 at 37°C.[19] A series of copolymers was prepared with R values varying from 2.6 ± 0.6 enzyme units (e.u.) to *ca.* 220 e.u. by control of the glutaraldehyde crosslinking step.

CG copolymers is this series were not seeded with cells as reported in a previous study.[4]

White female Hartley guinea pigs (Elm Hill Breeding Laboratories, Chelmsford, MA) were grafted using surgical procedures which have been described.[20] The excisional protocol used followed closely the standard mammalian free skin grafting model described by Billingham and Medawar.[21] An anatomically well-defined wound bed,[22] consisting of a layer of striped muscle, was thereby prepared for interaction with the CG copolymeric grafts. Nominal surface areas of wounds were usually 1.5 cm by 3.0 cm. In several controls similar results were obtained with 4.0 cm by 4.0 cm wounds. Animals in one control group were not grafted, but their wounds were treated simply with a Xeroform gauze.[20] The wound was photographed in the presence of a calibrated scale and its area calculated using measurements taken from the skin edges and not form the advancing edge of epithelial cell sheets.[20,21] The time required for the area to be reduced to 50% of its original value, ($t_{1/2}$, wound half life), was determined from the kinetics of contraction.

RESULTS

Ungrafted wounds first showed contraction by about Day 2 after surgery and continued contracting vigorously until about Day 30. At this time the wound edges were separated by a narrow strip of scar tissue. Thereafter, the area of scar tissue grew slowly, approximately following the growth of the animal.[23] The wound half life, $t_{1/2}$ = 8 ± 1 days, observed in our present study with ungrafted wound controls compares with $t_{1/2}$ values of 7 days which we estimated from independently obtained data with guinea pigs,[25] 9 days with rabbits,[22] and 11 days with guinea pigs.[20]

The degradation rate of the grafts affected the contraction rate significantly. As an example of the data obtained, Figure 1 shows that a decrease in R from 231 ± 20 e.u. (0 h crosslinking time) to 17 ± 4 e.u. (24 h crosslinking time) caused an increase in wound half life from 10 ± 1 to 17 ± 2 days.

CG copolymers which were uncrosslinked failed to increase $t_{1/2}$ significantly above the values observed with ungrafted controls. Significant increases in $t_{1/2}$, corresponding to $t_{1/2} \geq 15$ days, were observed when the *in vitro* degradation rate R was approximately 140 ± 25 e.u. or lower (Figure 2). Below this limiting value, $t_{1/2}$ remained sensibly unchanged down to the sensitivity limit of the assay, *ca.* 1 e.u.

DISCUSSION

The data show that CG copolymers do not delay wound contraction if they degrade sufficiently rapidly after being grafted (Figure 2). This conclusion suggests that the porous copolymers derive their biological activity partly from their persistence as insoluble matrices over a critical early period following contact with the freshly excised wound. The *in vitro* assay of degradation rate which we used in this work does not permit a direct estimate of the length of this critical period *in vivo*. However, independent observation of the contents of the wound by electron microscopy[25] has shown that fragments of the highly crosslinked CG copolymer matrix, measuring at least about 50 μm in length, persist in intimate contact with cells for a period of 10-15 days following grafting. Such fragments are not observed with uncrosslinked copolymers

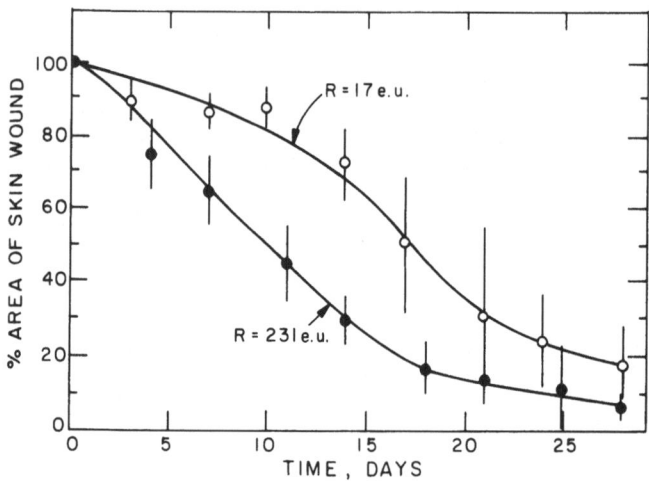

Figure 1. Kinetics of skin wound contraction in the presence of polymeric grafts which undergo enzymatic degradation at two different rates, R = 17 enzyme units (e.u.) and R = 231 e.u. The variation in R was achieved by controlling the duration of crosslinking of the collagen-*graft*-glycosaminoglycan in aqueous glutaraldehyde.

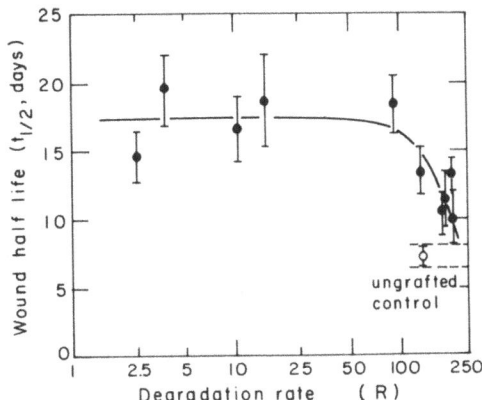

Figure 2. The wound half life, $t_{1/2}$, is shown to depend on the degradation rate, R, of collagen-*graft*-glycos-aminoglycan membranes which were contacted with the woundbed of fresh skin wounds in guinea pigs, prepared by full-thickness excision. R, expressed in enzyme units, was varied by controlling the residence time of the graft copolymer in aqueous glutaraldehyde.

under similar conditions. Obviously, additional studies are necessary to confirm directly the presumed necessity for a critical persistence period for a CG copolymer matrix which significantly delays wound contraction. However, our observations suggest that the CG matrix may remain active provided that it maintains a characteristic dimension several times the diameter of mesenchymal cells.

Previously, we have hypothesized that the lifetime of the CG matrix, expressed as the time constant for biodegradation t_b, is a critical quantity for biologically active matrices.[11,12] We also hypothesized that t_b is comparable to the time constant for normal healing of a skin incision, t_h, so that:[12]

$$\frac{t_b}{t_h} \approx 1$$

In such previous discussions we have assumed that t_h is about 25 days.[12] Although our data support the hypothesis of a minimal time constant for biodegradation, t_b probably lies in the range 10-15 range days rather than being closer to 25 days as hypothesized earlier.

Studies of developmental processes have stressed the importance of the extracellular matrix (ECM) in modulating such processes and several constituents of the ECM have been identified.[26] Substantially less attention has, however, been paid to a requirement for insolubility of the ECM over a specific period. Our data suggest the hypothesis that biologically active CG copolymers act as initially insoluble but eventually degradable catalytic surfaces which control the rate and possibly also the outcome of certain developmental processes. Future studies will address the question of the nature of catalytic phenomena involved and the timescale over which the presumed catalytic surface persists in the form of insoluble particles with a characteristic dimension several times that of a cell diameter.

ACKNOWLEDGMENT

This study was supported partly by an NIH grant GM23946, and partly by the office of the Associate Provost at MIT.

REFERENCES

1. I.V. Yannas in: "*Proc. Biomedical Materials Congress*", D.J. Lyman, Ed., Nat. Sci. Found., Brighton, UT, 1972, p. 133.
2. J. C. Houck, Ed., "*The Immunopathology of Inflammation*", Excerpta Medica, Amsterdam, 1971.
3. I. V. Yannas, D. P. Orgill, E. M. Skrabut and J. F. Burke in: "*Polymeric Materials and Artificial Organs*", C. G. Gebelein, Ed., Am. Chem. Soc., Washington, DC, 1984, Chap. 13.
4. I. V. Yannas, J. F. Burke, D. P. Orgill and E. M. Skrabut, Science **215**, 174 (1982).
5. I. V. Yannas, J. F. Burke, C. Huang and P. L. Gordon, Polymer Preprints, **16**(2), 209 (1975).
6. J. Gross in: "*Biochemistry of Collagen*", G. N. Ramachandran and A. H. Reddi, Eds., Plenum, NY, 1976, p. 275.
7. I. V. Yannas, J. F. Burke, C. Huang and P. L. Gordon, J. Biomed. Mat. Res., **9**, 623 (1975).
8. C. Huang and I. V. Yannas, J. Biomed. Mat. Res. Symp., **8**, 137 (1977).
9. A. V. Tobolsky, "*Properties and Structure of Polymers*", Wiley, NY, 1960, Ch. 5.
10. I. Mandl, J. D. Maclennan and E. L. Howes, J. Clin. Invest. **32**, 1323 (1953).
11. I. V. Yannas, J. F. Burke, M. Umbreit and P. Stasikelis, Fed. Am. Soc. Exp. Biol. **38**, 98B (1979).
12. I. V. Yannas and J. F. Burke, J. Biomed. Mater. Res., **14**, 65 (1980).
13. I. V. Yannas, J. F. Burke, P. L. Gordon, C. Huang and R. H. Rubenstein, J. Biomed. Mater. Res., **14**, 107 (1980).
14. I. V. Yannas and A. V. Tobolsky, Nature, **215**, 509 (1967).
15. I. V. Yannas, Revs. Macromol. Chem., **C7**, 49 (1972).
16. D. T. Cheung and M. E. Nimni, Connect. Tiss. Res., **10**, 201 (1982).
17. R. G. Dickinson and N. W. Jacobsen, Chem. Commun., 1719 (1970).
18. N. Dagalakis, J. Flink, P. Stasikelis, J. F. Burke and I. V. Yannas, J. Biomed. Mat. Res., **14**, 511 (1980).
19. Sigma Chemical Co., Enzymatic Assay of Collagenase, E.D. No. 3.4.24.3, St. Louis, MO, 1977.
20. I. V. Yannas in: "*The Surgical Wound*", P. Dineen, Ed., Lea & Febiger, NY, 1981, p. 171.
21. R. E. Billingham and P. B. Medawar, J. Anat., **89**, 114 (1955).
22. R. E. Billingham and P. S. Russell, Ann. Surg., **144**, 961 (1956).
23. R. E. Billingham and P. B. Medawar, J. Exp. Biol., **28**, 385 (1955).
24. H. C. Grillo, G. T. Watts and J. Gross, Ann. Surg., **148**, 145 (1958).
25. I. V. Yannas and J. F. Murphy, unpublished data.
26. E. D. Hay, Modern Cell Biol., **2**, 509 (1983).

CONTRIBUTORS

Y. T. Bao   85
Research Triangle Institute
Research Triangle Park, NC 27709

M. Dionne Bentz   313
Fibers and Polymers Laboratories
Massachusetts Institute of Technology
Cambridge, MA 02139

Christopher Bever, Jr.   205
Department of Neurology
University of Maryland Hospital
Baltimore, Maryland

Nancy J. Biegley   223
Florida Atlantic University
Department of Chemistry
Boca Raton, FL 33431

Cynthia Butler   175
Department of Biological Sciences
Florida Atlantic University
Boca Raton, FL 33431

J.A. Cameron   61
Institute of Materials Science
University of Connecticut
Storrs, Connecticut 06268

Charles. E. Carraher, Jr.   1, 139, 175, 223
Department of Chemistry
Florida Atlantic University
Boca Raton, FL 33431

David L. Cash   281
Material and Technology Division
Los Alamos National Laboratory
Los Alamos, NM 87545

Thomas Chandy   297
Division of Biosurface Technology
Sree Chita Tirunal Institute for
Medical Sciences and Technology
Poojapura, Trivandrum 695012, India

Mark Chapman   151
Department of Chemistry
Youngstown State University
Youngstown, OH 44555

William H. Daly   251
Department of Chemistry
Louisiana State University
Baton Rouge, Louisiana 70803

Laura J. DiBenedetto   61
Institute of Materials Science
University of Connecticut
Storrs, Connecticut 06268

David V. Duchane   281
Material and Technology Division
Los Alamos National Laboratory
Los Alamos, NM 87545

P. Dworjanyn   275
School of Chemistry
The University of South Wales
Kensington, N.S.W. Australia 2033

Norman Elliott   281
Material and Technology Division
Los Alamos National Laboratory
Los Alamos, NM 87545

Koji Enomoto   165
Faculty of Textile Science & Technology
Shinshu University
Ueda 386, Japan

Van Foster   1, 175
DAP, Inc.
P. O. Box 277
Dayton, OH 45431

Bruce P. Gaber   239
Bio/Molecular Engineering Branch, Code 6190
Naval Research Laboratory
Washington, D.C. 20375-5000

J. L. Garnett   275
School of Chemistry
The University of South Wales
Kensington, N.S.W. Australia 2033

Charles G. Gebelein   1, 151
Department of Chemistry
Youngstown State University
Youngstown, OH 44555

R. L. Gettings   91
Dow Corning Corp.
2200 West Salzburg Road
Midland, MI 48640-0994

320

Malay Ghosh   115
Department of Chemistry & Chemical Engineering
Stevens Institute of Technology
Hoboken, NJ 07030

David J. Giron   175, 223
Wright State University
Department of Microbiology and Immunology
Dayton, Oh 45435

Z-W Gu   85
Research Triangle Institute
Research Triangle Park, NC 27709

Kevin Hassett   17
Department of Entomology
Pesticide Research Laboratory
The Pennsylvania State University
University Park, PA 16802 USA

Masahiko Hayashi   45
Department of Agricultural Biochemistry
Tottori University
Tottori 680, Japan

Shigehiro Hirano   45
Department of Agricultural Biochemistry
Tottori University
Tottori 680, Japan

Samuel J. Huang   61
Institute of Materials Science
University of Connecticut
Storrs, Connecticut 06268

Yoshiaki Inaki   185
Faculty of Engineering
Osaka University
Suita, Osaka 565, Japan

B. Jansen   97
Hygiene-Institute
University of Cologne
Goldenfelsstr. 19 - 21
D-5000 Cologne 41, FRG

Yutaro Kaneko   165
Ajinomoto Co., Ltd.
1-5-8, Kyobashi, Chuo-ku
Tokyo 104, Japan

D.J. Kesler   125
Physiology Research Laboratory
Reproductive Biotechnology
Department of Animal Sciences
University of Illinois
Urbana, Illinois 61801

Ram Kossowsky   281
Penn State University
State College, PA 16801

David A. Kurtz   17
Department of Entomology
Pesticide Research Laboratory
The Pennsylvania State University
University Park, PA 16802 USA

E. Lee   313
Fibers and Polymers Laboratories
Massachusetts Institute of Technology
Cambridge, MA 02139

Soo Lee   251
Department of Chemistry
Louisiana State University
Baton Rouge, Louisiana 70803

Bruce E. Lehnert   281
Life Sciences Division
Los Alamos National Laboratory
Los Alamos, NM 87545

Hilton B. Levy   205
National Instutes of Allergy and Infectious Diseases
Bethesda, Maryland

Jerry E. London   281
Life Sciences Division
Los Alamos National Laboratory
Los Alamos, NM 87545

Kei Matsuzaki   165
Faculty of Textile Science & Technology
Shinshu University
Ueda 386, Japan

Tohru Mimura   165
Ajinomoto Co., Ltd.
1-5-8, Kyobashi, Chuo-ku
Tokyo 104, Japan

Tahseen Mirza   151
Department of Chemistry
Youngstown State University
Youngstown, OH 44555

Takashi Miyamoto   185
Faculty of Engineering
Osaka University
Suita, Osaka 565, Japan

Kakuko Murae   45
Department of Agricultural Biochemistry
Tottori University
Tottori 680, Japan

Philip D. Mykytiuk   175
Department of Chemistry
Wright State University
Dayton, OH 45435

Suguru Nagae   185
Faculty of Engineering
Osaka University
Suita, Osaka 565, Japan

Yoshinobu Naoshima   175
Okayama University of Science
Department of Chemistry
Ridaicho, Okayama 700 Japan

Takeshi Nishida   45
Department of Agricultural Biochemistry
Tottori University
Tottori 680, Japan

G. Peters   97
Hygiene-Institute
University of Cologne
Goldenfelsstr. 19 - 21
D-5000 Cologne 41, FRG

C. G. Pitt   85
Research Triangle Institute
Research Triangle Park, NC 27709

G. Pulverer   97
Hygiene-Institute
University of Cologne
Goldenfelsstr. 19 - 21
D-5000 Cologne 41, FRG

S. Schareina   97
Hygiene-Institute
University of Cologne
Goldenfelsstr. 19 - 21
D-5000 Cologne 41, FRG

F. Schumacher-Perdreau   97
Hygiene-Institute
University of Cologne
Goldenfelsstr. 19 - 21
D-5000 Cologne 41, FRG

Chandra P. Sharma   297
Division of Biosurface Technology
Sree Chita Tirunal Institute for
Medical Sciences and Technology
Poojapura, Trivandrum 695012, India

Tsuyoshi Shiio   165
Ajinomoto Co., Ltd.
1-5-8, Kyobashi, Chuo-ku
Tokyo 104, Japan

Alok Singh   239
Bio/Molecular Engineering Branch, Code 6190
Naval Research Laboratory
Washington, D.C. 20375-5000

H. Steinhauser   97
Institute of Physical Chemistry
University of Cologne
Luxemburger Str. 116
D-5000 Cologne 41, FRG

Rickey E. Strothers   139
Department of Chemistry
Florida Atlantic University
Boca Raton, FL 33431

Yoshihiko Sugiura   185
Faculty of Engineering
Osaka University
Suita, Osaka 565, Japan

Kiichi Takemoto   185
Faculty of Engineering
Osaka University
Suita, Osaka 565, Japan

Mary Trombley   223
Florida Atlantic University
Department of Chemistry
Boca Raton, FL 33431

Hisaya Tsuchida   45
Department of Agricultural Biochemistry
Tottori University
Tottori 680, Japan

Paul Y. Wang   75
Laboratory of Chemical Biology
Institute of Biomedical Engineering
University of Toronto
Toronto, Ontario, Canada   M5S 1A4

W. C. White   91
Dow Corning Corp.
2200 West Salzburg Road
Midland, MI 48640-0994

Debra A. Wrobleski   281
Material and Technology Division
Los Alamos National Laboratory
Los Alamos, NM 87545

Iwao Yamamoto   165
Faculty of Textile Science & Technology
Shinshu University
Ueda 386, Japan

I. V. Yannas   313
Fibers and Polymers Laboratories
Massachusetts Institute of Technology
Cambridge, MA 02139

J-H. Zhu   85
Research Triangle Institute
Research Triangle Park, NC 27709

Hemagglutination inhibition
  antibody response, 207
Hemolysis, erythrocytic, assay,
      285-286
Hemophilus influenzae vaccine, 207
Heparin, 282
  cofactor, *see* Antithrombin III
Heparinization, 282
Hexamethylphosphoric triamide
      (HMPT), 24, 25
1,6-Hexanediamine, 140
Higuchi
  equation, 154, 156, 157, 159
  kinetics, 5
Homo(alkyl amine), 257
Hormone, *see* separate hormones,
      Steroids
Horseradish peroxidase, 130
Human
  interferon response, 216, 217
  and poly(ICLC), 216-221
    in cancer, 216
    in multiple sclerosis, 216
  T-cell, 220
Hydrazinolysis, 266
Hydrocortisone acetate, 227
Hydrolysis, metal-promoted, 85-90
3-α-Hydroxy-5-α-androstan-17-one,
      see Esttone
2-Hydroxyethylmethacrylate, 102
Hydroxylamine, 253
Hydroxylapatite, 103
8-Hydroxyquinoline, 86
Hypersensitivity, delayed, 209
  in mouse, 209-211
Hypoxanthine, 186

Imidazole derivative, *see*
      Tetramisole
Immunoassay of hormone, 131
Immunogenicity
  and amino acid composition, 254
Implant device, biodegradable, 5
Infection, clinical
  due to foreign body, 97-98
Inflammation following surgery,
      313
Infusion
  apparatus, 284
  process, chemical, 282-294
  pump, 6
Insecticide strip, 5
Insulin, 6, 76, 77, 81-83
Interferon, 9, 205, 206, 209, 210,
      215-217, 223, 226, 227,
      232, 233
Iron overload, 85
  and desferrioxamine B, 85
Irradiation, 276
2-Isocyanatoethylmethacrylate,
      152

Isofoam PE-*20*, 20
Isolan, 21
Isopropyl(E,E)-11-methoxy-3,7,11-
      trimethyl-2,4-
      dodecadienoate,
      see Methoprene

Japanese radish
  seed germination, 45-59

Kidney, artificial, 297
Komeen, 36
Klebsiella pneumoniae, 179, 181
Krestin, 165, 166

Lactide, 30
Leaching, 26
  pesticide formulation for, 27
Lentinan, 165
Leukocyte adherence assay,
      284-285, 293
Levamisole, 223-227, 232
Lindane, 19
Lipid, 241-246
  polymerization, 243-245
Lithium alkylamide, 258
Lithium borohydride, 253
Lithium perchlorate, 276-278
Lymphocyte, 225
Lymphokine, 226
Lysozyme, 45

Macroinitiator of polymer, 256,
      262
Macromolecule, bioactive, 3
Macrophage, 232
  activating factor, 225
  colony stimulating factor,
      in vitro, 209
  cytotoxicity activation
      in vitro, 210, 211
Malathion, 19, 20
Maleic anhydride, 76, 78
Mandelic acid mixture, racemic,
      261
MAS polymer, 36
Material bioactive
  encapsulated, listed, 2
  immobilized, listed, 2
Matrix
  combined, concept of, 75-84
  and delivery of polypeptide,
      bioactive, 75-84
  entrapment of pesticide, 18
  extracellular, 317
Membrane
  biomedical, 261
  for hemodialysis, 297-311
    permeability, 300-310
    preparation, 298-299
Metal-promoted hydrolysis, 85-90

Metalochlor, 30
Methacrylate, 102
Methanol, 20
  -treated sludge, *see* MAS
Methomyl, 21
Methoprene, 20
Methotrexate, 139-150
  -platinum polymer, 143-149
Methyldopa complex, 297-311
  preparation, 299
Methylene blue, 76-81
γ-Methyl-L-glutamate, 257
Methyl methacrylate, 102, 315
Methyl parathion, 28
Methyl pirimiphos, 29
Methyl quinaldate, 88
6-Methylthiopurine, 8, 151
Metribuzin, 31
  formula, 32
Microcapsule, 6-7
Microencapsulation, 28
Migration inhibitory factor, 225
Mixture, racemic
resolution methods, 261
Monkey
  and interferon, 215
  and poly(ICLC), 213-216
  vaccinated, 207-208
  virus diseases listed, 206
Monocyte in human, 217, 218
Monomer, steroid
  preparation, 117-122
  properties, physical, 118-121
Mouse, 209-213, 223-238
Mulch, plastic, 38
Multiple sclerosis in human
  and poly(ICLC), 216-221
Mushroom polysaccharide, 165
Mycobacterium tuberculosis
  cell wall polysaccharide, 167
    structure, 167

Nalco-trol, 36
Naled, 19, 37
Naloxone, 3
Naltrexone, 3
Neisseria mucosa, 179, 181
Nickel acetate, 89
Nitrocellulose, 255
Nitroglycerin, 6
Nomate, 29
Nucleic acid analog, 8, 185-204
Nucleoside, 1990201
  bonded to silica gel, 188, 190
Nucleotide, 199, 201
Nucleotide phosphodiesterase,
    cyclic, 224

Oligoethyleneimine, 191
  and nucleic acid bases, 191, 197

Oligonuceotide, 199
Organostannane, *see* Tin
  and xylan, 177
Organotin, 39
Orthophosphate, 77
Oxacillin, 105, 109

Palmitic acid, 76, 77, 82, 83
Pancreas, artificial, 6
Paraquat, 38
Patch, transdermal
  for nitroglycerine, 6
  for scopolamine, 6
Pellet disc, 75-84, 126
  methylene blue release from,
      76-81
  preparation, 76
Penncap M, 28, 30
Pentachlorophenyl acetate, 31
Permethrin, 29, 37, 38
Pesticide
  adsorption to polymer, 19
  application, 17
  bonded physically to polymer,
      19-30
    release, 21-29
  carreir
    lecithin, 25
    soybean oil, 25
  on devices, 37-39
    ear tag, 37
    leg band, 37
    mulch, plastic, 38-39
    strip, plastic, 38
    wrap, military, 37-38
  immobilization, 18
  matrix entrapment of, 18-21
    microencapsulation of, 18,
        28-29
  polymer
    formation, 18, 30-35
    release from, 33-35
    research review (1976-1987),
        17-43
  solubilization, 33-35
Phagocyte, 226
Phagocytosis, 226
Phenoxyacetic acid, 33
Pheromone, 23, 38
Phosamidon, 21
Phosphatidylcholine
  acetylenic, 240
  diacetylenic, 239-249
  dialkanoyl, 240
  polymerization, 246
  structure, 240, 245
Phospholipid, short-chain,
    239-249
Phosphorothioate, 33
Phytoagglutinin, 225